Praise for *Life Lines*

"In *Life Lines*, the graphic-storytelling form becomes its own language of care – a place where images invite us into the intimate, everyday moments of both fragmentation and connection. Roth's drawings are full of vulnerability, wonder, and a playfulness in a touching tribute to his dad's lifetime oeuvre of mysterious markings. A rare and moving work that shows how art helps us understand what it means to be together, through the most trying times of illness, uncertainty, and the end of life."

Jason Danely, author of *Aging and Loss: Mourning and Maturity in Contemporary Japan*

"As an intimate and collaborative work of graphic ethnography, *Life Lines* offers a powerful contemplation of what it means to give care, to create together, and to be present for each other in the landscape of very old age. Through a rich life history, Roth and his father collaborate to highlight a life-long artistic practice that beautifully disrupts our comfortable boundaries between communicative language and aesthetic expression."

Mitra Emad, Associate Professor of Cultural Studies, University of Minnesota Duluth

"*Life Lines* is a moving, intimate biography and family history that provides a welcome antidote to the utilitarian cynicism of our day and age. Joshua Hotaka Roth demonstrates that art can be caring, and that care is a form of art – as is life itself."

Steven Van Wolputte, Professor of Anthropology, KU Leuven and co-author of *In the Land of the Lacandón: A Graphic History of Adventure and Imperialism*

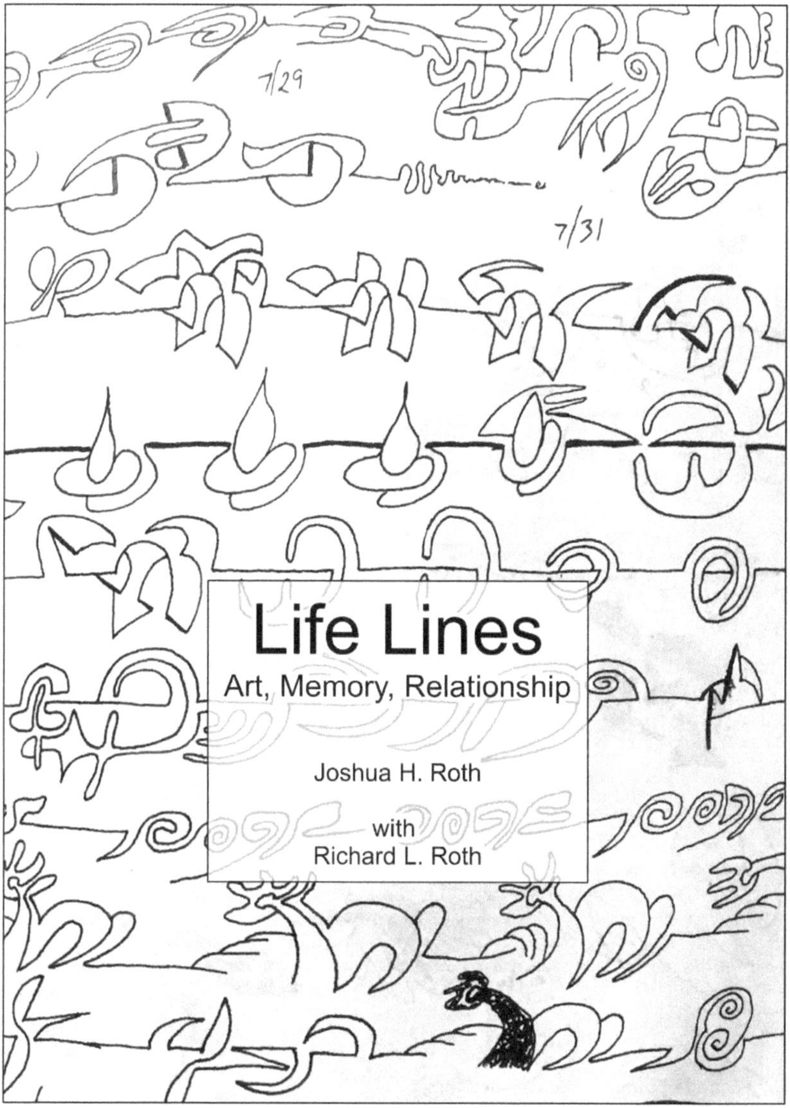

Life Lines
Art, Memory, Relationship

Joshua H. Roth

with
Richard L. Roth

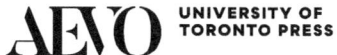
UNIVERSITY OF TORONTO PRESS

Aevo UTP
An imprint of University of Toronto Press
Toronto Buffalo London
utppublishing.com

© Joshua Roth 2026

All rights reserved. No part of this publication may be reproduced, stored in or introduced into a retrieval system, or transmitted in any form or by any means (electronic, mechanical, photocopying, recording, or otherwise) without the prior written permission of both the copyright owner and the above publisher of this book.

Library and Archives Canada Cataloguing in Publication

Title: Life lines : art, memory, relationship / by Joshua H. Roth with Richard L Roth.
Names: Roth, Joshua Hotaka, author | Roth, Richard Lewis, 1927– author, artist Description: Includes bibliographical references.
Identifiers: Canadiana (print) 20250325977 | Canadiana (ebook) 20250326027 | ISBN 9781487562830 (paper) | ISBN 9781487562854 (EPUB) | ISBN 9781487562847 (PDF)
Subjects: LCSH: Roth, Joshua Hotaka – Comic books, strips, etc. | LCSH: Roth, Richard Lewis, 1927– – Comic books, strips, etc. | LCSH: Aging parents – Care – Comic books, strips, etc. | LCSH: Fathers and sons – Comic books, strips, etc. | LCSH: Art and older people – Comic books, strips, etc. | LCSH: Adult children of aging parents – Comic books, strips, etc. | LCGFT: Nonfiction comics. | LCGFT: Autobiographical comics. | LCGFT: Graphic novels.
Classification: LCC HQ1063.6 .R68 2026 | DDC 306.874084/6 – dc23

ISBN 978-1-4875-6283-0 (paper)   ISBN 978-1-4875-6285-4 (EPUB)
                                       ISBN 978-1-4875-6284-7 (PDF)

Printed in the USA

Cover design: Alan Jones
Cover image: Joshua Roth

The manufacturer's authorised representative in the EU for product safety is Mare Nostrum Group B.V., Doelen 72, 4831 GR Breda, The Netherlands. Email: mailto:gpsr@mare-nostrum.co.uk

We wish to acknowledge the land on which the University of Toronto Press operates. This land is the traditional territory of the Wendat, the Anishnaabeg, the Haudenosaunee, the Métis, and the Mississaugas of the Credit First Nation.

University of Toronto Press acknowledges the financial support of the Government of Canada, the Canada Council for the Arts, and the Ontario Arts Council, an agency of the Government of Ontario, for its publishing activities.

Canada Council   Conseil des Arts
for the Arts   du Canada

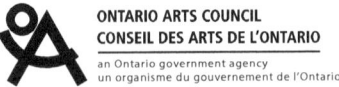

ONTARIO ARTS COUNCIL
CONSEIL DES ARTS DE L'ONTARIO
an Ontario government agency
un organisme du gouvernement de l'Ontario

Funded by the   Financé par le
Government   gouvernement
of Canada   du Canada

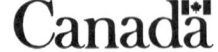

Contents

Introduction   vii

1 MOOPs and Bones   1

2 Changes   13

3 I Am the Giver   33

4 The Hero of the Story   53

5 Kluwital   67

6 Everyday Rituals   87

7 Text and Image   109

8 Documenting the Progress of My Decrepitude   135

9 What Am I Doing Here?   151

10 Epilogue   191

Afterword   201

Acknowledgments   205

References   209

Introduction

In the Japanese folktale of Obasuteyama, those reaching the age of seventy are carried by their adult children to the top of a sacred mountain where they are left to die, freeing the younger generations from the burden of care of elders in their declining years. While there is little evidence that such a practice ever actually existed in Japan, it is clear that this story, retold over the years in a variety of genres including kabuki theater and cinema, continues to be compelling to Japanese audiences not so much as a document of a harsh past, but as commentary on the present (Danely 2014). In the tale, the mother herself insists that she be taken to the mountain. The adult son does not abandon her there in an act of heartless cruelty. The mother is beloved by her son, who reluctantly carries out his duties as an act of filial piety. Even in the twenty-first century, older Japanese people can identify with the mother's desire not to be a burden on her family (Allison 2023; Kawano 2005; Long

2005; Traphagan 2000). Generational succession can be emotionally fraught whether in premodern or modern times, in times of scarcity as well as affluence. And not just in Japan.

Anthropologists have long been fascinated with generational succession. Mark Auslander, who worked with the Ngoni of eastern Zambia in the late 1980s, wrote that, when a member of the community died, it was required that a full accounting of the person's life be made, reciting their lineage and accomplishments, and details of their individual lives all the way to the moment of their last breath — or else the dead would not remain buried and would roam the village (Auslander 2011, 276). Auslander was especially interested in rituals and acts of documentation that give voice to the dead, who have no means of speaking for themselves. But documentation and remembrance may also be important in helping to ease transitions before the end of life, as well as for those who are stepping down from positions of authority, or those who are giving up a degree of autonomy. In such cases, the act of documentation itself may serve as an important form of care. This graphic memoir, *Life Lines*, served this purpose. Documenting my dad's life and accomplishments honored him and eased his transition into a new stage of life, but it also kept us both engaged in a positive way, a welcome reprieve from the necessary but sometimes oppressive care that focuses exclusively on health and safety.

Transitions in old age happen over a period of years, but there are certain moments that may mark the change in status in dramatic fashion — giving up the car keys and control over finances, accepting home care or moving into assisted living.

Remarkably, Dad didn't seem to experience any of these too severely. He did not insist on what Sarah Lamb has called the "permanent personhood" of the successful aging paradigm prevalent in the United States (Lamb 2014, 2017). Dad drove an old blue Honda Civic. Compact and low to the ground, it was a good size for parking on crowded New York City streets, where alternate side of the street parking regulations forced him to move the car twice per week. But he willingly gave up the car keys as this routine became increasingly burdensome by the time he was getting into his mid-eighties and had developed hip pain.

Similarly, Dad was aware that he was having trouble managing both his finances and the health care bureaucracy. Things came to a head when, after a partial hip replacement, we realized that Medicare would not pay for home care. He would have to qualify for Medicaid to get help for home care services, and to do so Dad and Mom would have to divest themselves of their modest savings. Although he couldn't quite understand the necessity, Dad agreed to have my brother and me serve as executors of what would be in effect their Medicaid trust, using that money to pay their rent and any other expenses not covered by Medicaid.

Finally, Dad was willing to give up the private space of his apartment, welcoming the presence of care workers at home once he was released from rehab. Many of us think of our home as our castle, a private realm where we are free to do as we please, free from the prying eyes of others. Yet, it can also be a space of isolation. In her graphic non-fiction work *Seek You: A Journey Through American Loneliness*, Kristen Radtke writes about her dad's ham radio obsession. He would send out "CQ" (Seek You) signals every night:

> A CQ call is a reaching outward, an attempt to make a connection across a wavelength with someone you've never met. It means, essentially, "Is there anyone out there?" and invites anyone listening to answer. In morse code, it looks like:
>
> $$-\cdot-\cdot--\cdot-$$
>
> (2021, 19)

Maybe reaching out to strangers over ham radio allowed him to connect to others more easily than he could in face-to-face relationships. Radtke describes her father as "stoic, religious, and extraordinarily strict" (2021, 23). My dad was the opposite of stoic. He loved indulgences — food, music, art. He was not religious; he was a humanist. He was not strict; he was permissive. We had good relations in the family. He and Mom were well liked in the building and the neighborhood. But he had only a couple of friends who came over from time to time, and I think he was lonely much of his life. In some ways, his artwork — the impenetrable script that was the basis for his MOOP series — was self-isolating. At the same time, they were works of art, of beauty, and thus, a reaching outwards. His CQ could be any excerpt of his mysterious script:

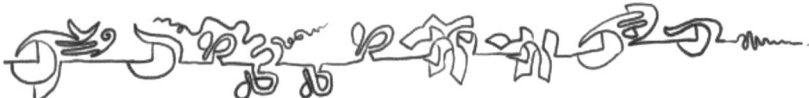

In his nineties, Dad enjoyed having the care workers around. They were there to attend to the activities of daily living — toileting, bathing, clothing, laundry, food prep, etc. But they also provided him with company and conversation and the attention that Dad relished. In doing so, they did what anthropologist-philosopher Annamarie Mol describes as "tinkering with care" (Mol et al. 2010), figuring out what was the most effective, sustainable, and meaningful way of engaging with each other, and being willing to adjust and improvise to respond to changing circumstances and needs. Our caretakers' tinkering — the human connection that they were able to forge with Dad — made all of the daily activities easier and more pleasant to accomplish. Most of the time, he didn't see them as outsiders invading his private space.

Likewise, I tinkered with care, finding that the MOOP graphic memoir project engaged Dad in a way that he seemed to appreciate, different from what the care workers provided. Dad and Mom had had some modest successes in their art careers, but by the time he was in his nineties, it had been some years since he'd been actively painting. He'd really slowed down in his eighties when a tremor in his right hand made it difficult to draw, and cataracts and a blood clot in one of his eyes degraded his vision. Dad's claim to fame was the fifty-meter mural he did in a corridor at Lincoln Center connecting what had been called Avery Fisher Hall to the State Theater. But he never got representation at a prestigious gallery and rarely sold any of his works. Mom had some greater success with sales through her Japanese university alumni network in New York City, many of whom appreciated the beauty of her landscapes. Dad may have made the transition to advanced old age somewhat more smoothly compared to others, but it would be wrong to suggest that it was easy, and I like to think our MOOP graphic memoir project helped ease the transition. He enjoyed our sessions, for they allowed him to rediscover his work. Tinkering with care, our project allowed us to engage with each other in a way that was gratifying, and in some ways revelatory.

Dad lived to ninety-seven, and I spent the last six years getting to know him better as we worked on the graphic memoir project. In the process, I discovered some things about him that he had kept to himself for decades. Although I knew he had been stationed near Nuremberg, Germany, during the American occupation after World War II and was able to attend the war crime trials there in 1946, and that he later volunteered and served with an English-speaking regiment of the Haganah (the Jewish paramilitary organization) in Palestine in 1948, I didn't know any details of these experiences and how they may have affected the course of his life and his work as an artist.

While Dad resisted any easy explanation for his art, the context of his life experience raised intriguing questions about his later creative work. Dad's art suggests language, and in fact, his long-lasting series of paintings, what he called his "MOOP" series, features a set of five distinct writing systems comprised of idiosyncratic shapes. His visual compositions have a playful quality that evokes certain quotidian aspects of his everyday life. But I can't get away from the question of why Dad would devise systems of writing that he alone could read. In his art, writing is transformed into visual images whose meaning is dense and opaque. I wondered: What connection might exist between Dad's earlier wartime experiences and his art that embodies emotional depth and power without communicating explicitly? Could his work be a sublimation of trauma?

Scholars who have explored care in recent years have offered several definitions that push beyond most taken-for-granted understandings of the term. Berenice Fisher and Joan Tronto have written that care is "everything we do to maintain, continue, and repair our world so that we can live in it as well as possible in a complex, life sustaining web" (1990, 40, quoted in Allison 2023, 7). This definition encompasses a broad range of caretaking action, including the kind of collaborative documentation project that Dad and I undertook. Other scholars have suggested moving beyond a binary of categories of care givers and care recipients, and recognizing the reciprocal dimensions of care, even if they are asymmetrical rather than balanced (Shohet 2013). In her research on the children of immigrants who often act as translators for their parents, Inmaculada Garcia-Sanchez describes care as a "reciprocal distributed interactional achievement" (2018, 176). She writes that children and parents bring different knowledge and skills together to collaboratively create knowledge. That was certainly the case between Dad and me, in that we were both beneficiaries of our care relationship. Our project made me into a graphic artist. It was often challenging but cathartic, and frequently enjoyable.

The "interactional achievement" between me and my dad wouldn't have been possible, however, without being a part of a larger network of other care relationships and institutional support. In our case, it was a combination of Medicaid support for home care, and the presence of middle-aged immigrant women — in our case from Jamaica and Guyana — working in the home care field. Despite taking six months to navigate the bureaucratic hurdles of qualifying for Medicaid, and another six months before we were approved for the necessary number of hours of care work, Medicaid eventually did cover the cost of home care, allowing us to use the remaining savings to pay the rent and other expenses, the most important being some extra pay for the generally underpaid care workers. Our care workers were officially on duty thirteen hours per day (8 a.m. to 9 p.m.), but at night when they heard the sounds of Dad's walker, they would check in to make sure he wouldn't fall. They would urge him to get back into bed, and help him if he had to go to the bathroom. The extra stipend we provided was insufficient to compensate for all of this, but it was a meaningful expression of our appreciation, strengthening the bond that had formed among us, an acknowledgement of our interdependence. When I apologized to one of our care workers that we weren't giving as much as they deserved, she told me that she knew it came "from the heart."

The authors of *The Care Manifesto* write that "if the neoliberal defunding and undermining of care has led to paranoid and chauvinist caring imaginaries — looking after 'our own' — adequate resources, time and labor would make people feel secure enough to care for, about and with strangers as much as kin" (Chatzidakis et al. 2020, 42). Our care workers had come to love my parents. Within a social context in which we depended on the marketplace and on bureaucratic institutions to access care, we were able to mold this care into something more than the disinterested and fragmented variety endemic of the market, and more like the care motivated by love that might be expected of family members (Fisher and Tronto 1990).

Life Lines is an account of one small effort to create a caring community within a sea of carelessness. Hopefully, it provides some useful caregiving strategies that others can make use of. And yet, every human life is unique, and every case requires its own set of approaches, and outcomes rarely fully satisfy. For much of her adult life, Mom had thought of herself as a care giver, and she had a much harder time accepting others' care than Dad did. Care giving was deeply engrained in her identity, and she resented the presence of paid care givers, who she saw as usurping her own role. How I wished Mom and I could have found our way towards a "reciprocal distributed interactional achievement," as Dad and I had done, but that would have required both of us to be givers and to be receivers, which was hard to do when our roles had long been defined — Mom the giver, me (and everyone else in the family) the receiver. Born in Japan in 1928, fiercely independent and hard-working but also loving, she was the pillar of the family. I cannot but help think that her unwillingness to receive care until after she was struck by illness in March 2020 may have contributed to her debilitation.

Like the mother in the Japanese folktale of Obasuteyama, Mom provided for her family and did not wish to be a burden. Unlike in Obasuteyama, I did not take my parents to the mountain and leave them there, nor did they expect me to. Although Mom may have feared abandonment when we asked her and Dad to divest themselves of their modest savings in order to qualify for Medicaid, this is what allowed us to build a loving community of care for them in their final years. My brother Abe and I did our part to care for our parents, but it was the three care workers who performed the tasks of daily living.

Filial piety cannot be the answer for the modern version of Obasuteyama — the mass abandonment of older people in nursing homes or other forms of impersonal care. Most of us will need a broader network of care to support us in our advanced old age, and for some of us an institutional context will be the best option, especially if the reform movement can succeed in establishing more caring institutions (Gawande 2014). The efforts documented here suggest that home care can also be refashioned to be more loving and humane. The difficult transitions at the end of life will continue to be hard on the younger generations, but given some luck and handled with imagination, these transitions can be turned into opportunities for celebration and deeper mutual understanding. And as Arthur Kleinman has written, caregiving is an opportunity to "become more human" (2009).

MOOPs and Bones

Chapter 1

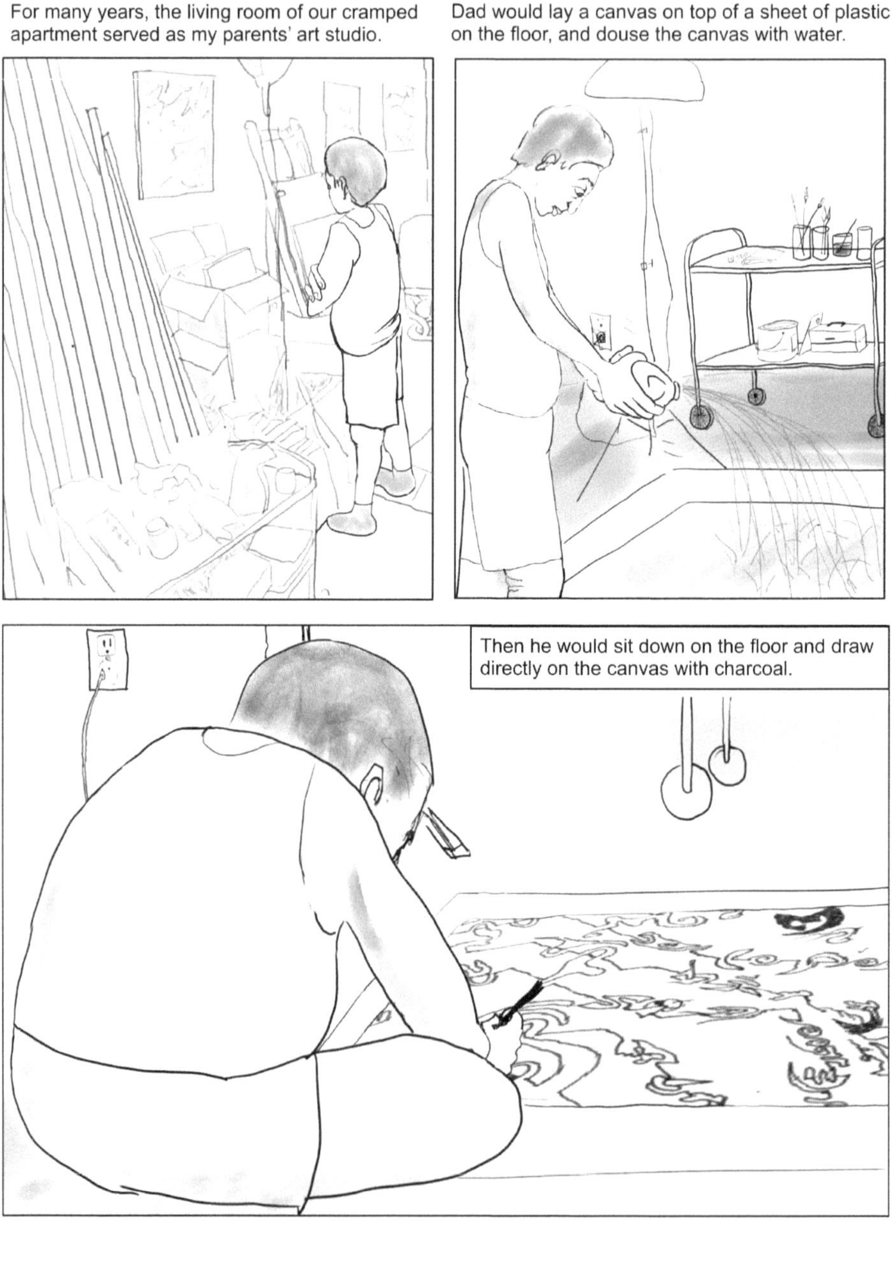

For many years, the living room of our cramped apartment served as my parents' art studio.

Dad would lay a canvas on top of a sheet of plastic on the floor, and douse the canvas with water.

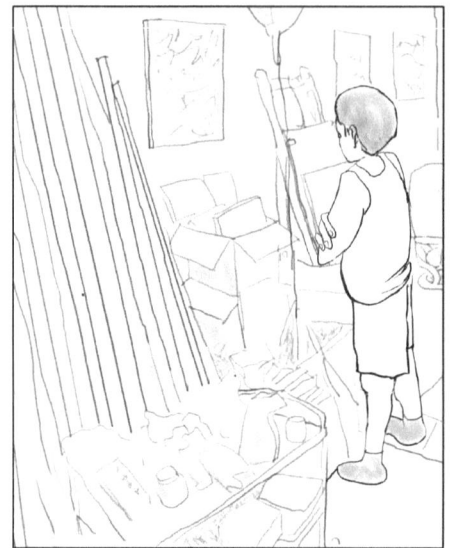
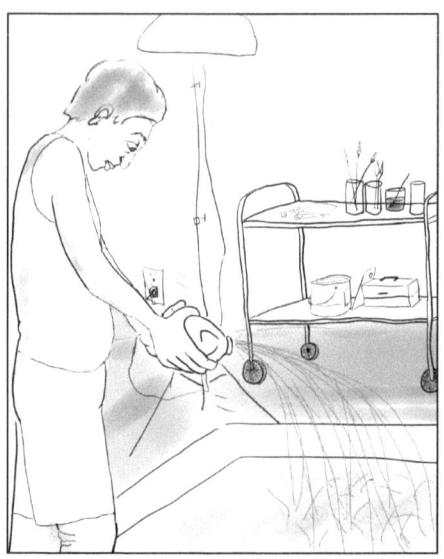

Then he would sit down on the floor and draw directly on the canvas with charcoal.

He spent 30 years on a series of paintings he called MOOPs. He gave shapes sound values, and created several alphabets with which he spelled out messages that only he could read.

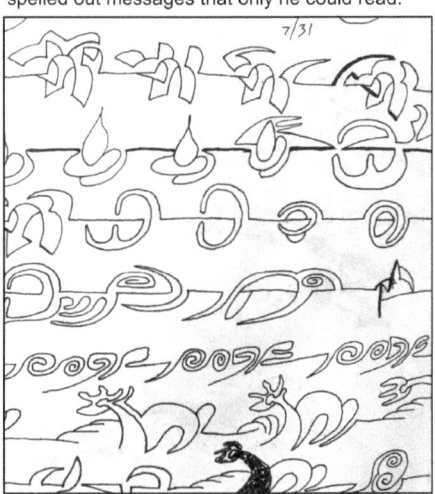

Before working with the canvas on the floor, he would draw in his notebook.

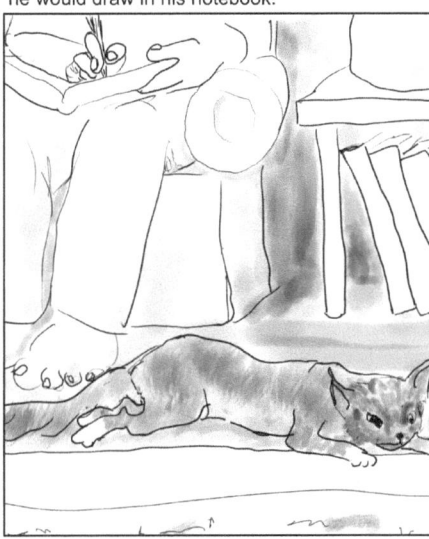

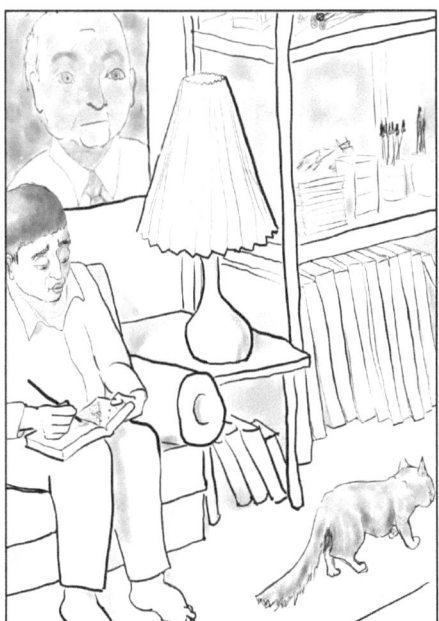

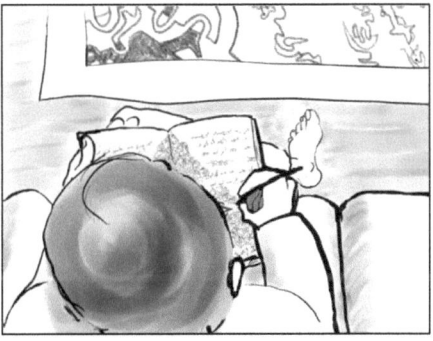

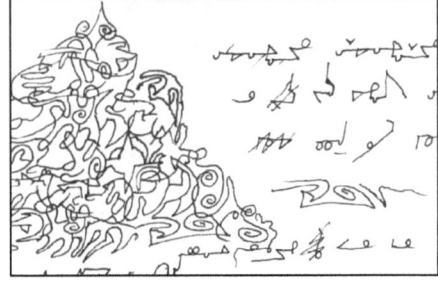

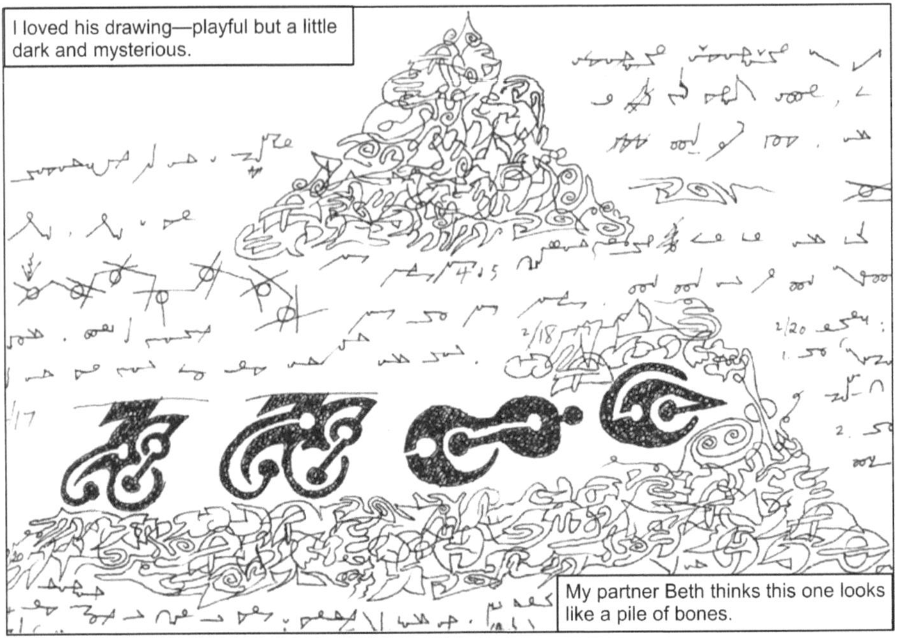

I loved his drawing—playful but a little dark and mysterious.

My partner Beth thinks this one looks like a pile of bones.

Dad did love bones...

ME AT AGE 8

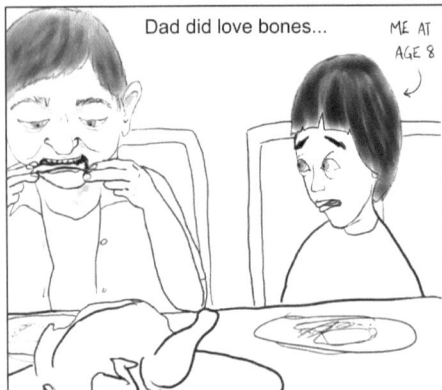

Dad would gnaw everything away, crush the top, and suck out the marrow.

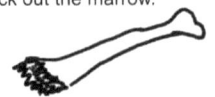

When I ate a drumstick, I'd leave cartilage and skin at the ends.

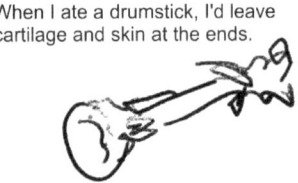

MY DAD'S DAD.

GRANDPA SAM ATE CHICKEN BONES SO CLEANLY...

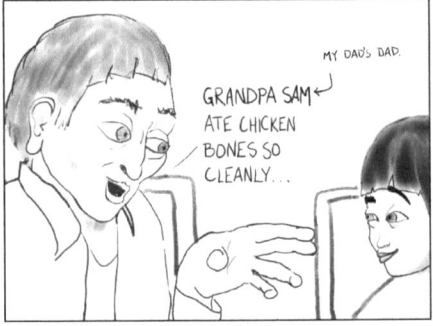

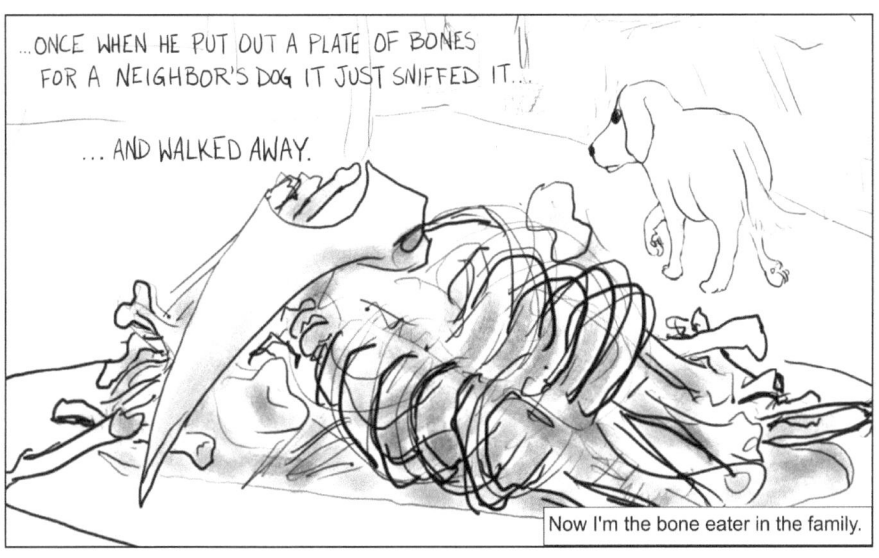

...ONCE WHEN HE PUT OUT A PLATE OF BONES FOR A NEIGHBOR'S DOG IT JUST SNIFFED IT...

...AND WALKED AWAY.

Now I'm the bone eater in the family.

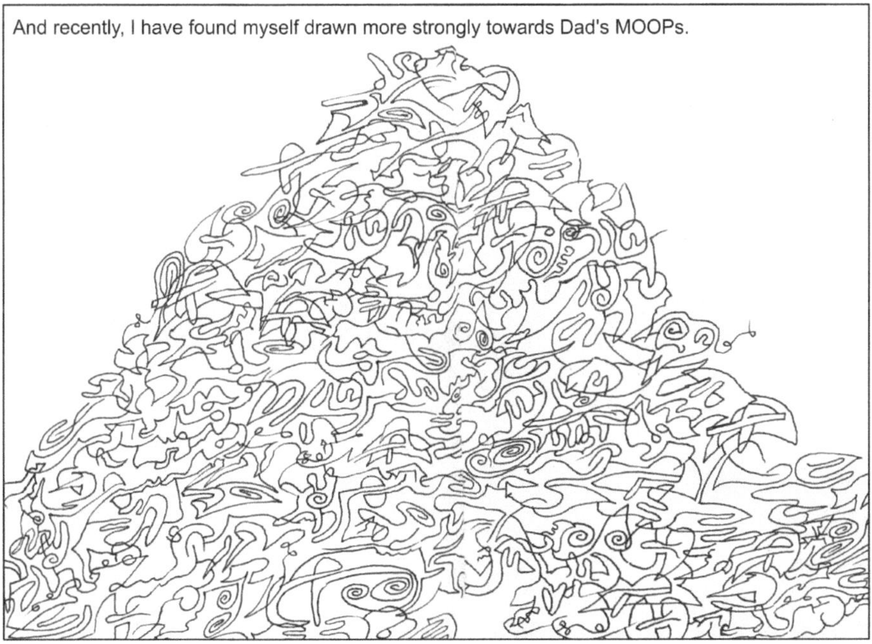

And recently, I have found myself drawn more strongly towards Dad's MOOPs.

Dad and Mom were living on their own in their apartment into their early 90s.

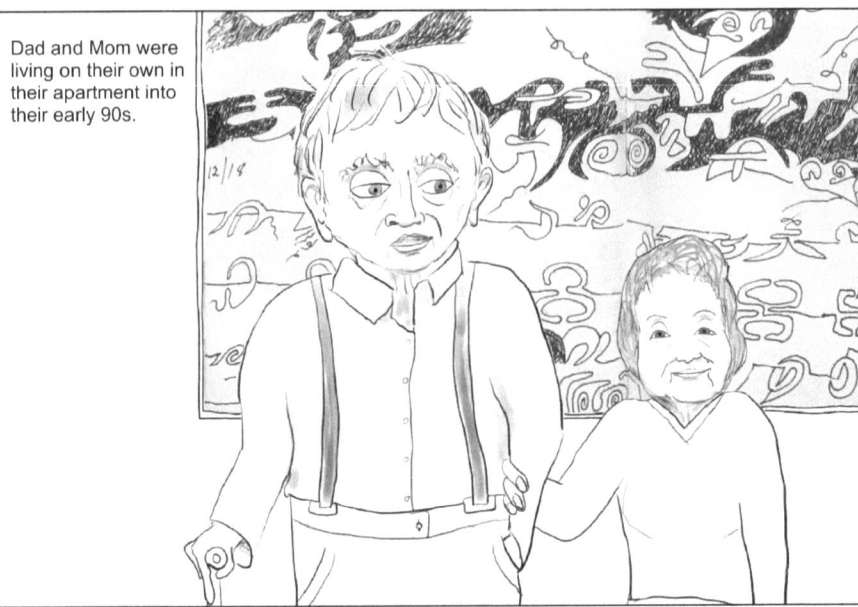

I live in Western Massachusetts.

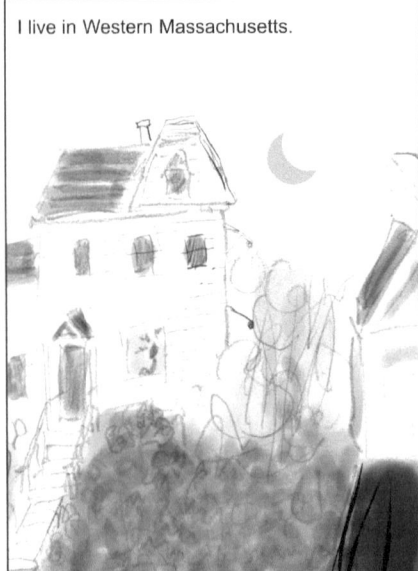

It's a little under three hours by car to my parents' apartment in NY.

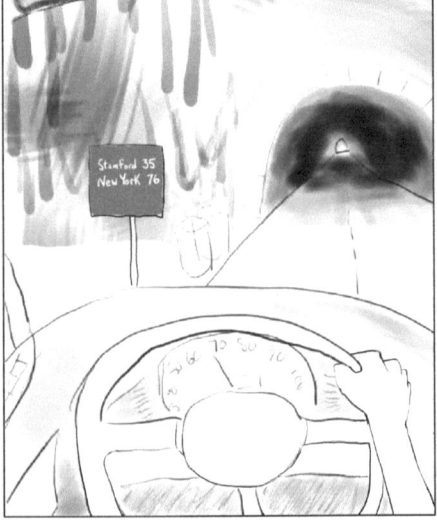

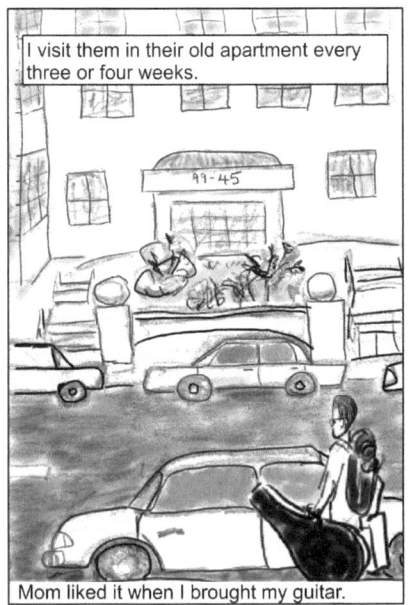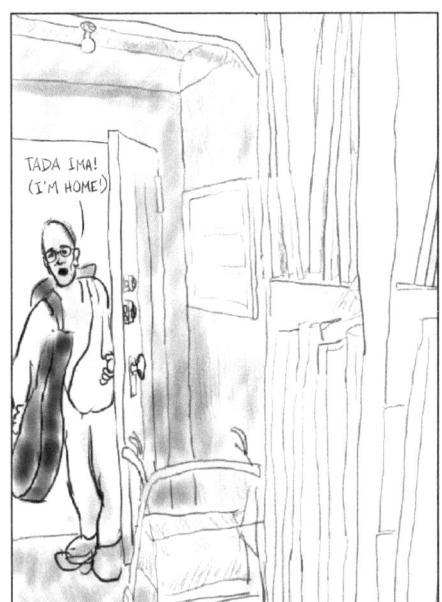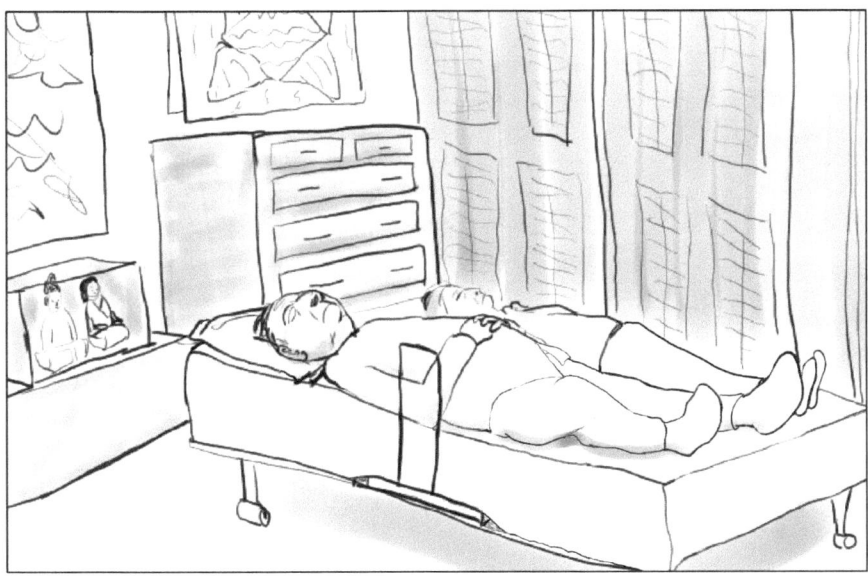

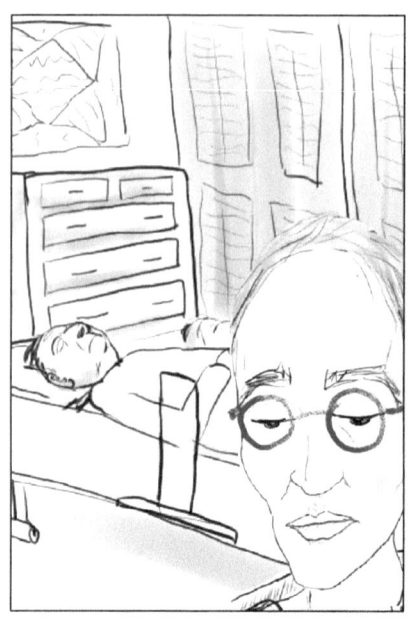 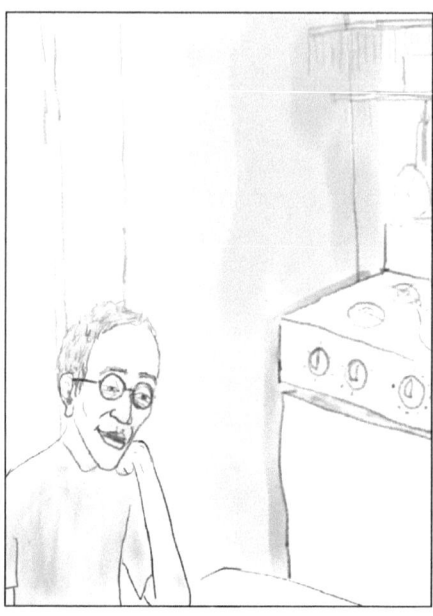

When I am waiting for Dad and Mom to get up from their frequent naps, I do some shopping, try to clear some clutter. In the past I put in grab bars, and arranged for a new higher toilet. There was some drama about that.

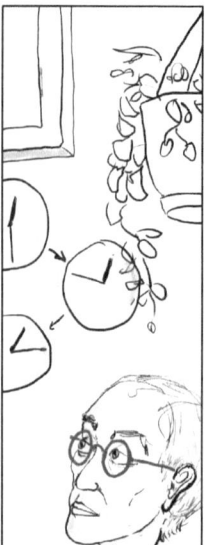 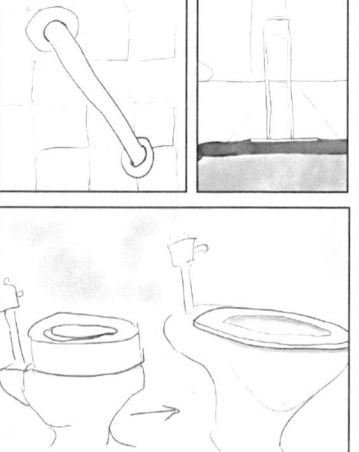

Mom glimpsed the gaping hole in the floor when the plumber was installing the new toilet and it scared her.

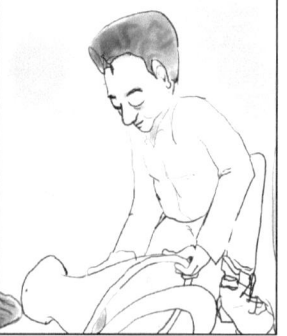

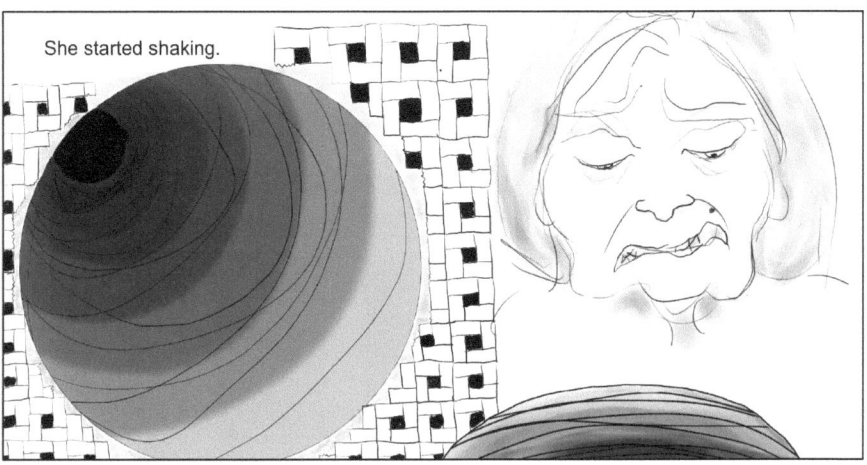

My efforts were rarely appreciated, but what else could I do, especially after the "menorah incident"?

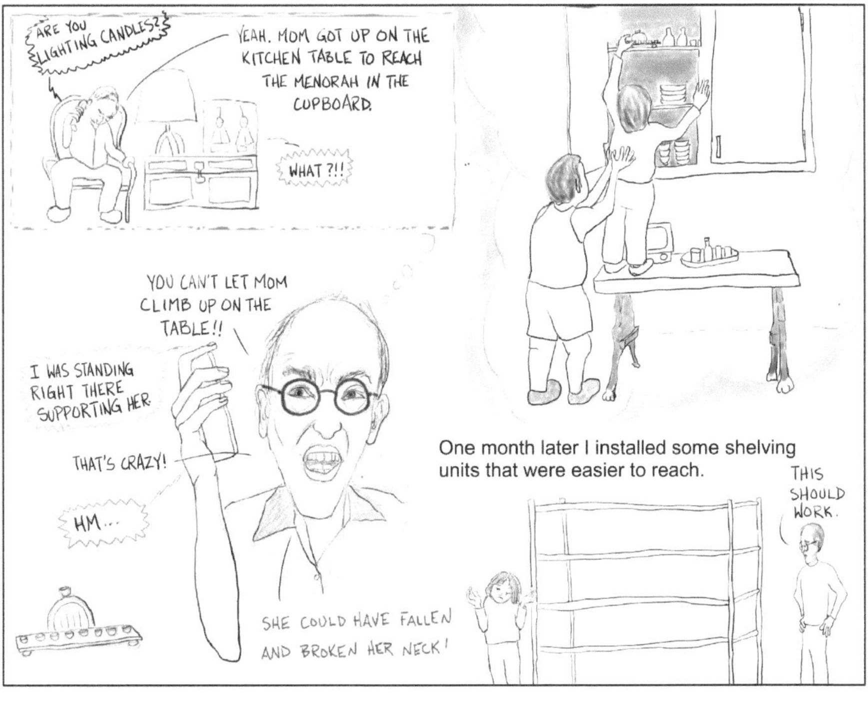

One day, I pulled out one of Dad's old MOOP notebooks. It had been 15 years since he last made an entry. I sat down with Dad and leafed through it with him.

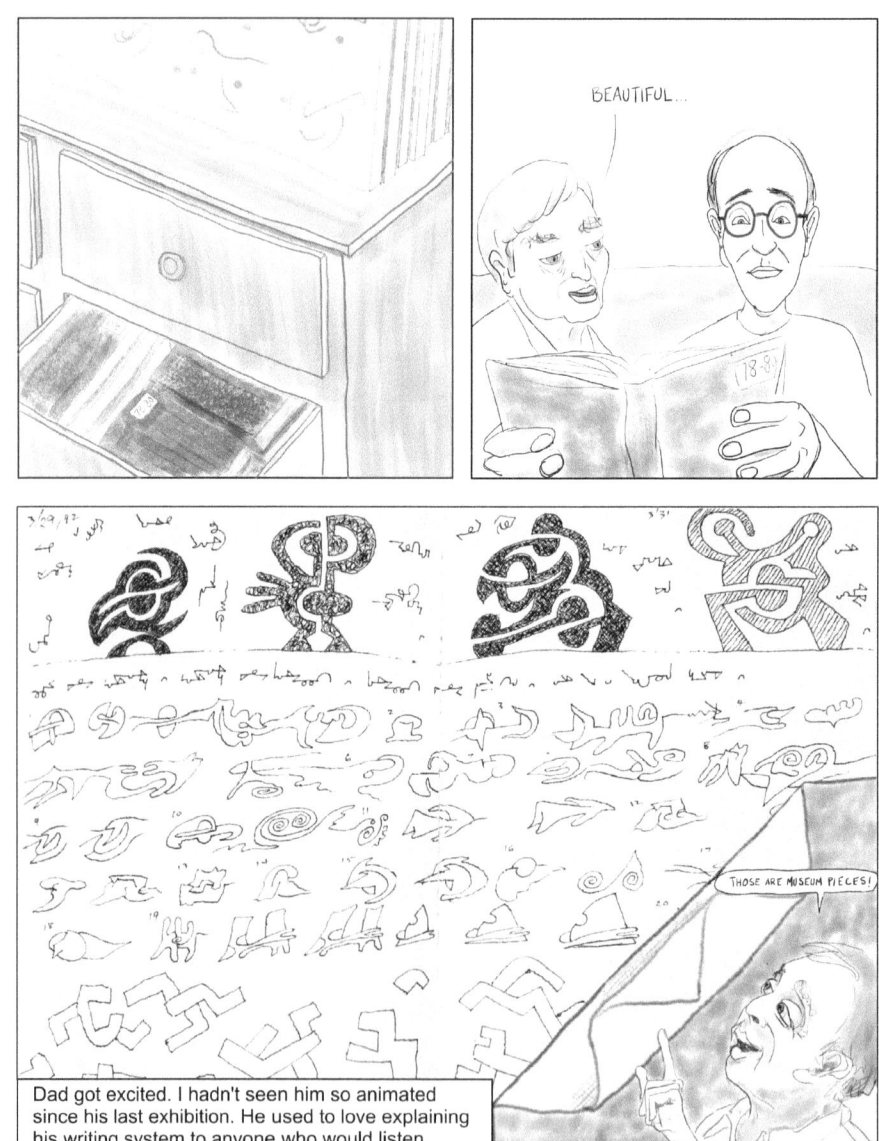

Dad got excited. I hadn't seen him so animated since his last exhibition. He used to love explaining his writing system to anyone who would listen.

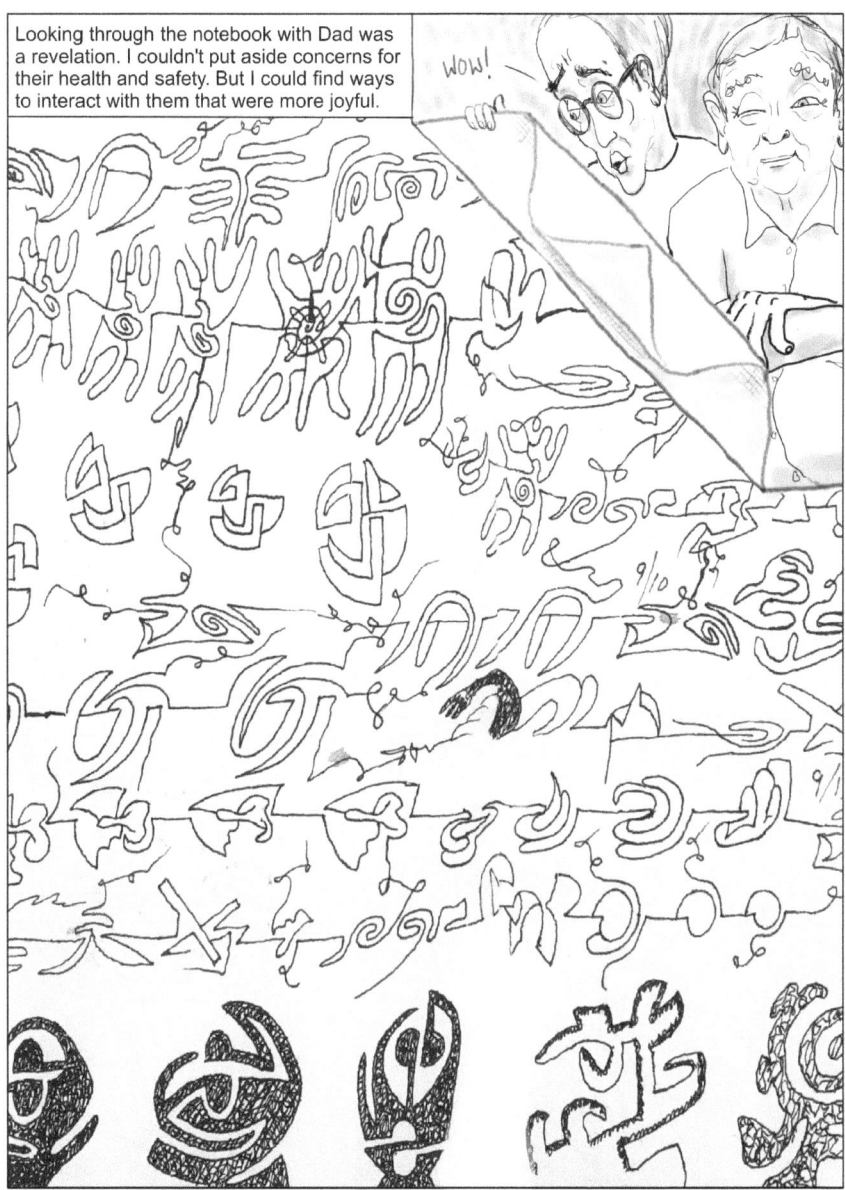

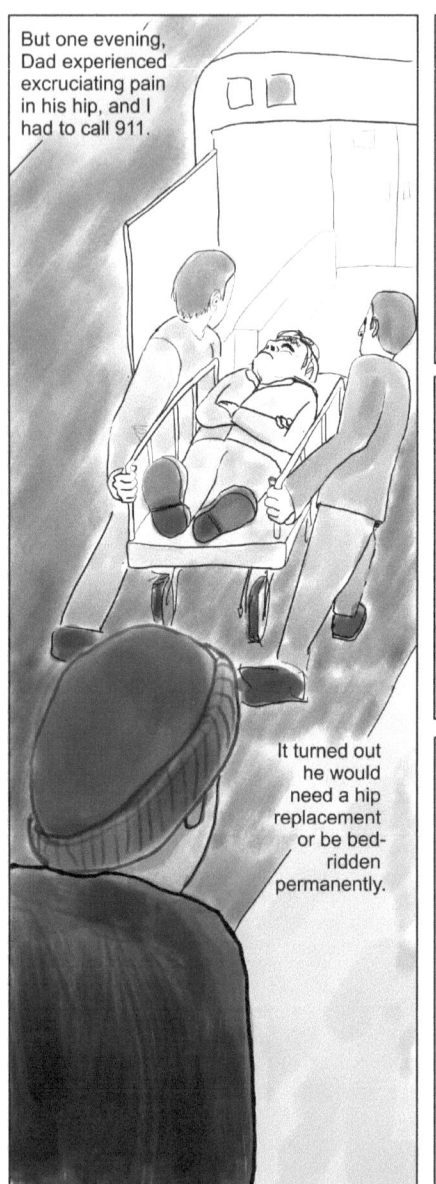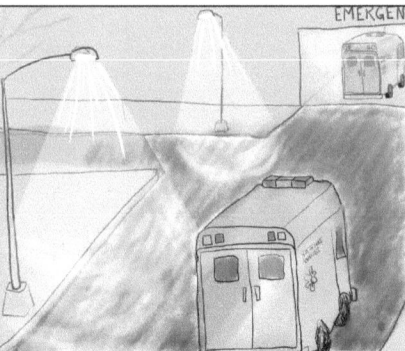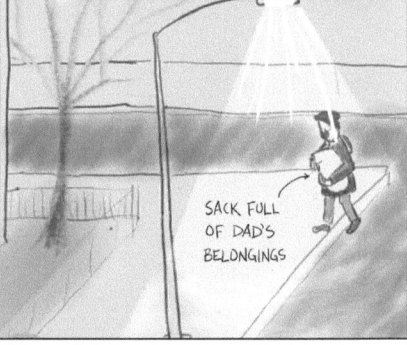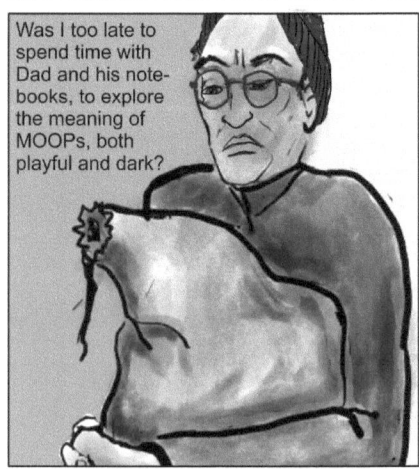

Changes

Chapter 2

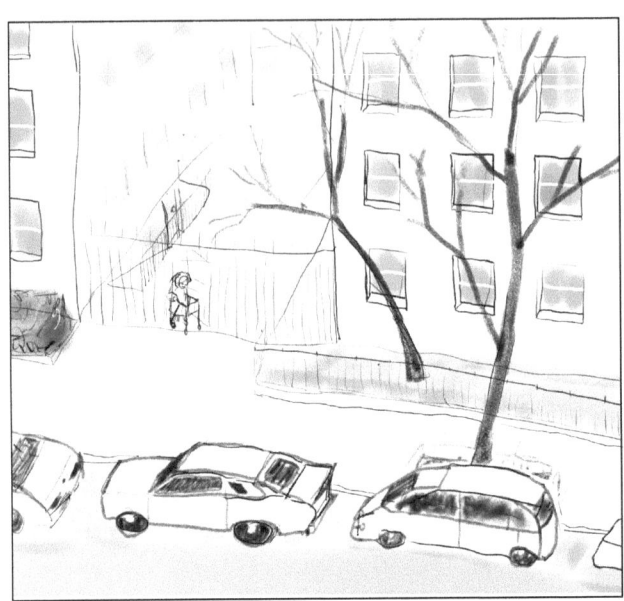
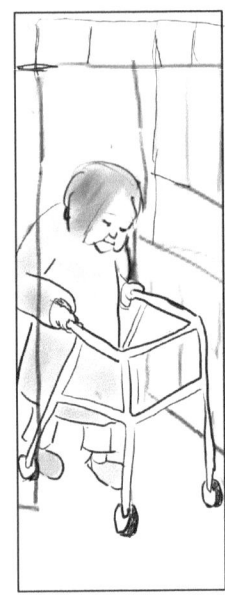

For three months, Mom walked the half mile every day to the rehab center where Dad was staying. Rain...

...or shine.

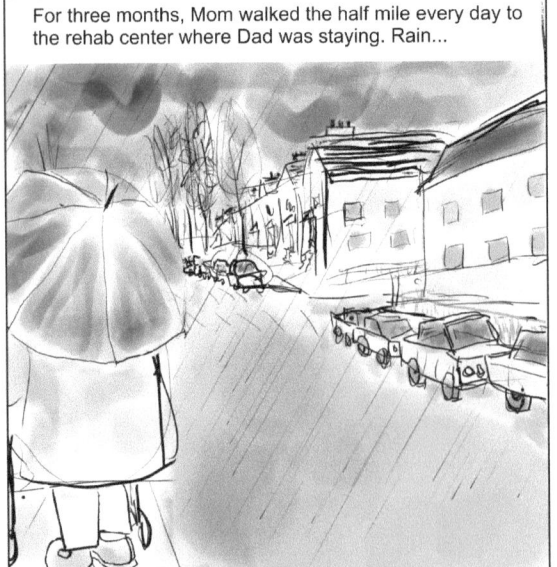
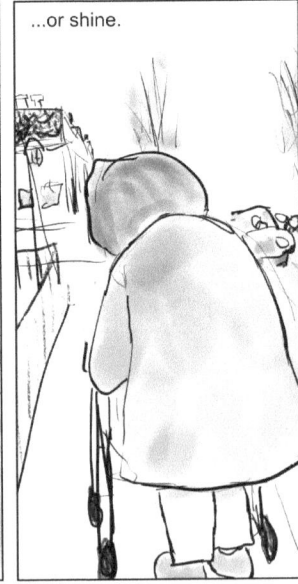

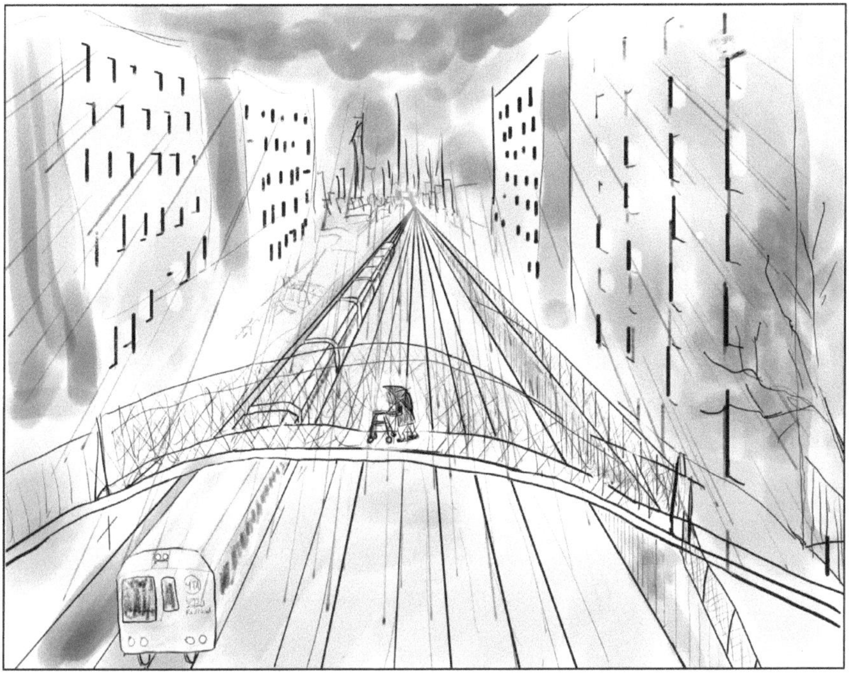

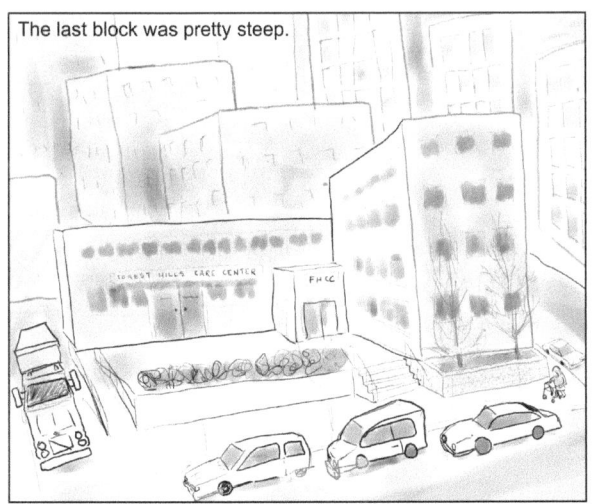

The last block was pretty steep.

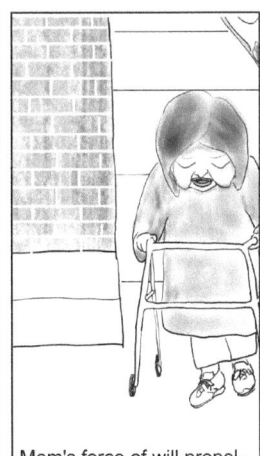

Mom's force of will propelled her to the rehab center.

Mom had spent a couple of months at this center ten years ago when Dad had tripped on a rug at a doctor's office and fallen on her, breaking her leg.

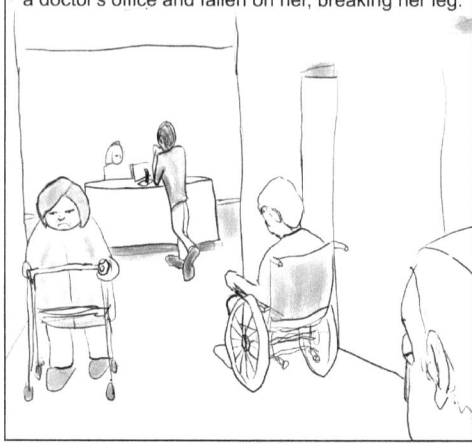

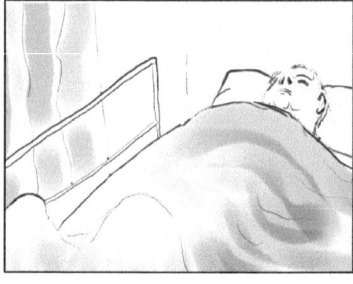

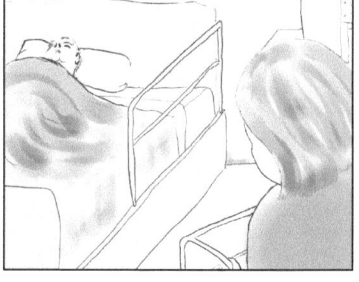

Aside from her own time at the care center, Mom had been the one caring for my dad. Until recently, she'd done most of the cooking and cleaning.

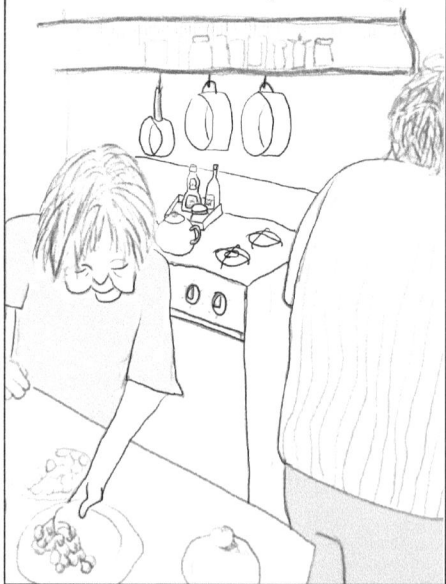

HOW MANY TIMES DO I HAVE TO GO BACK AND FORTH ON THIS?

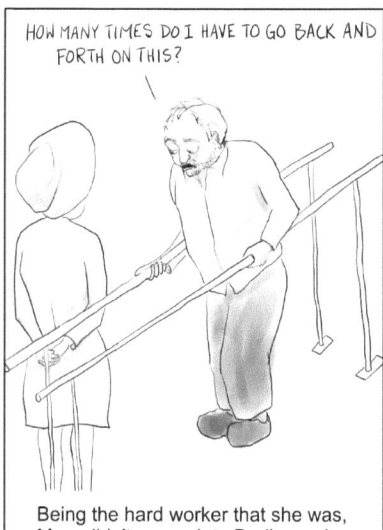

Being the hard worker that she was, Mom didn't appreciate Dad's mock complaints about physical therapy.

When I was growing up, we'd take two-week vacations to Maine every summer.

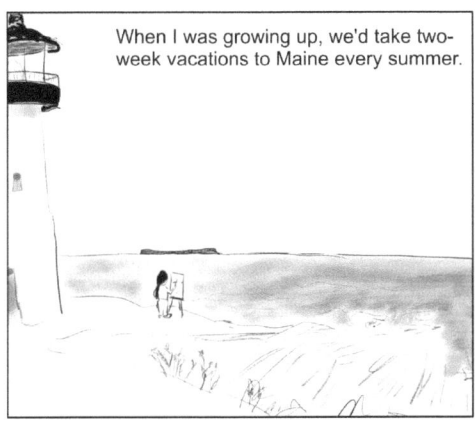

They were working vacations for Mom.

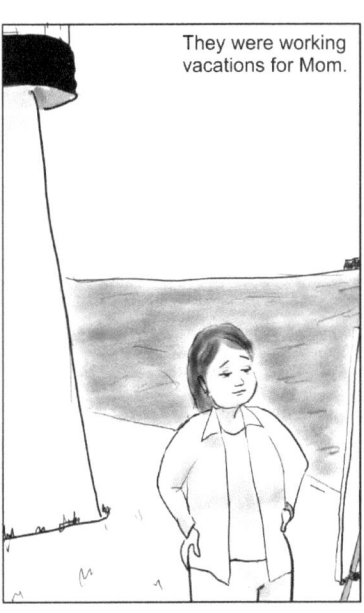

She would make a promising start on one sizable painting every day, and complete them over the next several months at home.

Dad called Mom the "pillar of the family."

He referred to himself as the "pillow of the family."

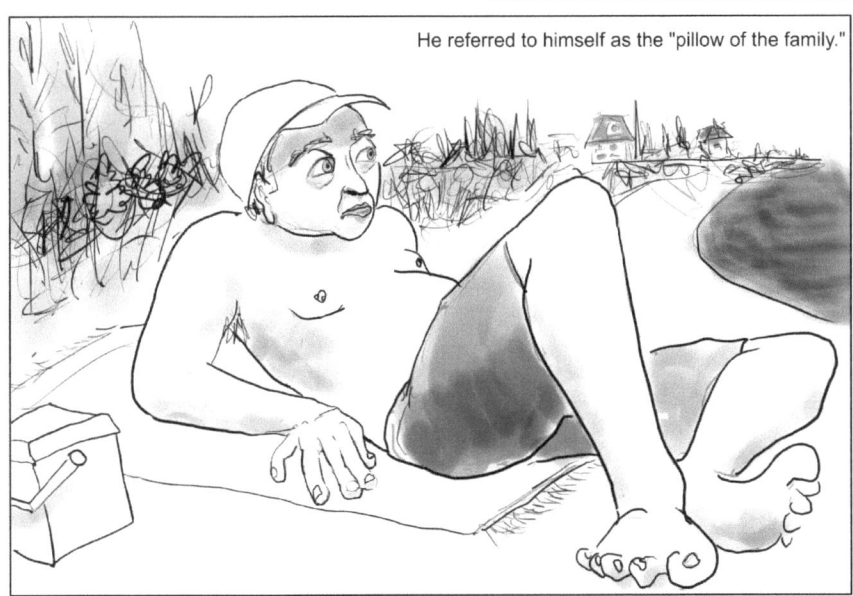

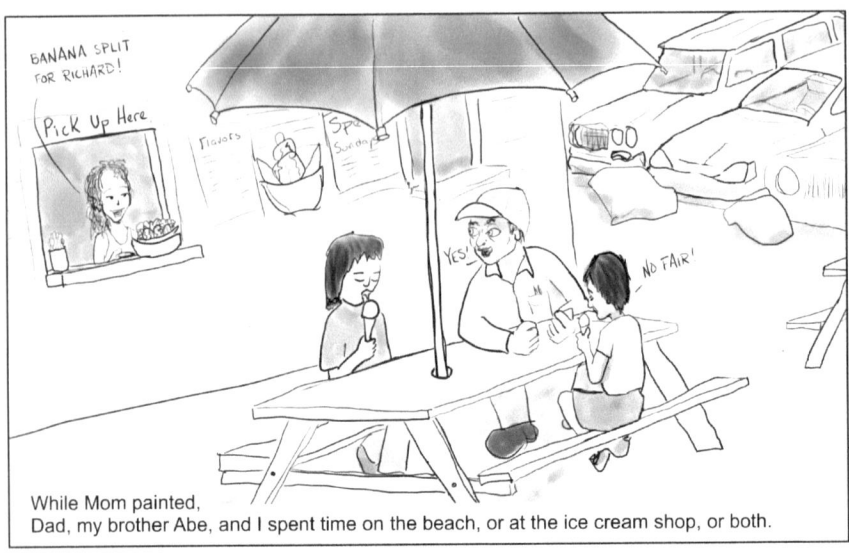

While Mom painted,
Dad, my brother Abe, and I spent time on the beach, or at the ice cream shop, or both.

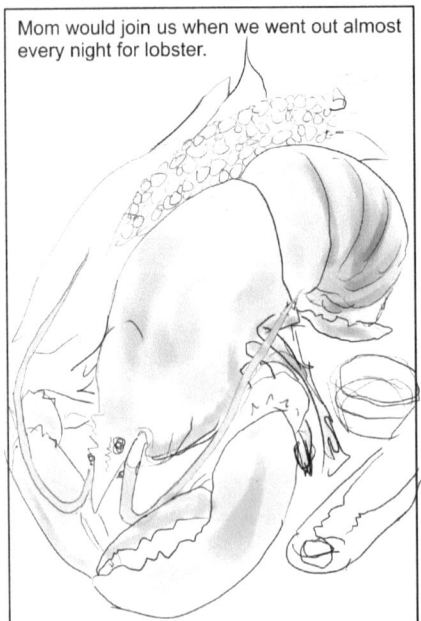

Mom would join us when we went out almost every night for lobster.

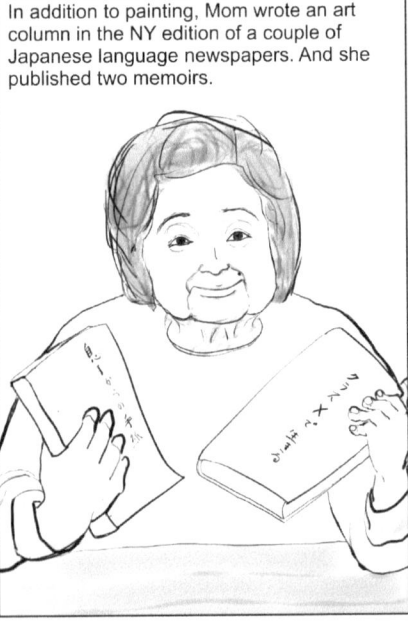

In addition to painting, Mom wrote an art column in the NY edition of a couple of Japanese language newspapers. And she published two memoirs.

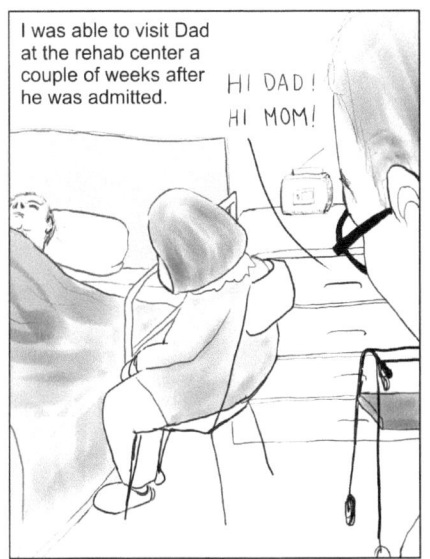
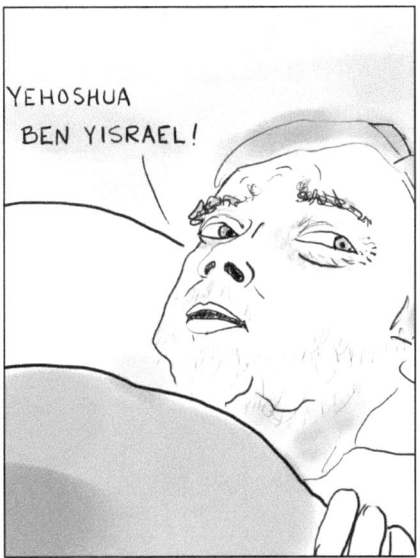

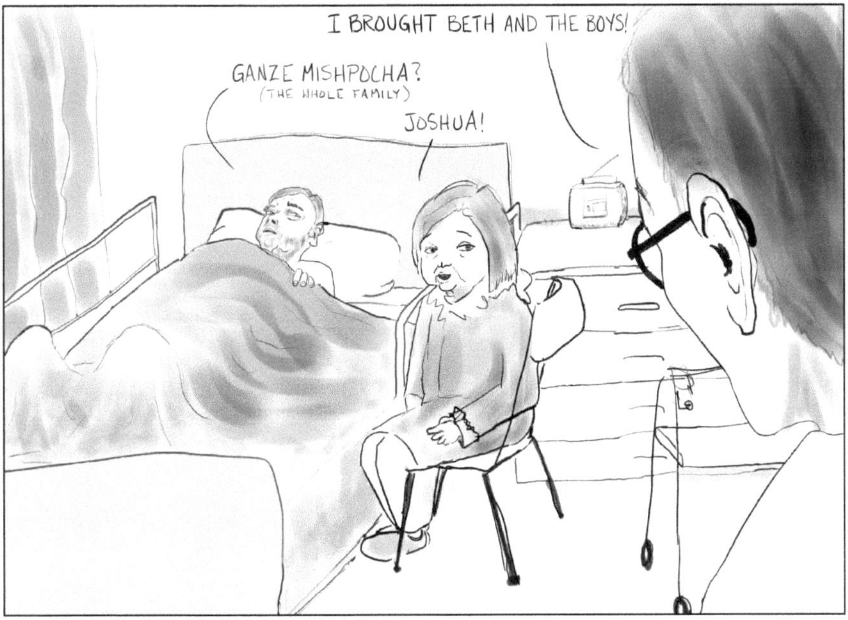

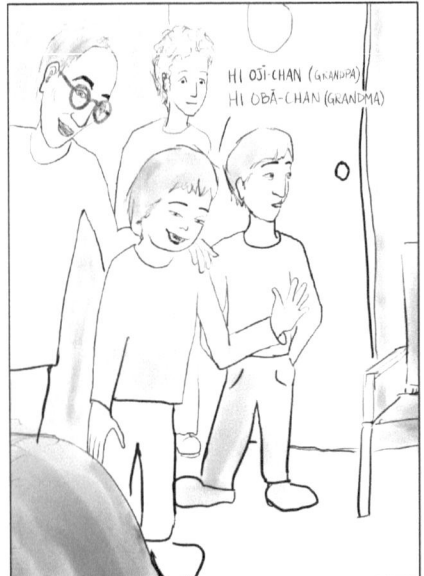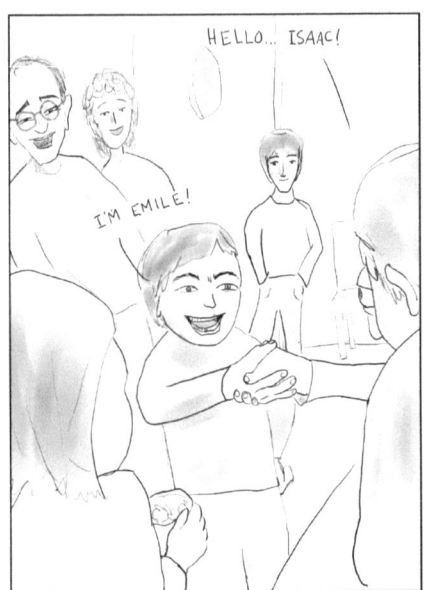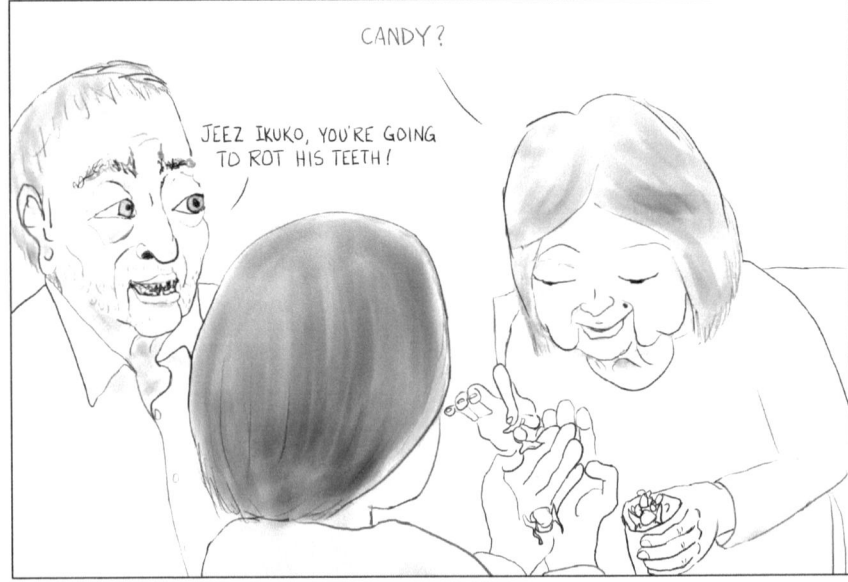

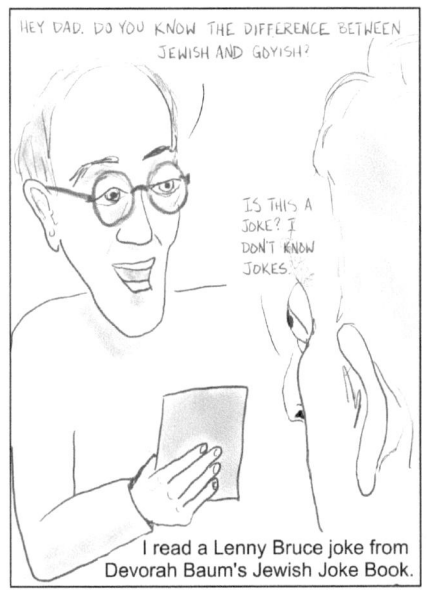
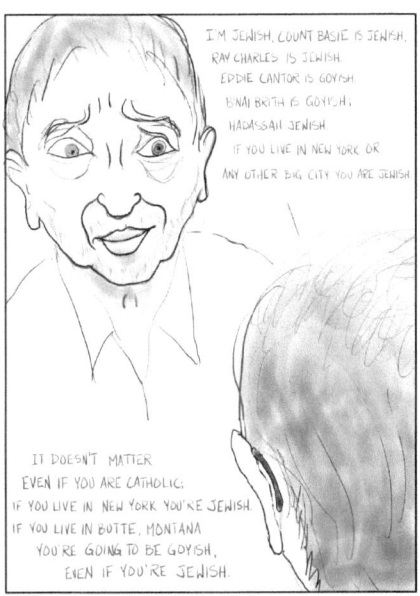
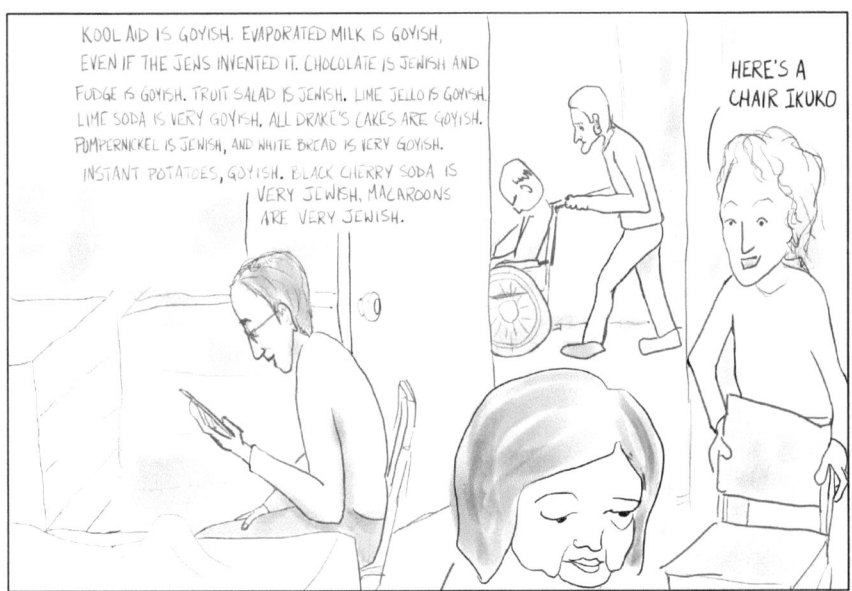

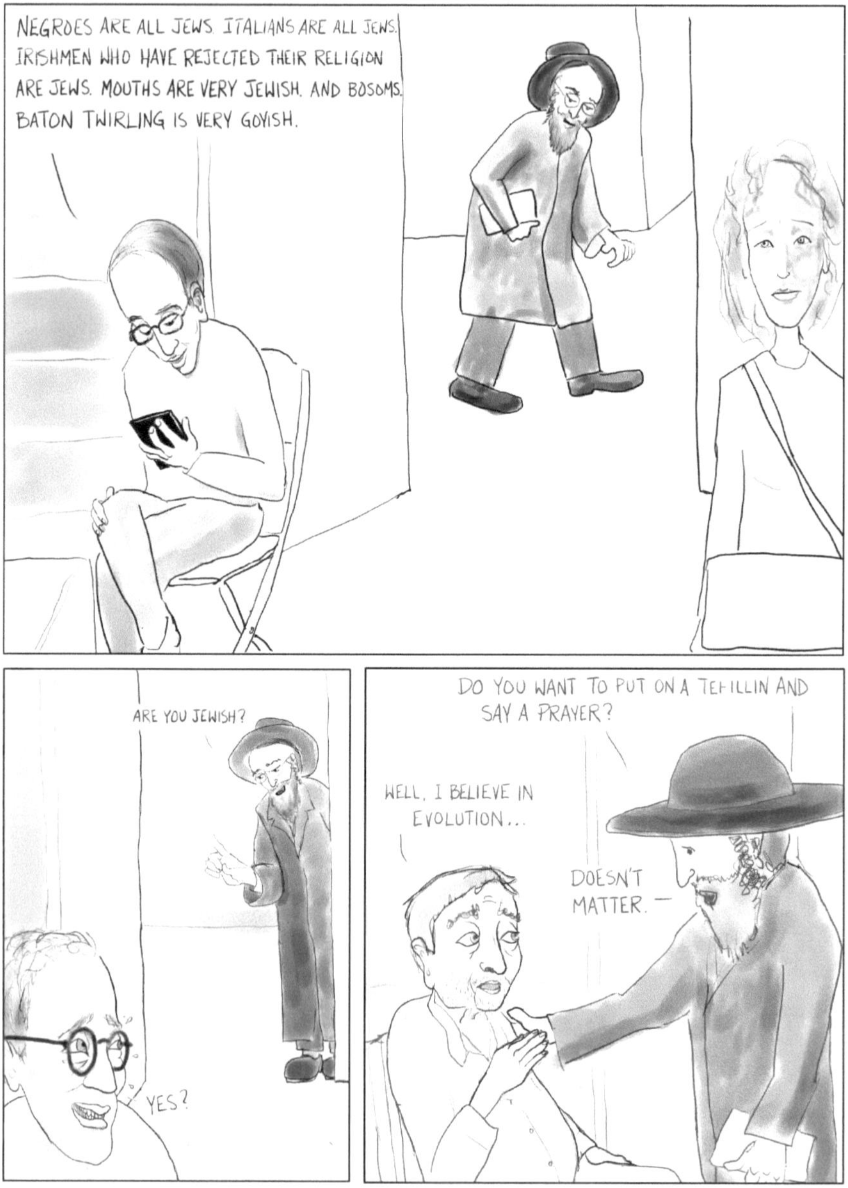

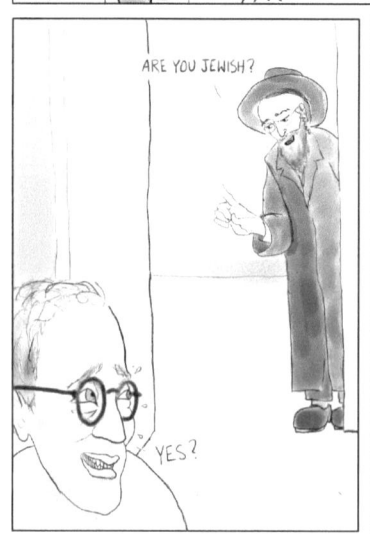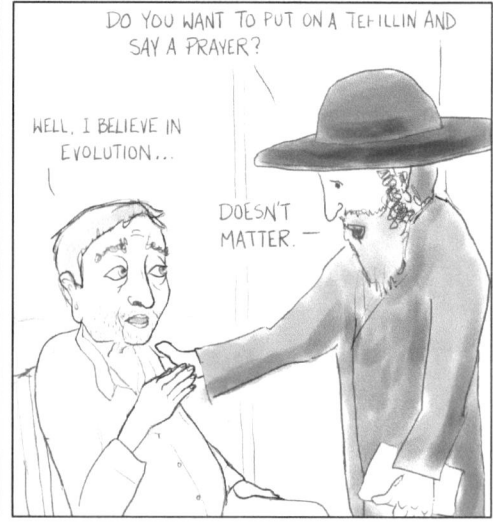

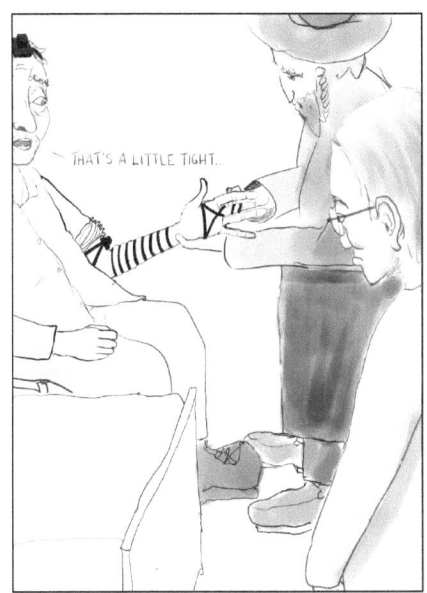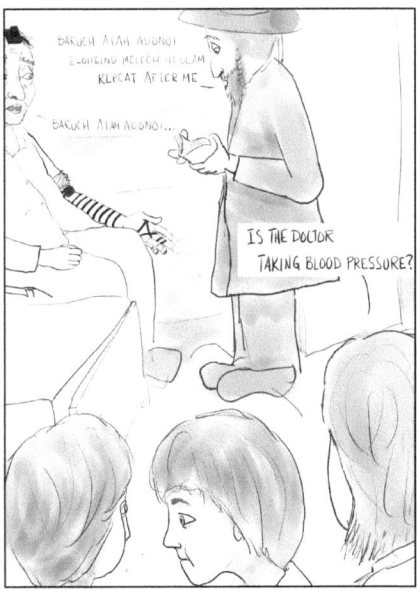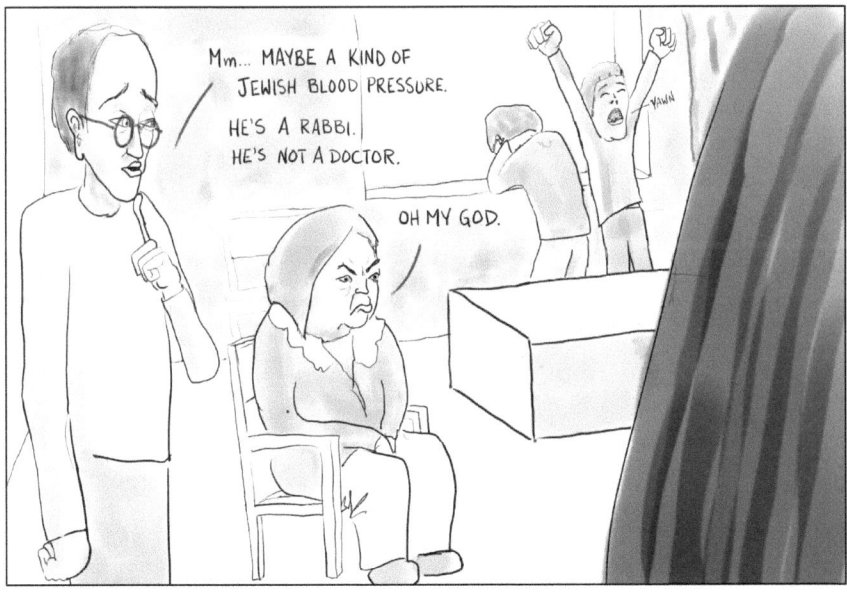

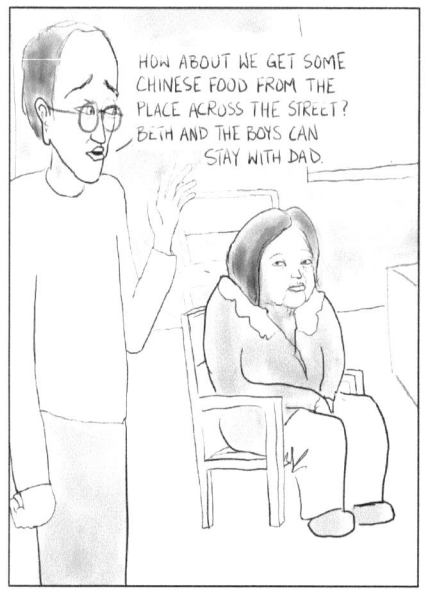
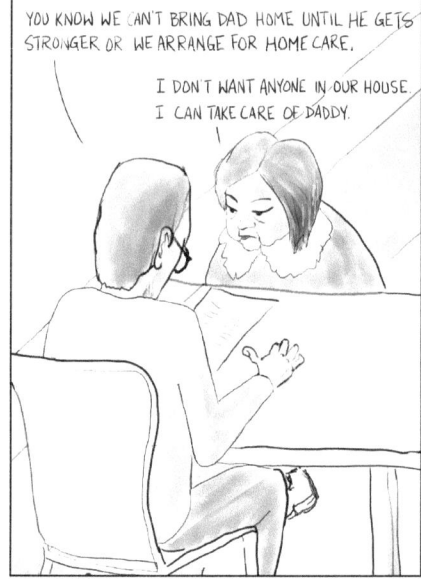
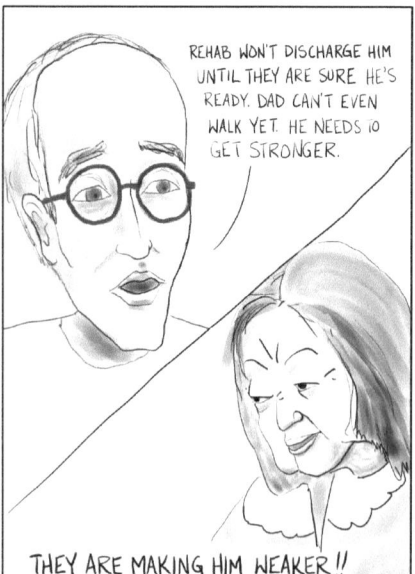
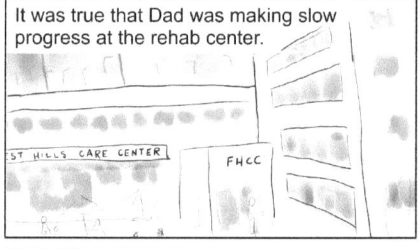

It was true that Dad was making slow progress at the rehab center.

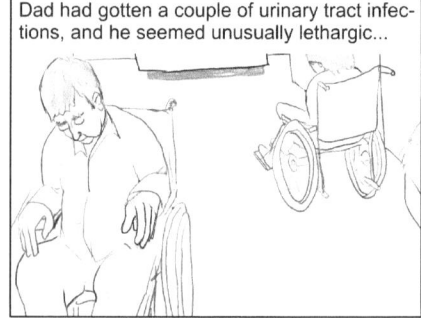

Dad had gotten a couple of urinary tract infections, and he seemed unusually lethargic...

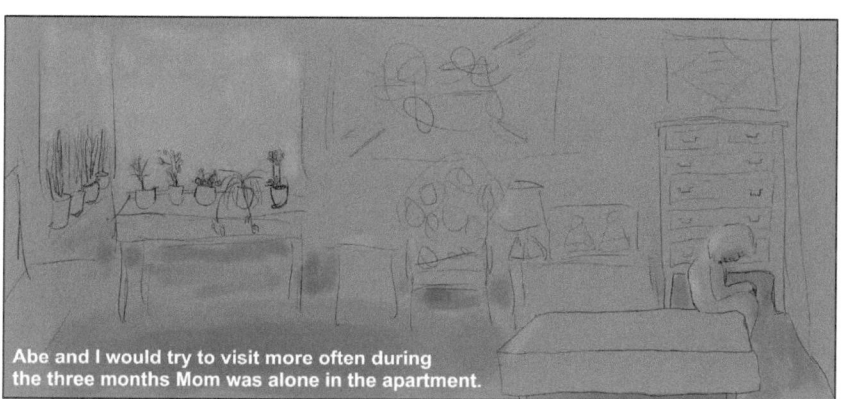

It was a much bigger trip for Abe, who lives in Columbus, Ohio.

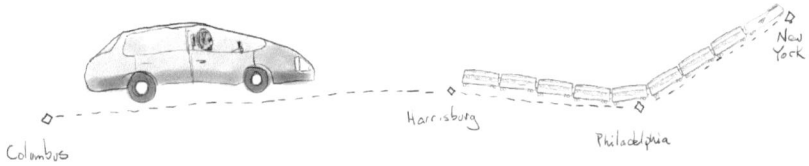

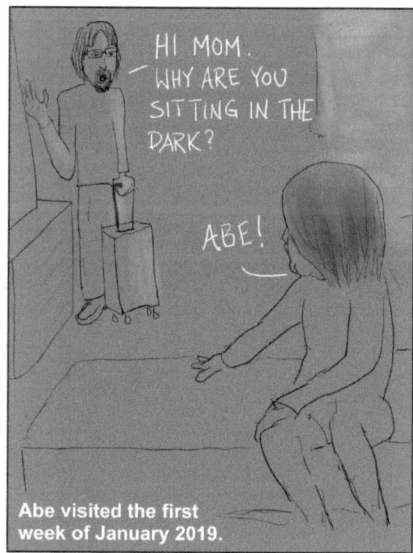

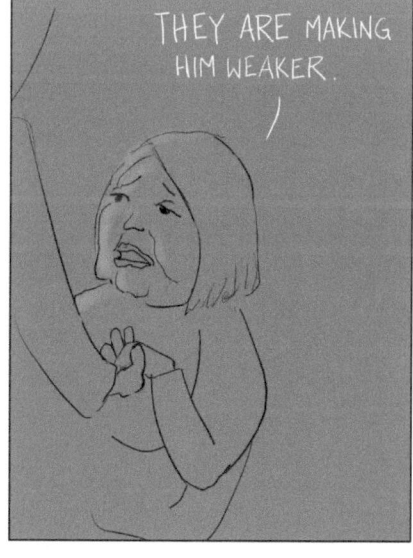

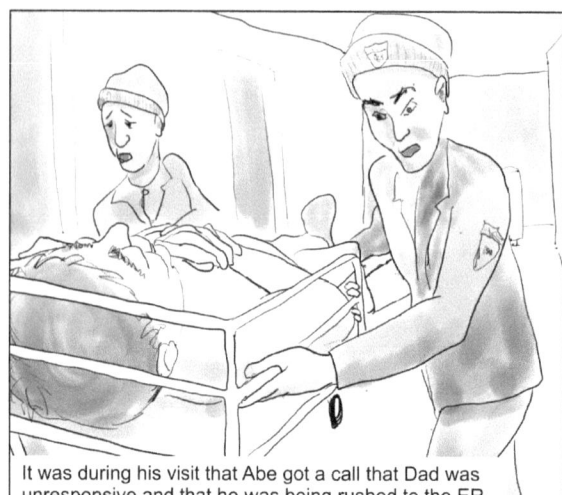
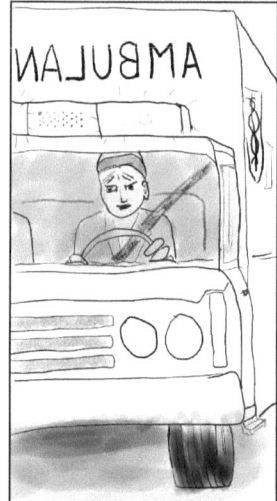

It was during his visit that Abe got a call that Dad was unresponsive and that he was being rushed to the ER.

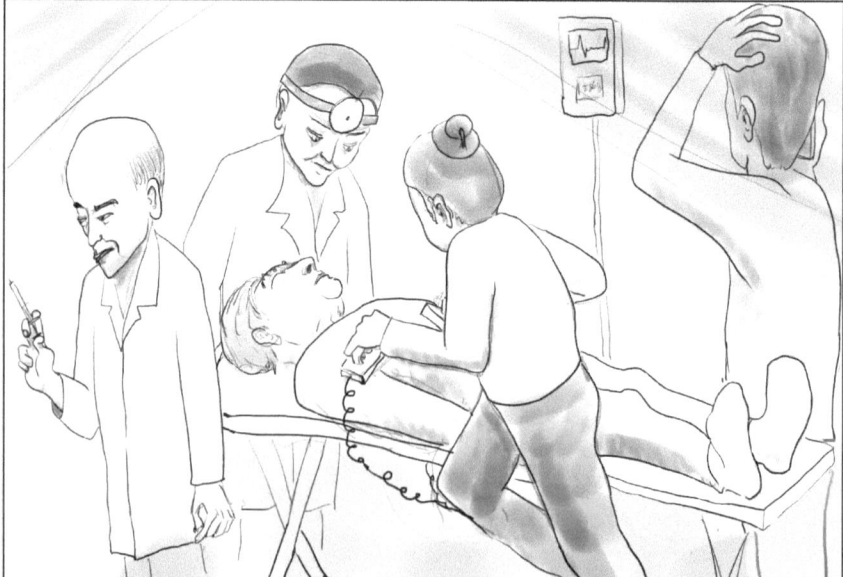

The ER docs couldn't revive Dad, and asked Abe if we should let him go. Abe was desperate to reach me but it was a rare Saturday that I went to shul and I didn't have my phone on me. Then one doctor tried administering a dose of Narcan.

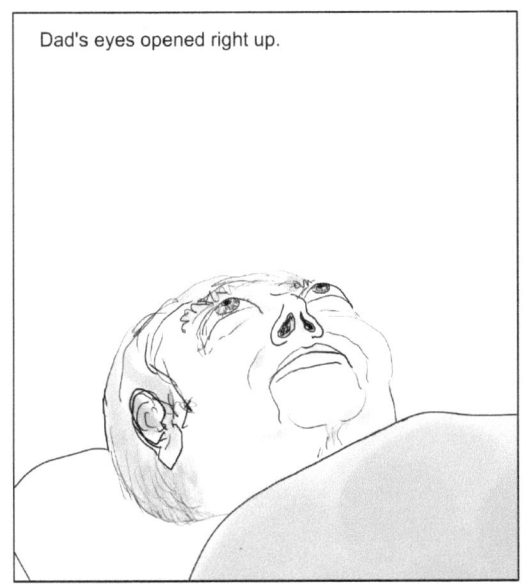
Dad's eyes opened right up.

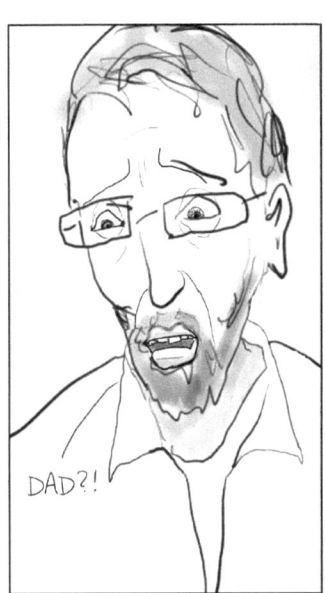
DAD?!

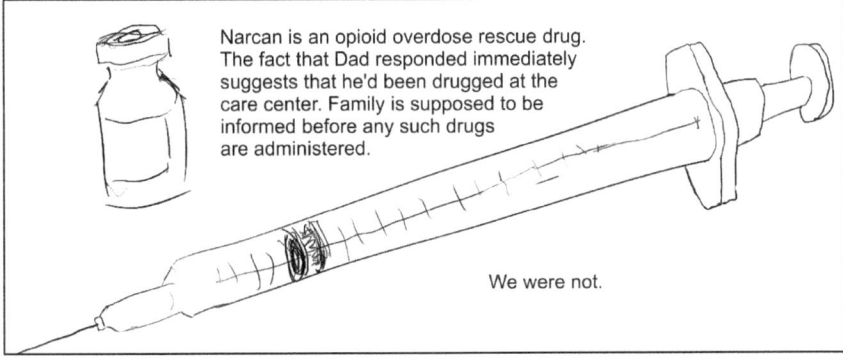
Narcan is an opioid overdose rescue drug. The fact that Dad responded immediately suggests that he'd been drugged at the care center. Family is supposed to be informed before any such drugs are administered.

We were not.

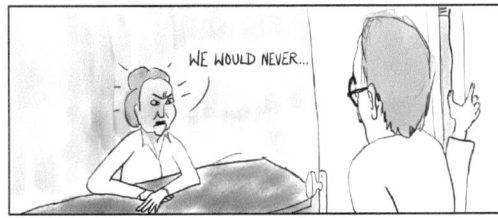
WE WOULD NEVER...

The care center denied giving Dad any opioids, but it seems to be something nursing homes do to sedate agitated patients, especially during the night when the centers are short staffed.

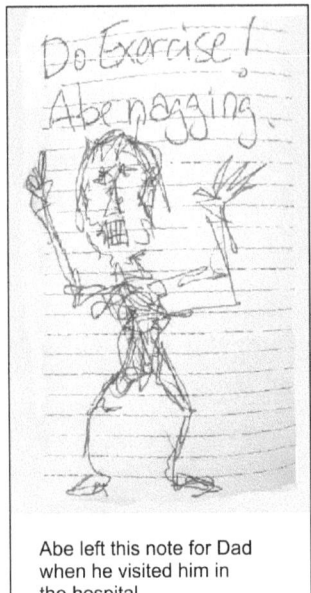

Abe left this note for Dad when he visited him in the hospital.

Dad was kept at the hospital for a week, and received very little physical therapy. I had Dad do some shadow boxing.

One day, when I was visiting Dad at the hospital, a doctor was going over Dad's chart with a nurse and mentioned that Dad had dementia.
I was aware that Dad's short term memory was deteriorating, but it was a shock to overhear the formal diagnosis.

When was it made? Why wasn't I told directly?

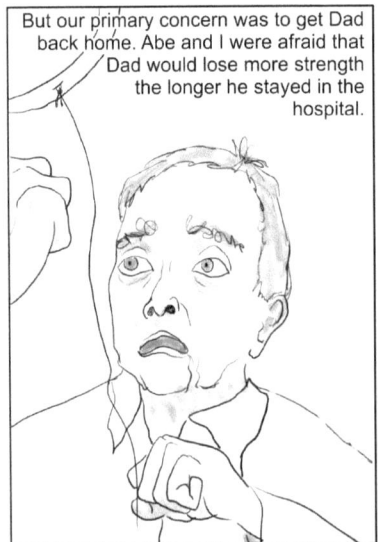

But our primary concern was to get Dad back home. Abe and I were afraid that Dad would lose more strength the longer he stayed in the hospital.

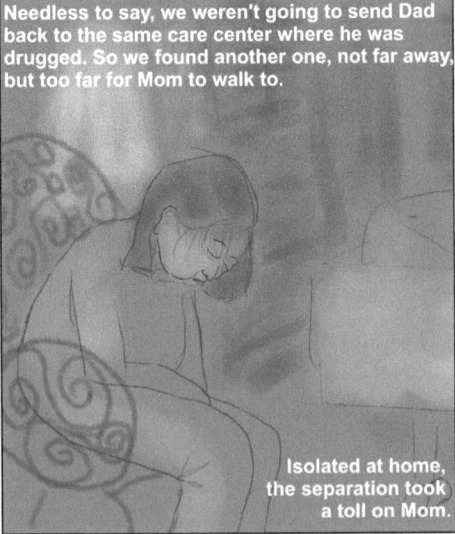

Needless to say, we weren't going to send Dad back to the same care center where he was drugged. So we found another one, not far away, but too far for Mom to walk to.

Isolated at home, the separation took a toll on Mom.

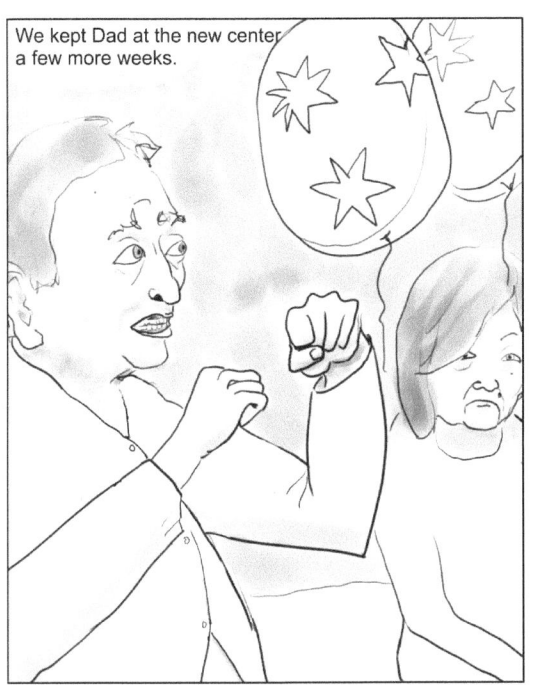

We kept Dad at the new center a few more weeks.

In the meantime, I called around to see if I could set up home care and Medicaid to cover its costs.

HOW MUCH PER HOUR? 27? WE DON'T HAVE MEDICAID YET. WE'RE APPLYING.

NY State assessed Medicaid eligibility for home care with a a three month look back at bank accounts, compared to a five year look back for nursing home care.

nystateofhealth

Now is the time to enroll.
Call us: 1-855-355-5777

Individuals & Families

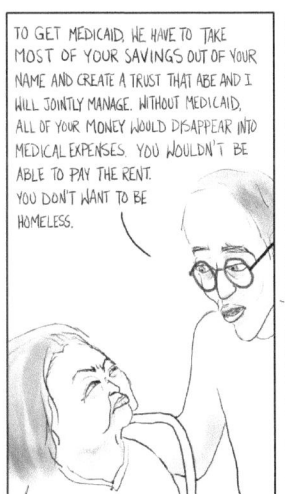

TO GET MEDICAID, HE HAVE TO TAKE MOST OF YOUR SAVINGS OUT OF YOUR NAME AND CREATE A TRUST THAT ABE AND I WILL JOINTLY MANAGE. WITHOUT MEDICAID, ALL OF YOUR MONEY WOULD DISAPPEAR INTO MEDICAL EXPENSES. YOU WOULDN'T BE ABLE TO PAY THE RENT. YOU DON'T WANT TO BE HOMELESS.

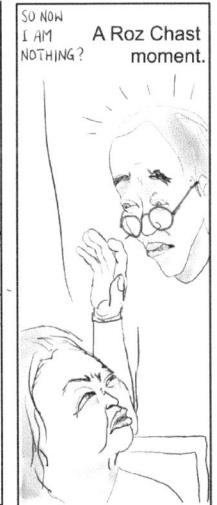

SO NOW I AM NOTHING?

A Roz Chast moment.

Years ago Mom had given Abe and me money to start our children's college education funds. She wanted to be able to give, and once divested, that would be impossible. She wanted to care for Dad, but soon professional care workers would usurp that role.

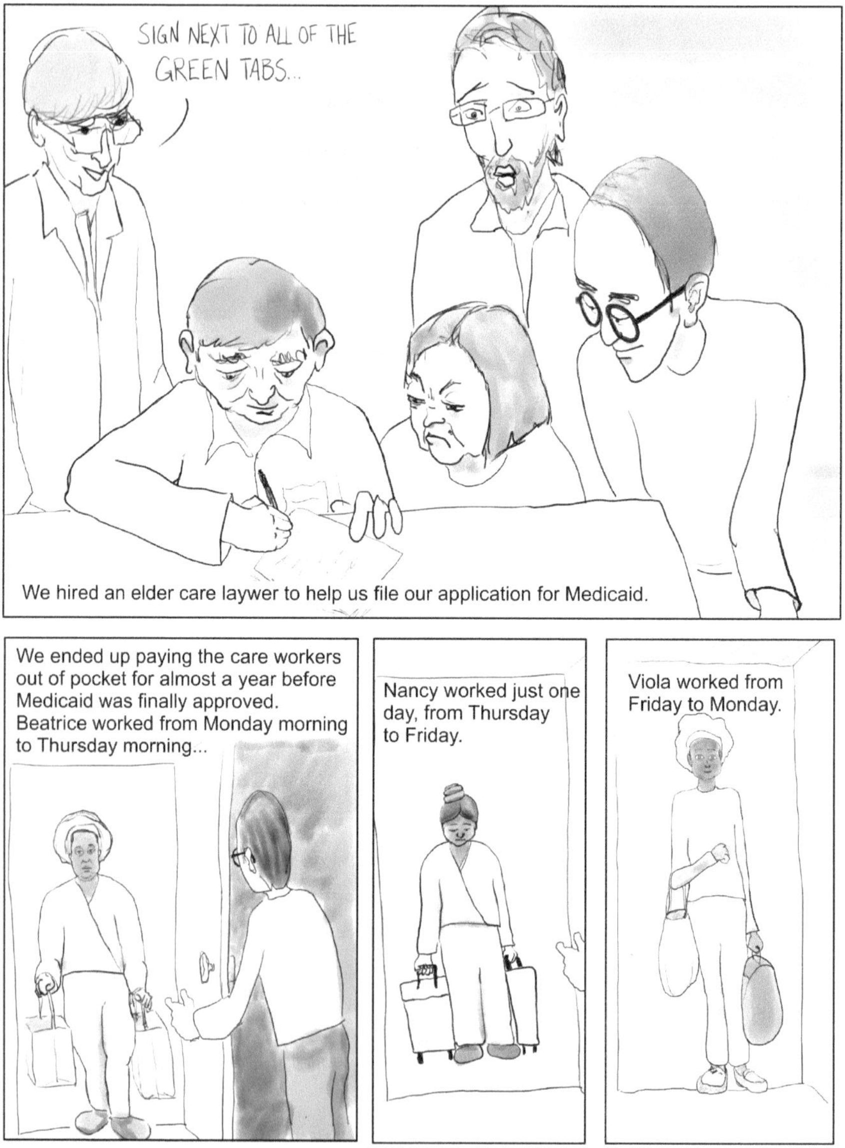

We hired an elder care laywer to help us file our application for Medicaid.

We ended up paying the care workers out of pocket for almost a year before Medicaid was finally approved. Beatrice worked from Monday morning to Thursday morning...

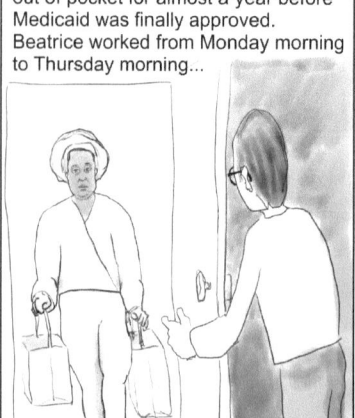

Nancy worked just one day, from Thursday to Friday.

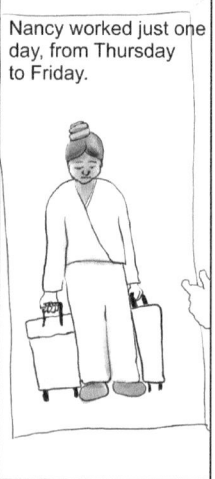

Viola worked from Friday to Monday.

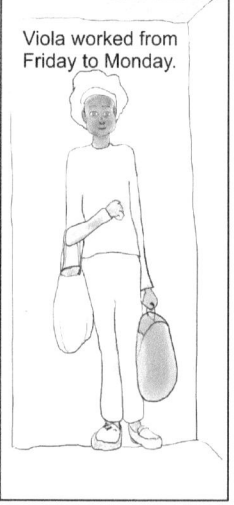

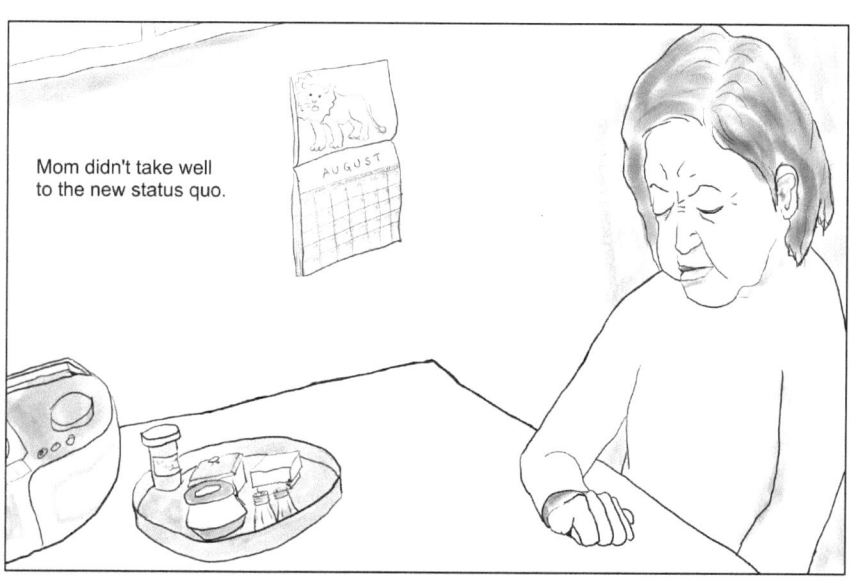
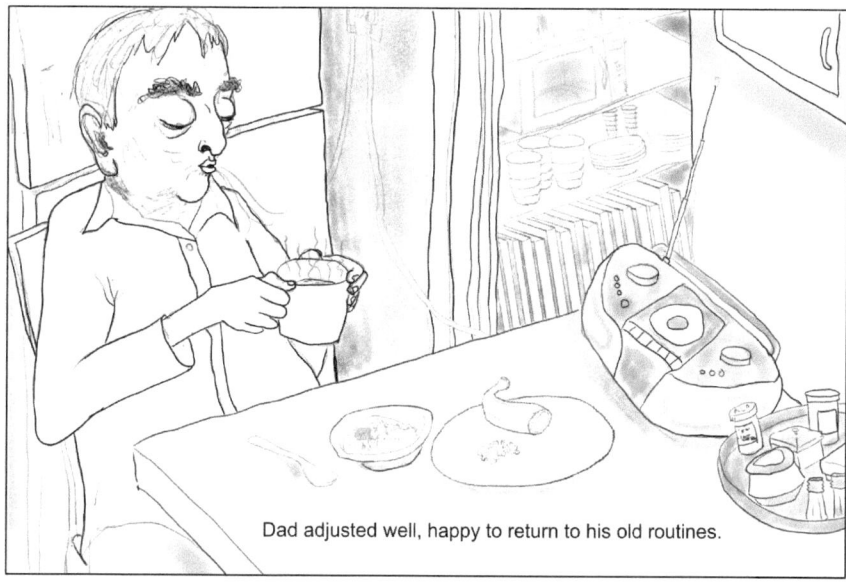

I Am the Giver

Chapter 3

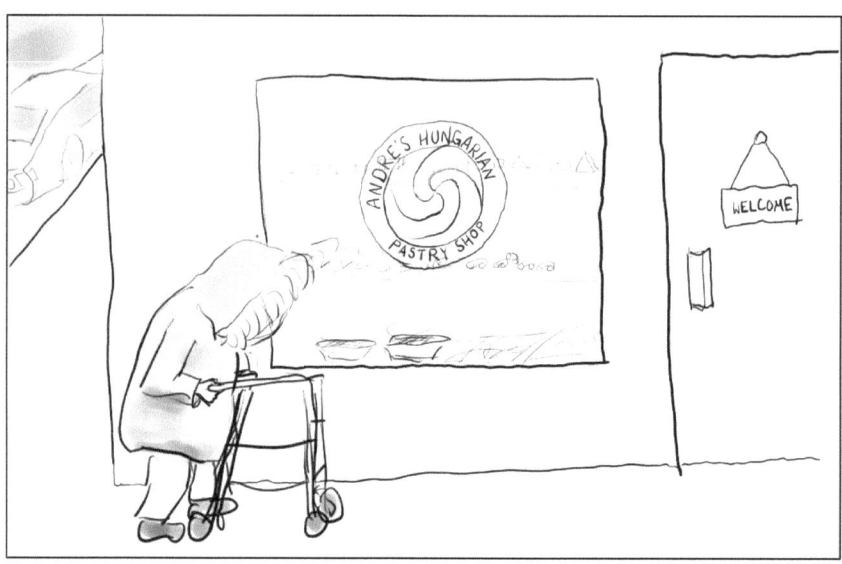
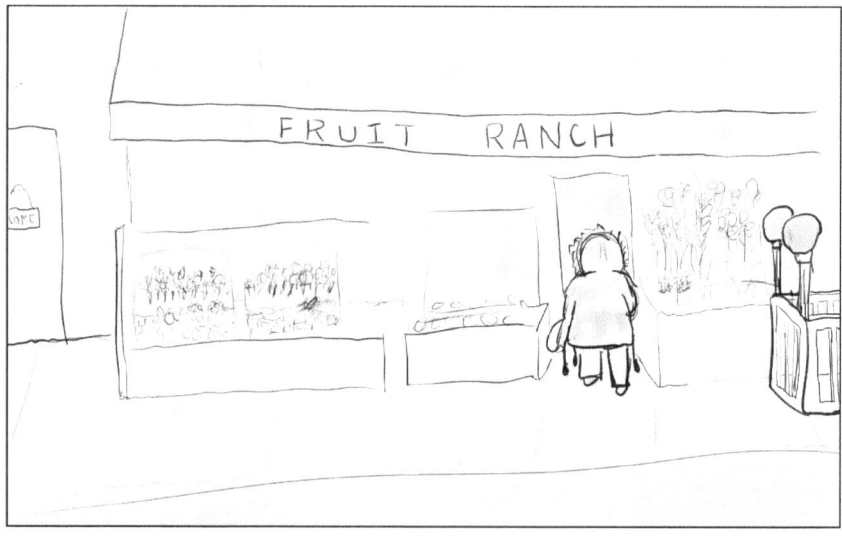

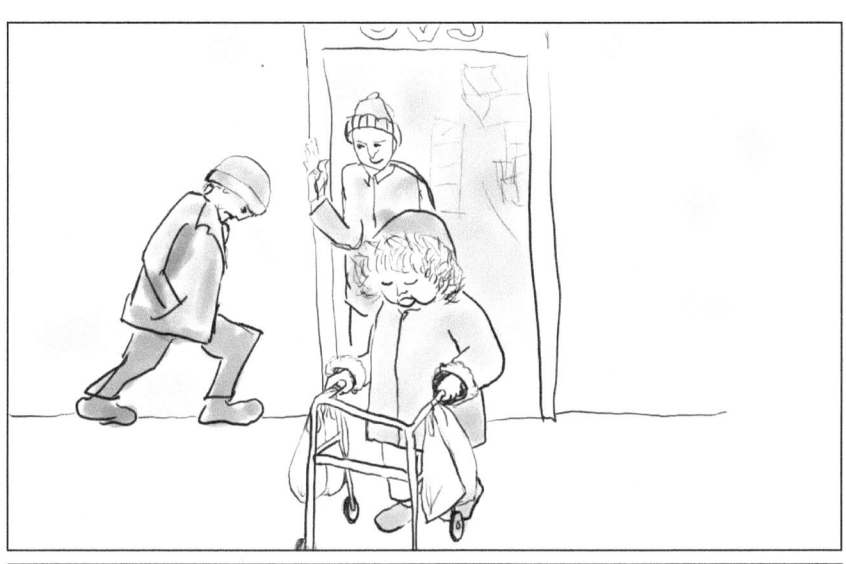
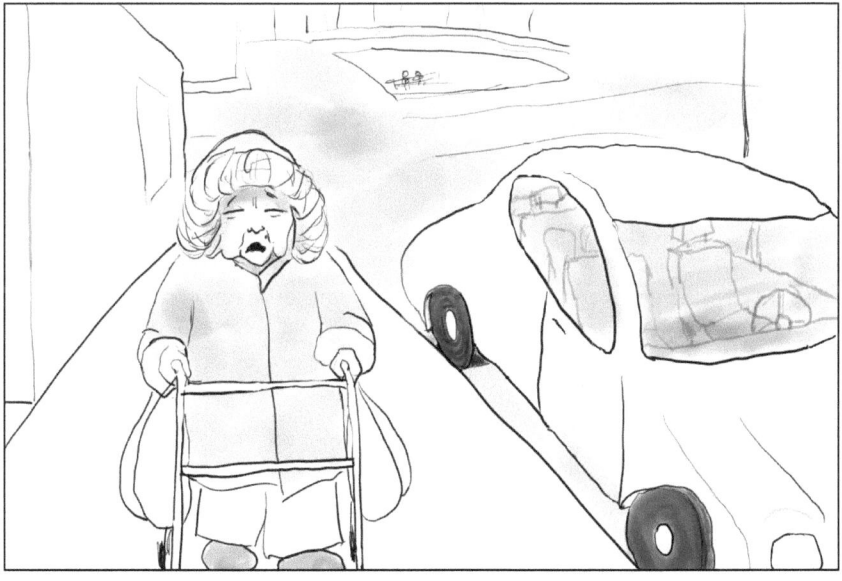

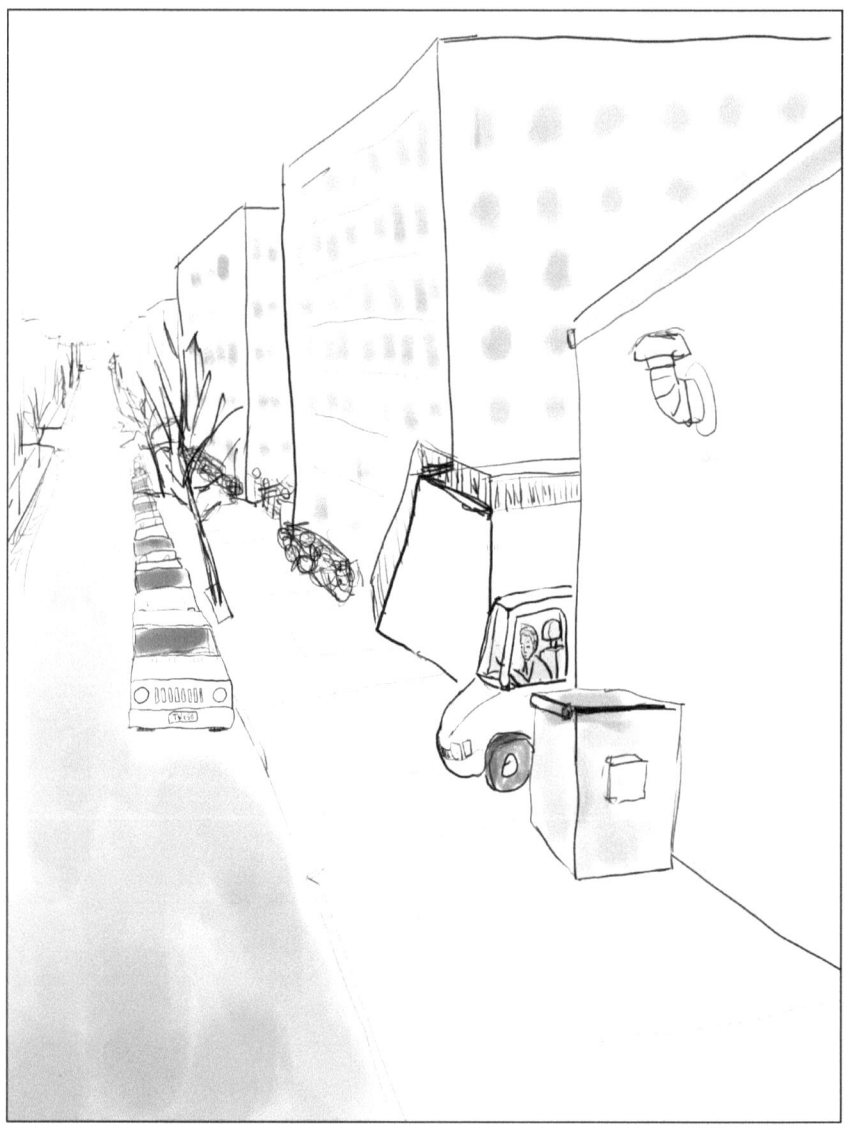

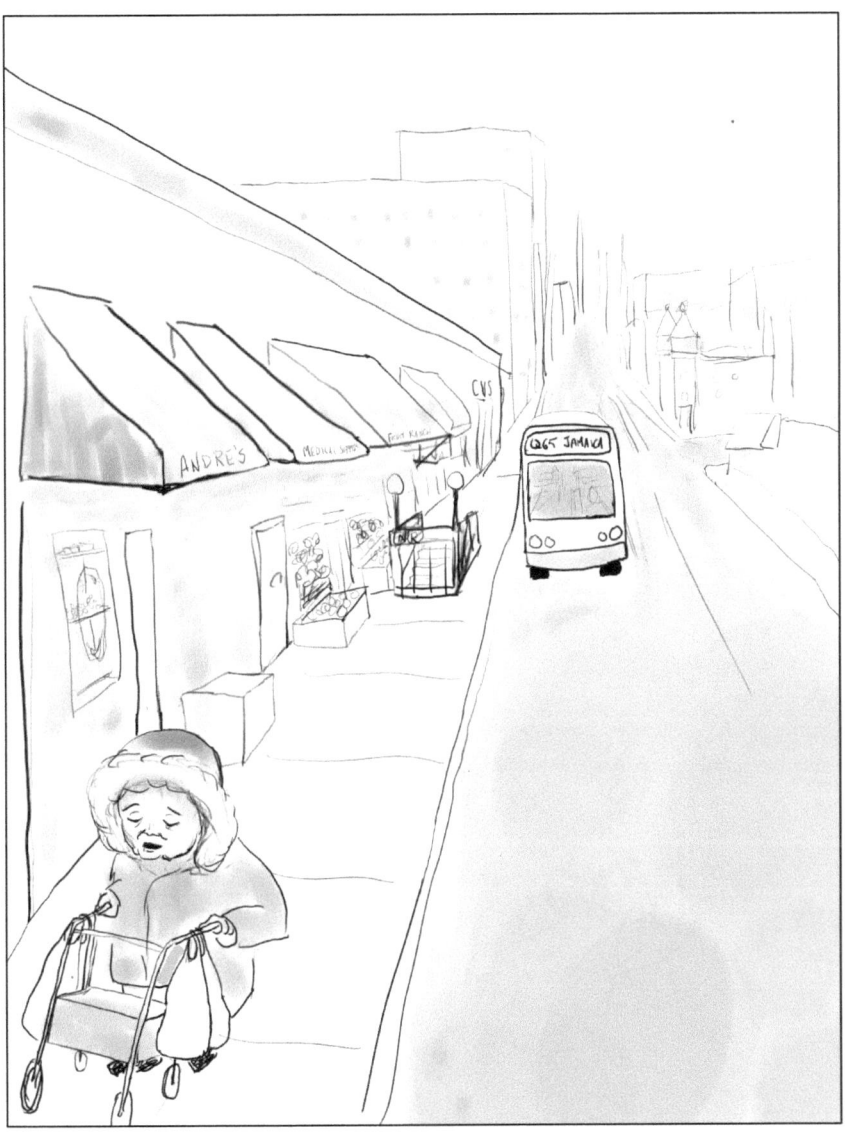

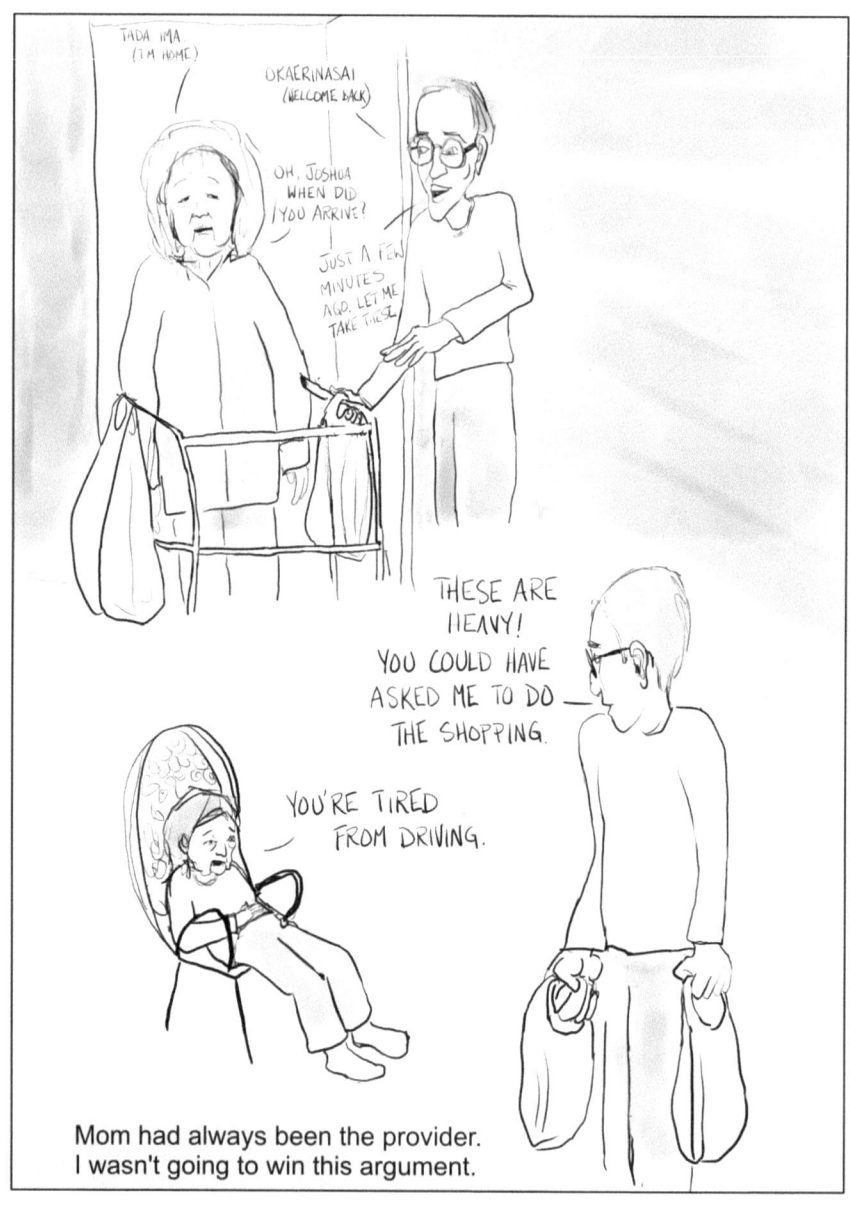

When I was growing up, we would say the standard Japanese phrases at the start and end of meals.

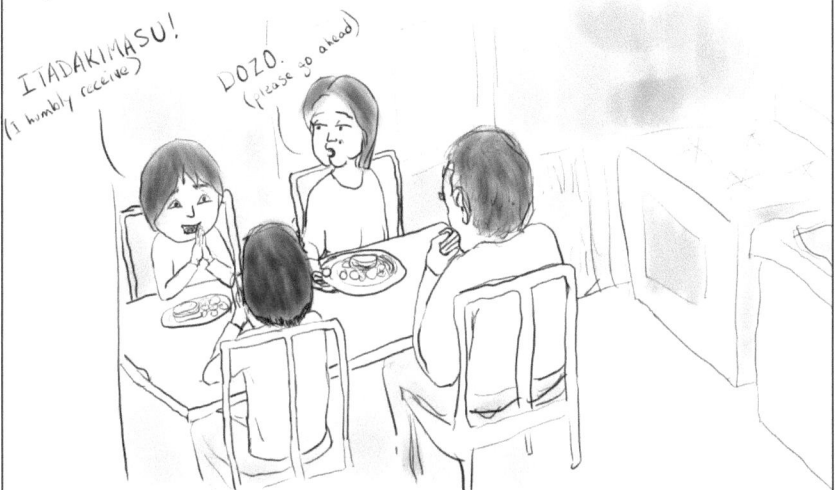

Sometimes Abe or I would flip the script, which never failed to provoke Mom to clarify who had the right to say what.

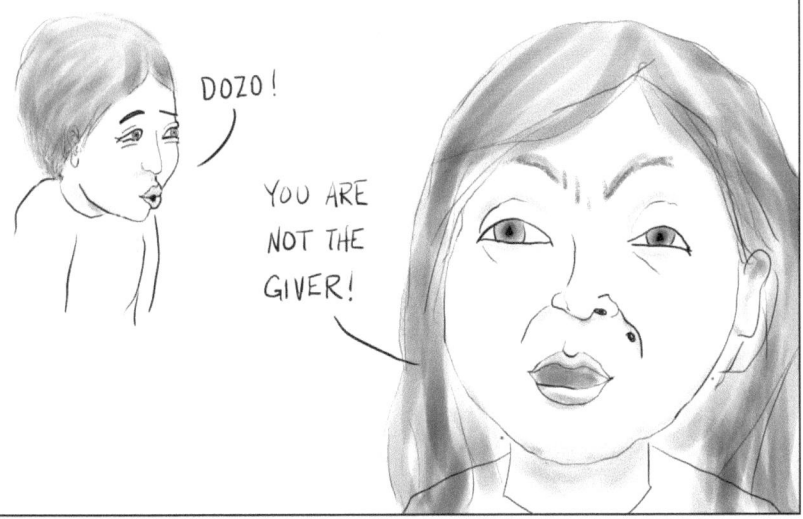

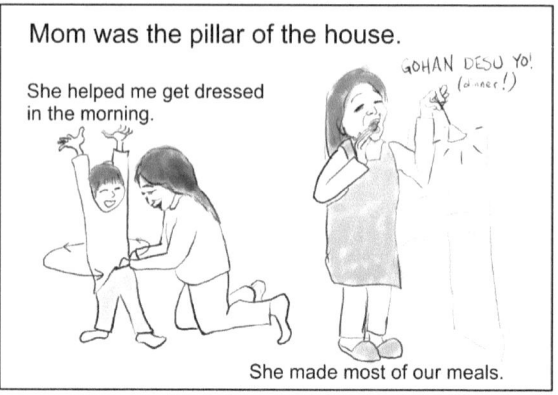
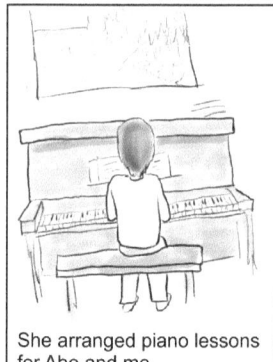
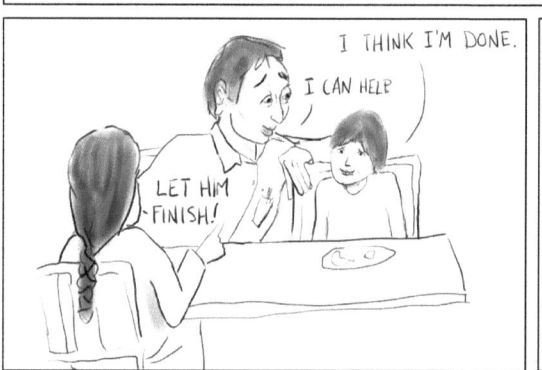
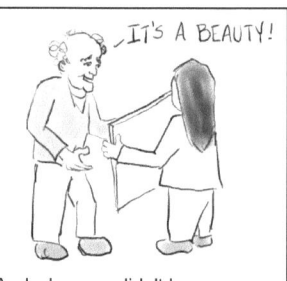
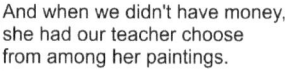
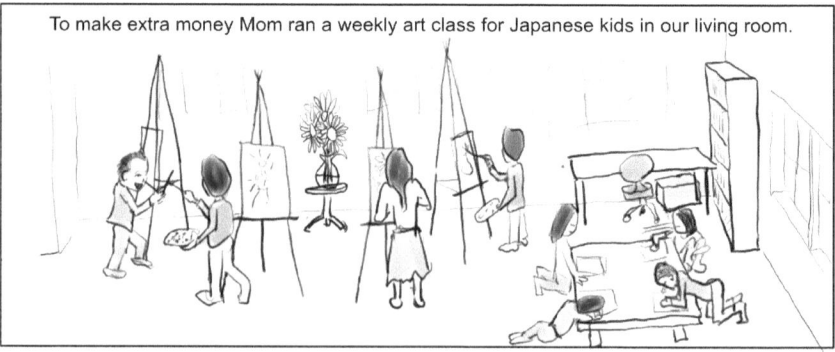

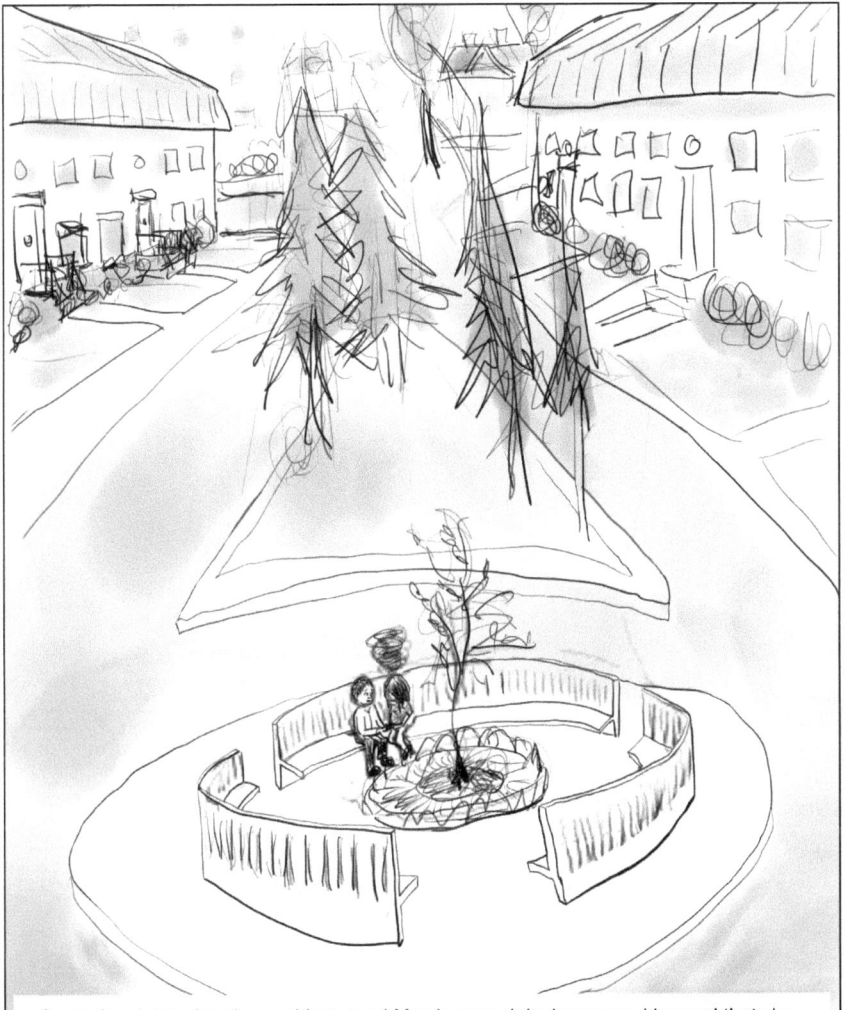

Some time later when I was able to read Mom's memoir in Japanese, I learned that she suffered a long period of depression, starting soon after her father died in 1972, and that during that period, Dad was a compassionate support for her. So Mom was able to accept help in moments of need. But she had trouble recognizing such moments.

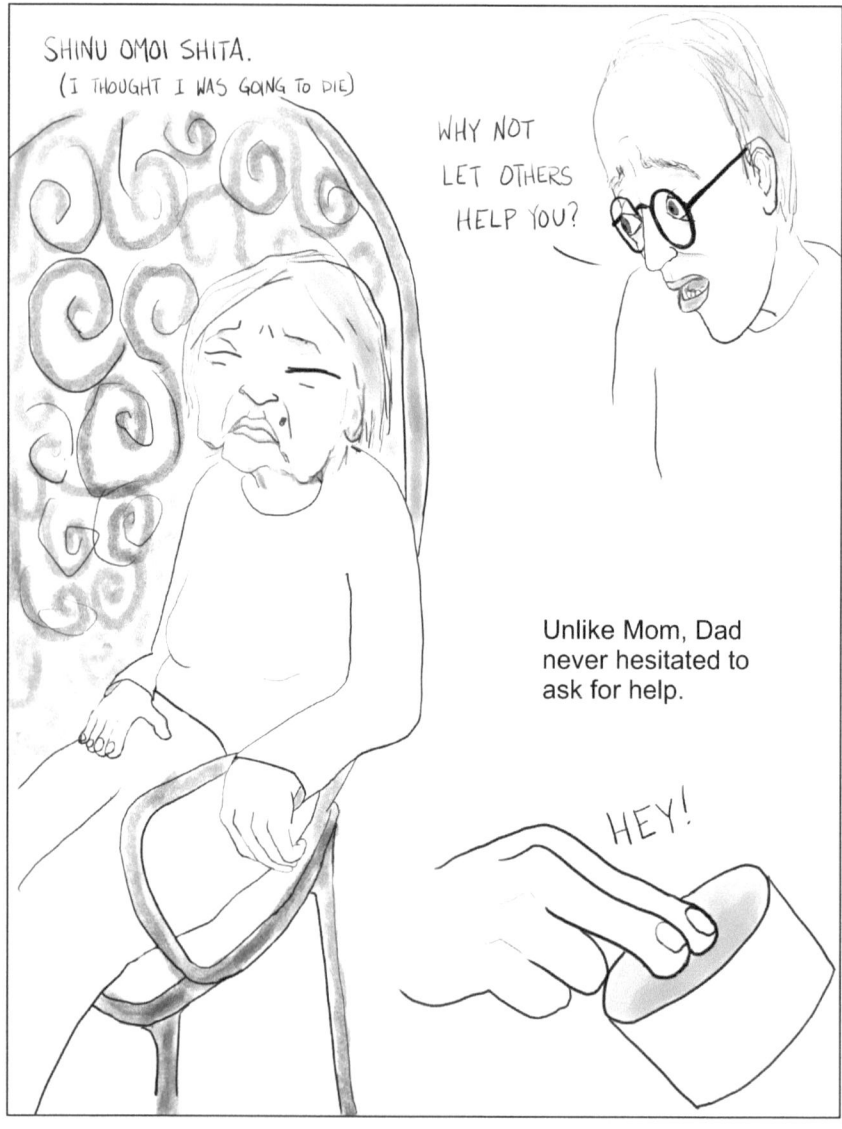

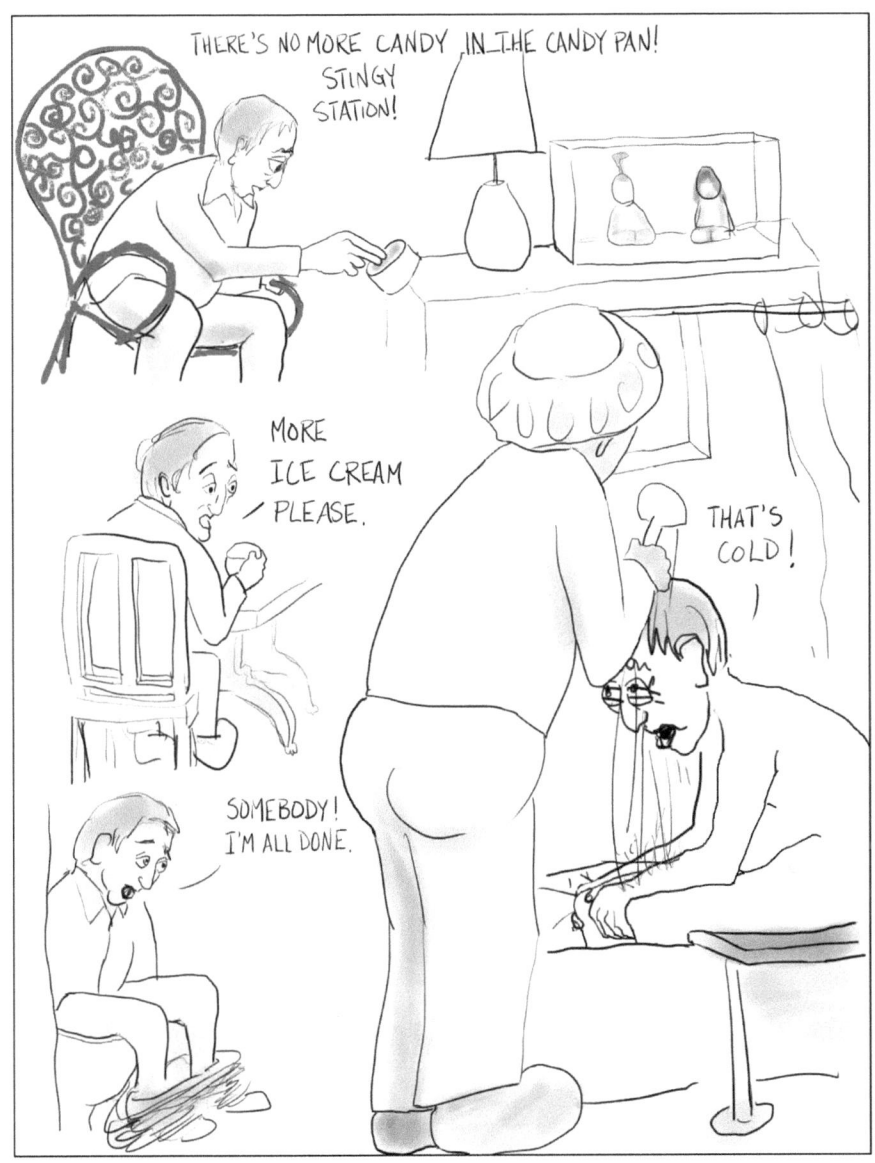

The care workers were especially careful about controlling urinary tract infections (UTIs) and falls. UTIs could be controlled by helping with wiping clean after toilet use, regular changing of diapers, and hydration. They had both Dad and Mom drinking a lot of liquids throughout the day, but Mom took care of toileting on her own.

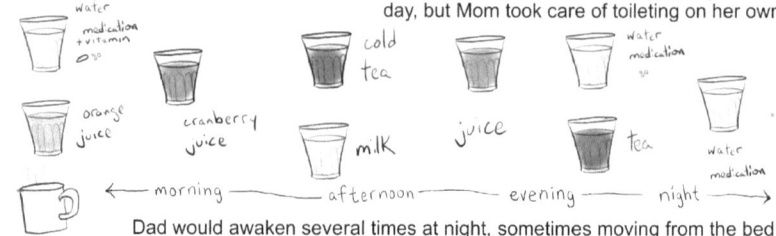

Dad would awaken several times at night, sometimes moving from the bed to the reading chair. Concerned about falls, the care workers would always check in on him when they heard the sound of the walker. Plus they did a diaper change at about 3:30 a.m.

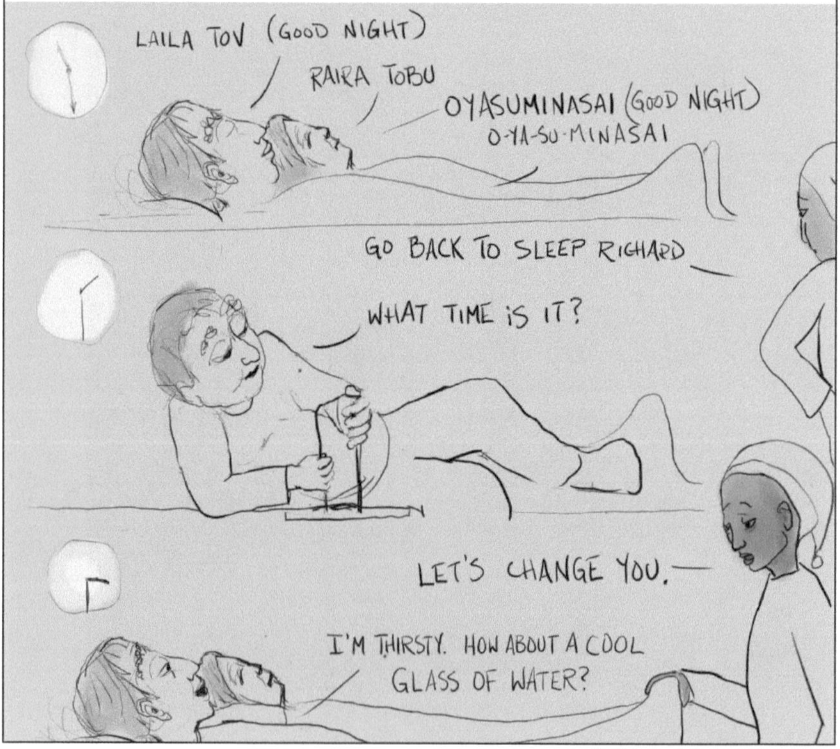

LAILA TOV (GOOD NIGHT)
RAIRA TOBU
OYASUMINASAI (GOOD NIGHT)
O-YA-SU-MI-NA-SAI

GO BACK TO SLEEP RICHARD

WHAT TIME IS IT?

LET'S CHANGE YOU.

I'M THIRSTY. HOW ABOUT A COOL GLASS OF WATER?

Despite being high maintenance, the care workers really liked Dad.

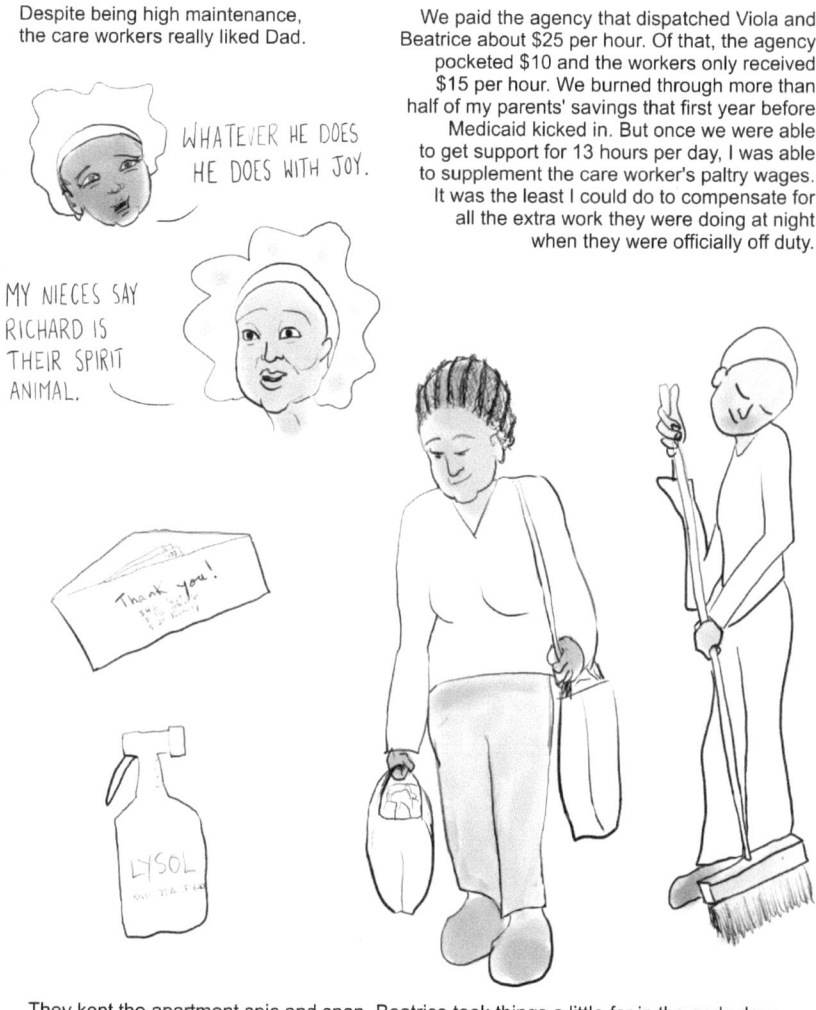

WHATEVER HE DOES HE DOES WITH JOY.

MY NIECES SAY RICHARD IS THEIR SPIRIT ANIMAL.

We paid the agency that dispatched Viola and Beatrice about $25 per hour. Of that, the agency pocketed $10 and the workers only received $15 per hour. We burned through more than half of my parents' savings that first year before Medicaid kicked in. But once we were able to get support for 13 hours per day, I was able to supplement the care worker's paltry wages. It was the least I could do to compensate for all the extra work they were doing at night when they were officially off duty.

They kept the apartment spic and span. Beatrice took things a little far in the early days of Covid, going through an entire container of Lysol in three days, even spraying down a nurse at the entrance of the apartment. But she was proud that the apartment didn't have the dreaded "old person smell."

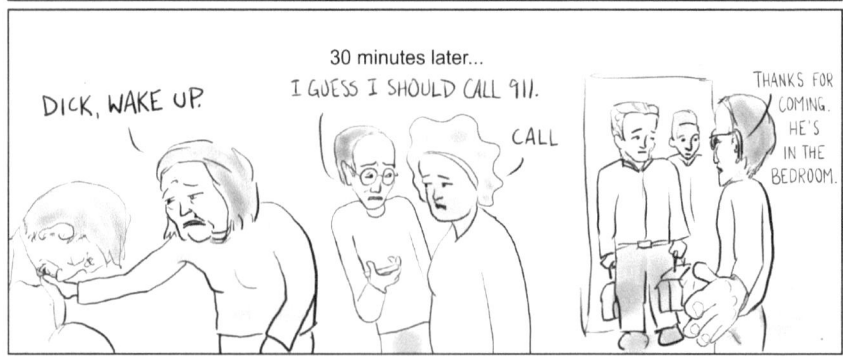

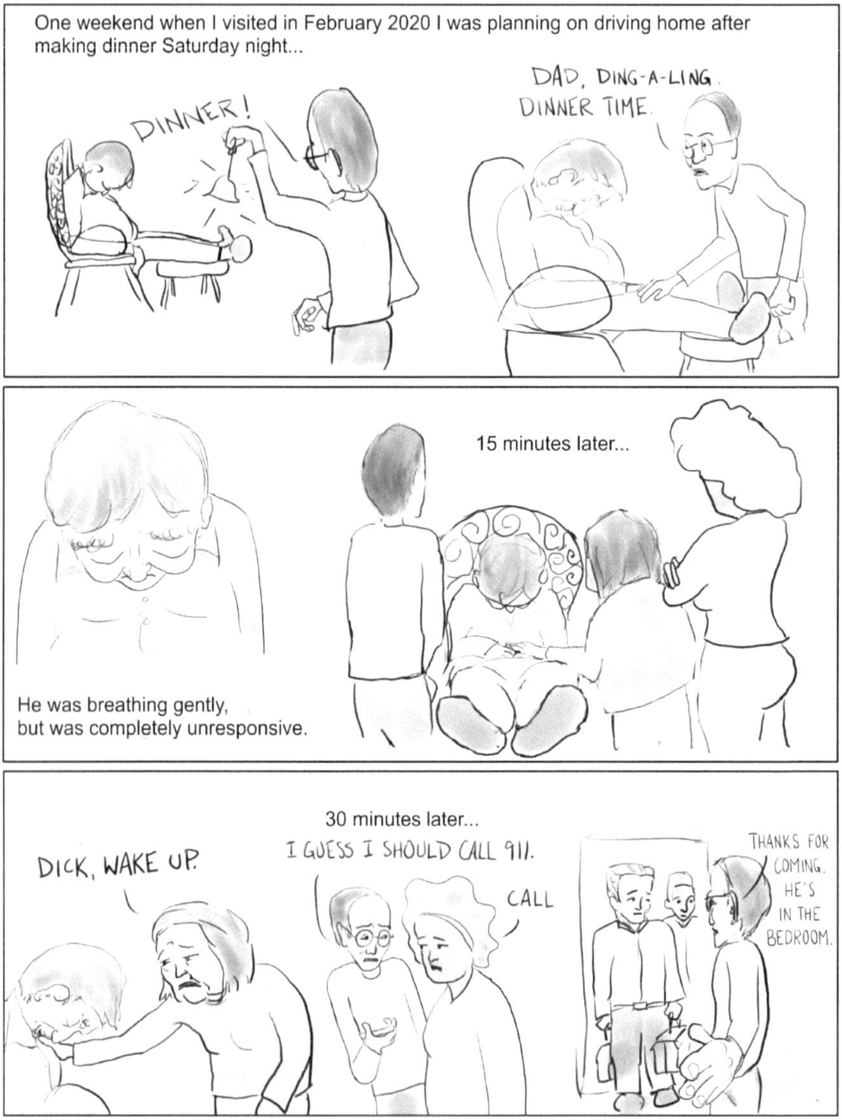

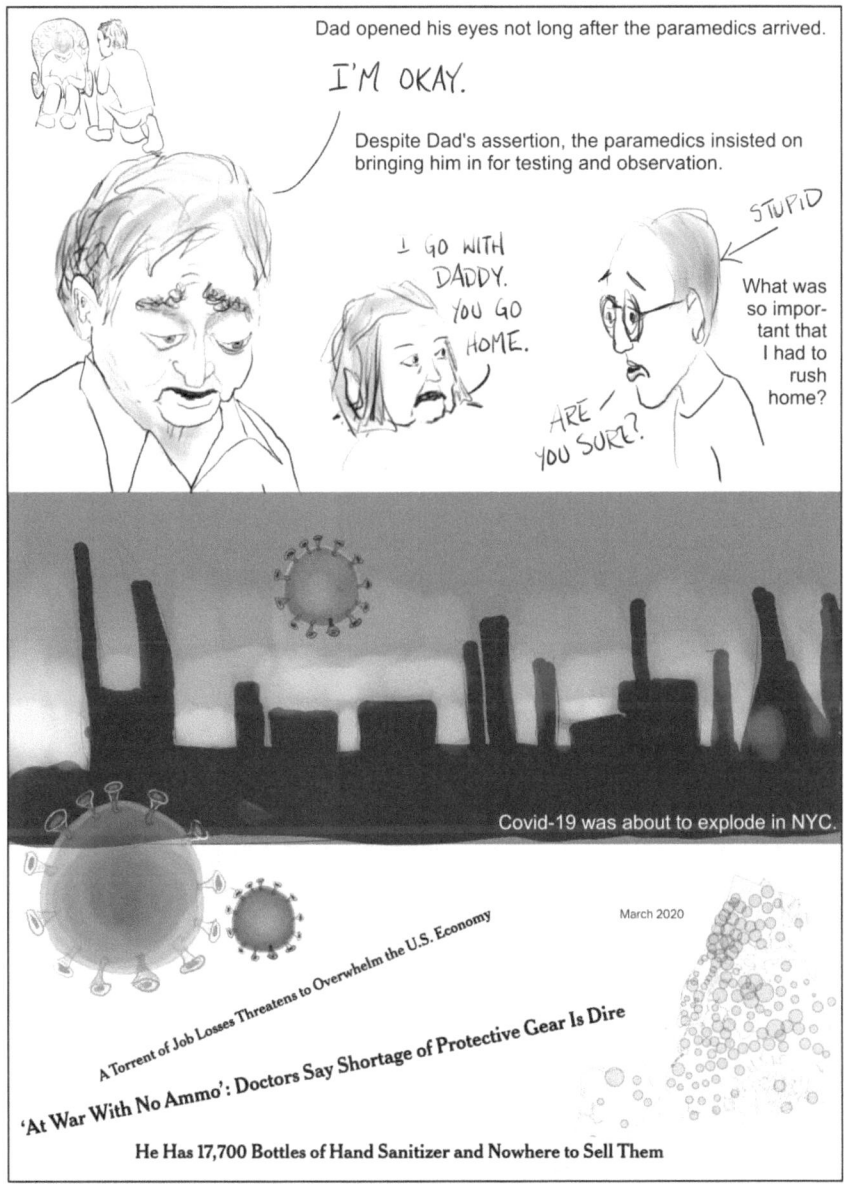

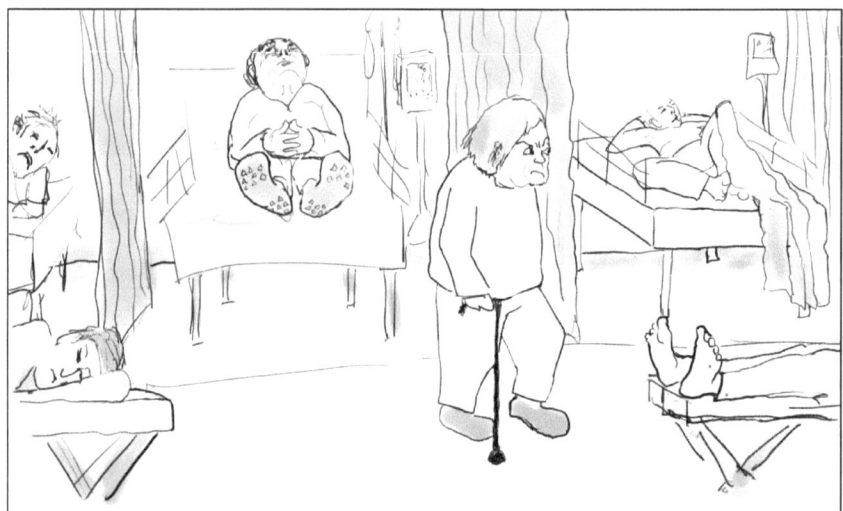

This was a 12 hour stint in the ER for Dad before getting admitted to a room.
A fierce frigid wind greeted Mom and Ophelia as they exited the hospital at 2 a.m.

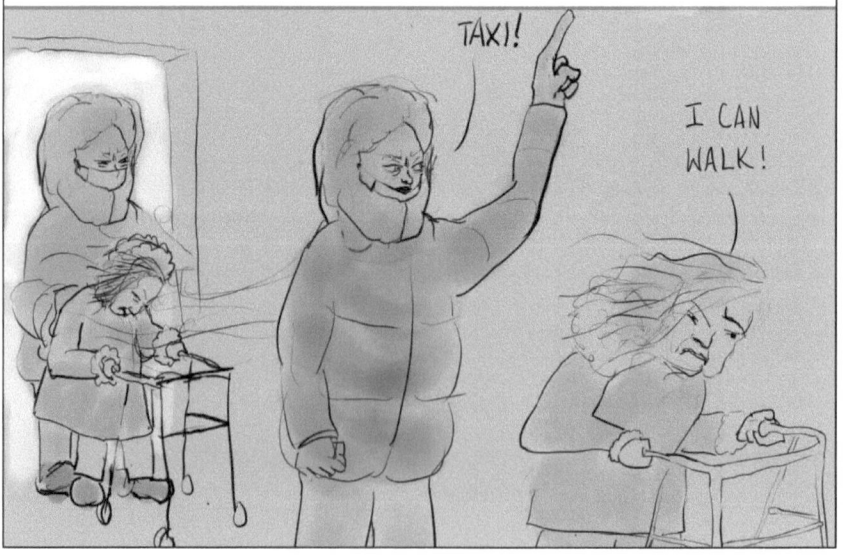

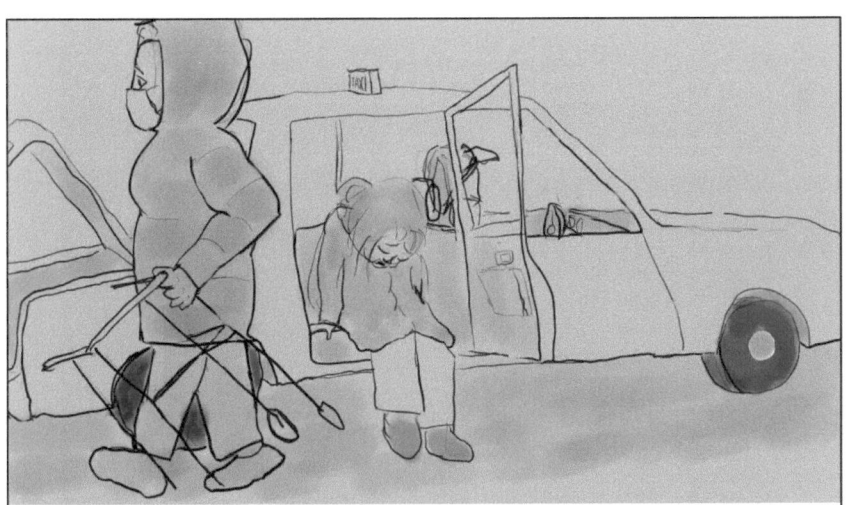

By the time Dad checked out of the hospital a few days later he was fine, but Mom had become deathly ill. Had she contracted an early case of Covid? Testing wasn't readily available in those initial weeks, and we never found out. She tested positive for a bacterial infection, so maybe she just had a severe urinary tract infection. When I FaceTimed with the care workers and they put Mom on, her face was swollen and strangely immobile. And she couldn't speak. With Covid raging in NYC, I stayed away for three months.

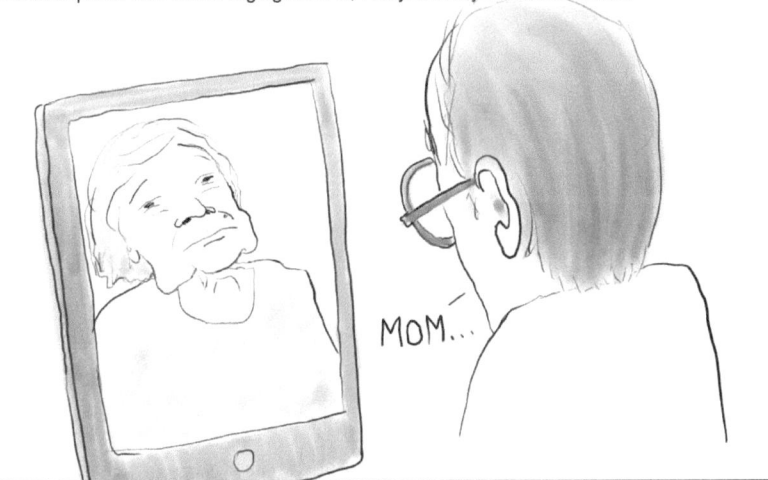

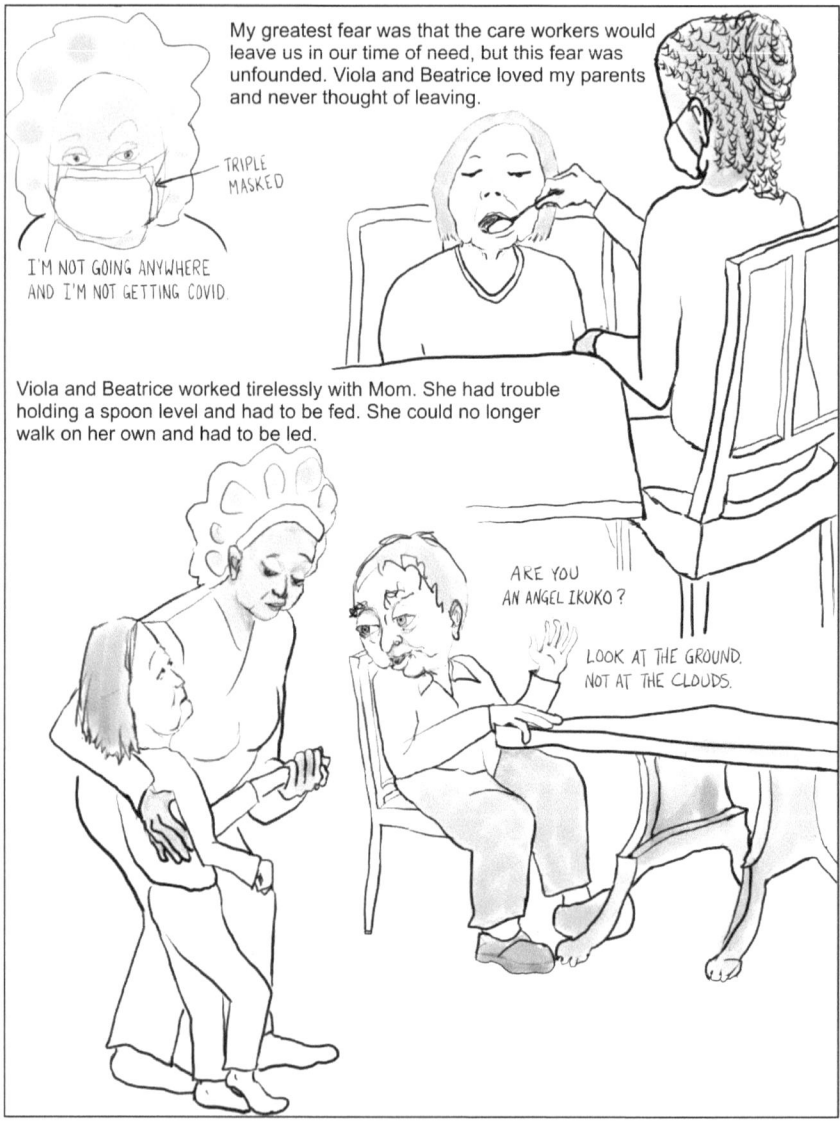

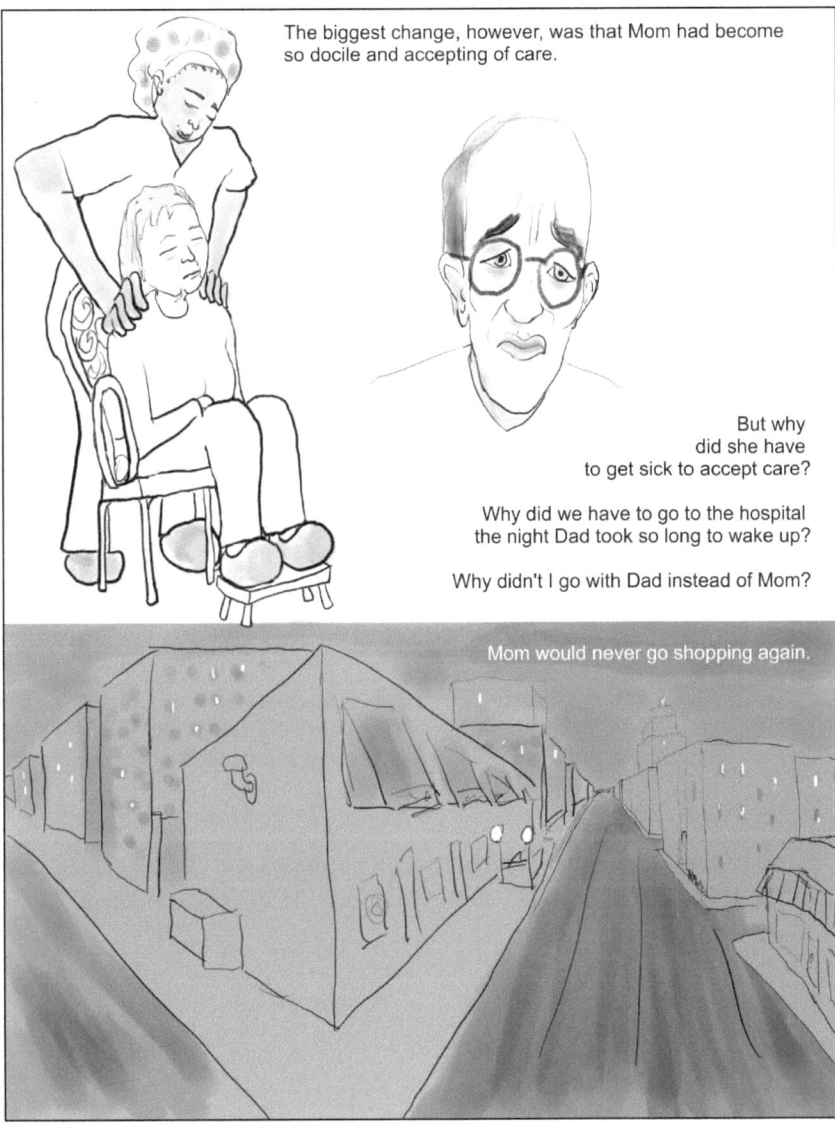

The Hero of the Story

Chapter 4

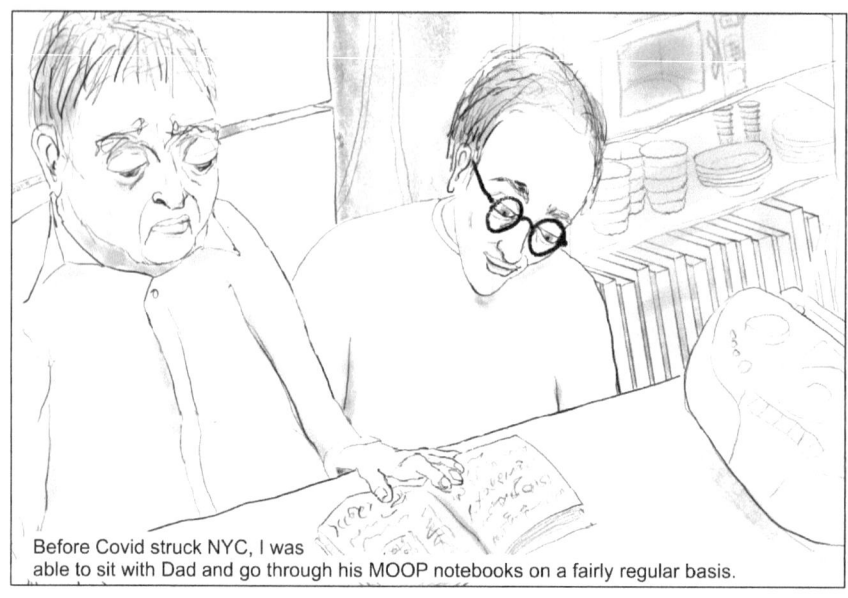

Before Covid struck NYC, I was able to sit with Dad and go through his MOOP notebooks on a fairly regular basis.

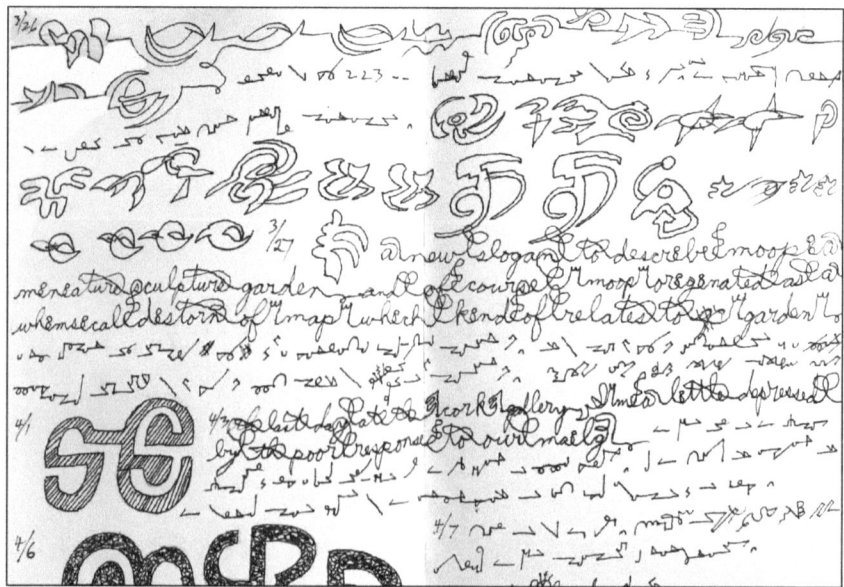

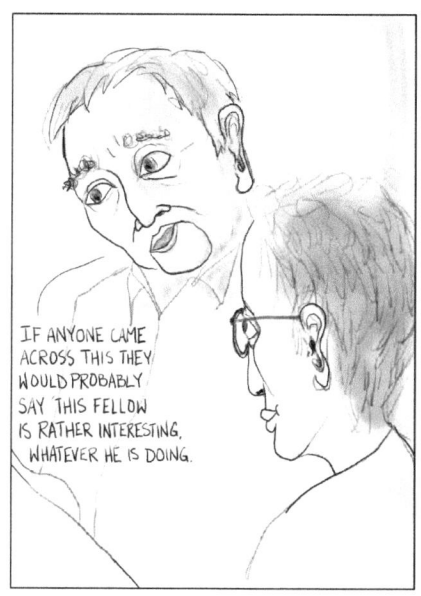
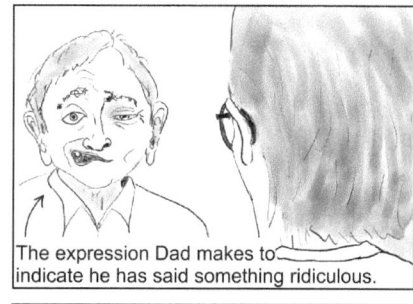
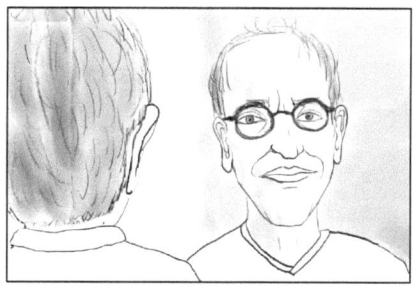
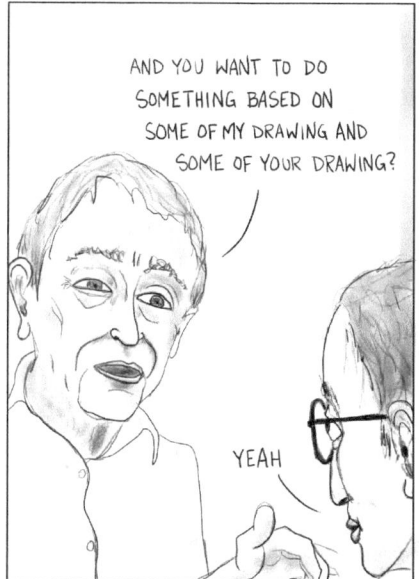
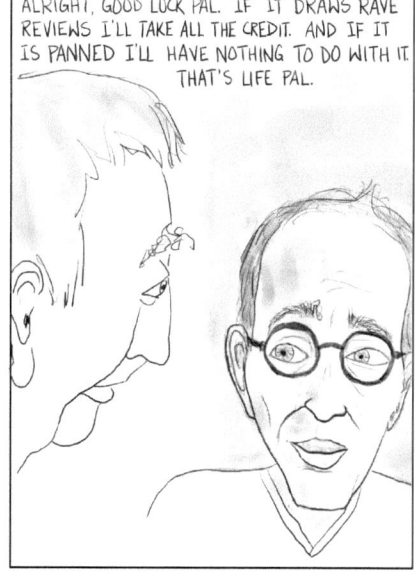

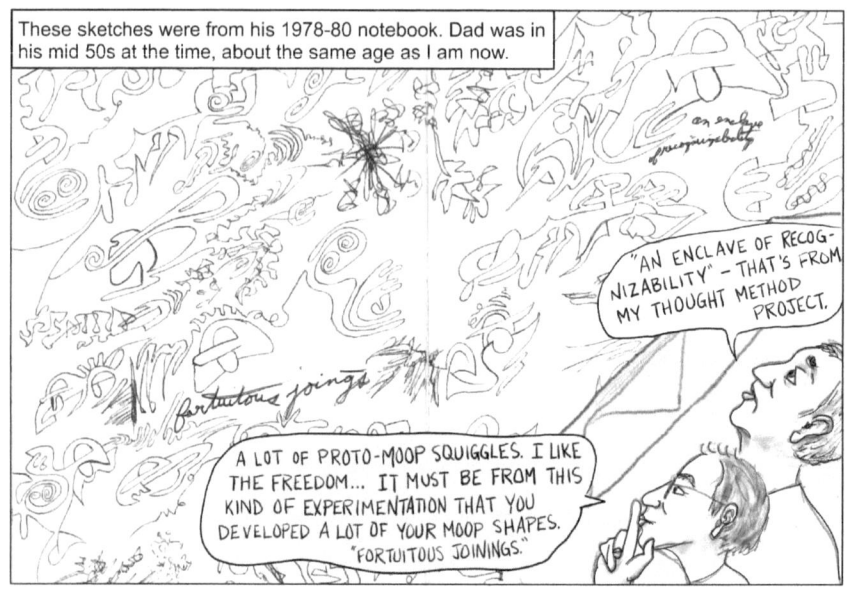
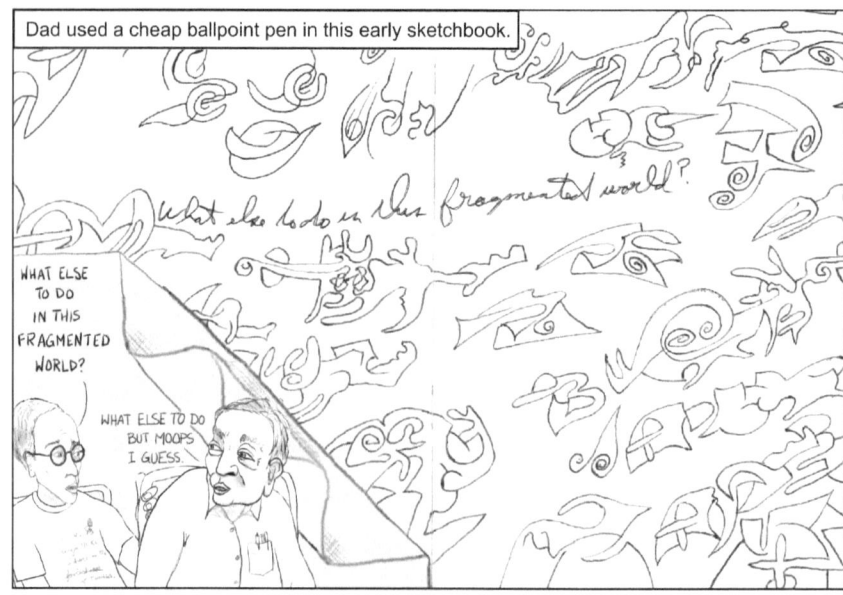

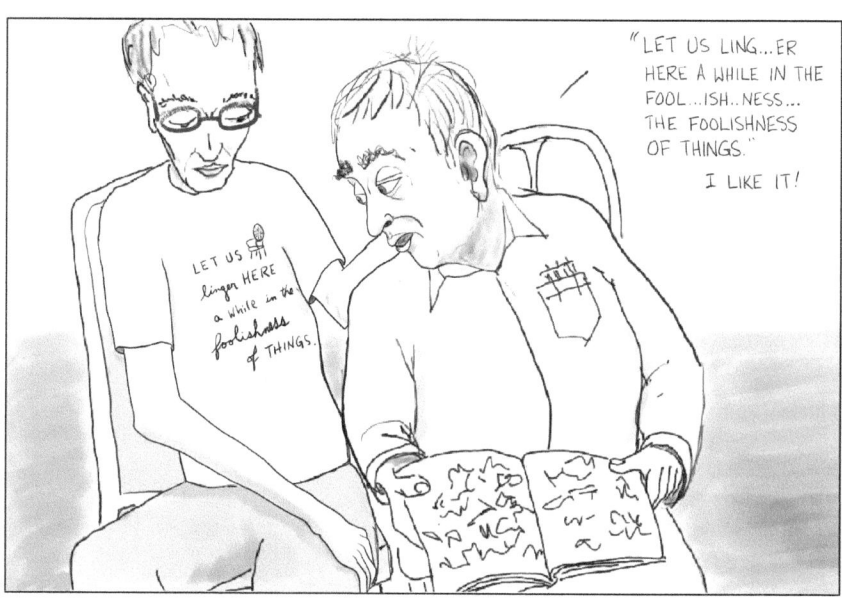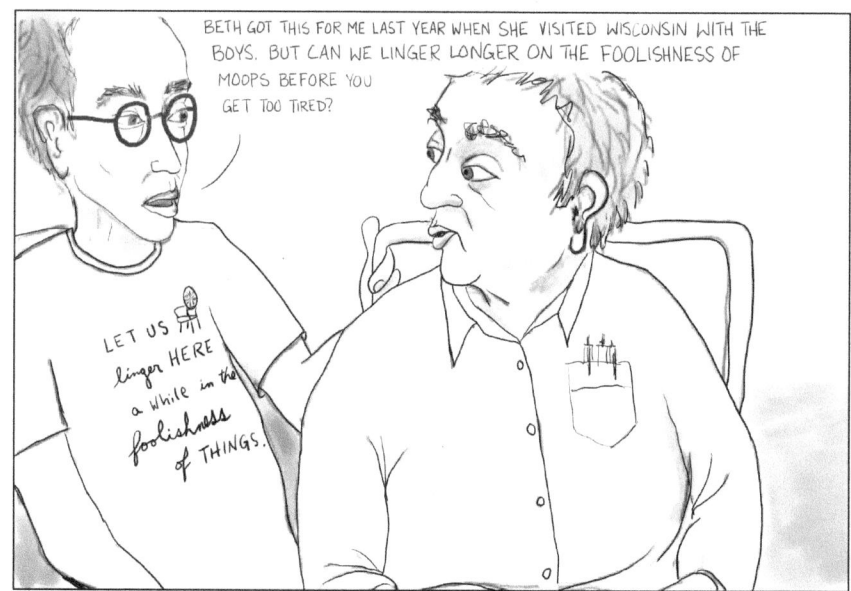

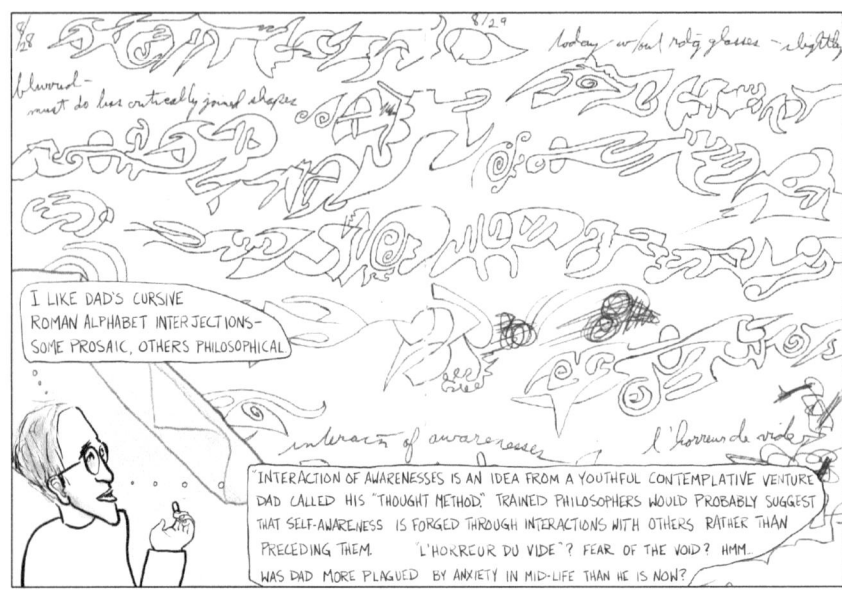

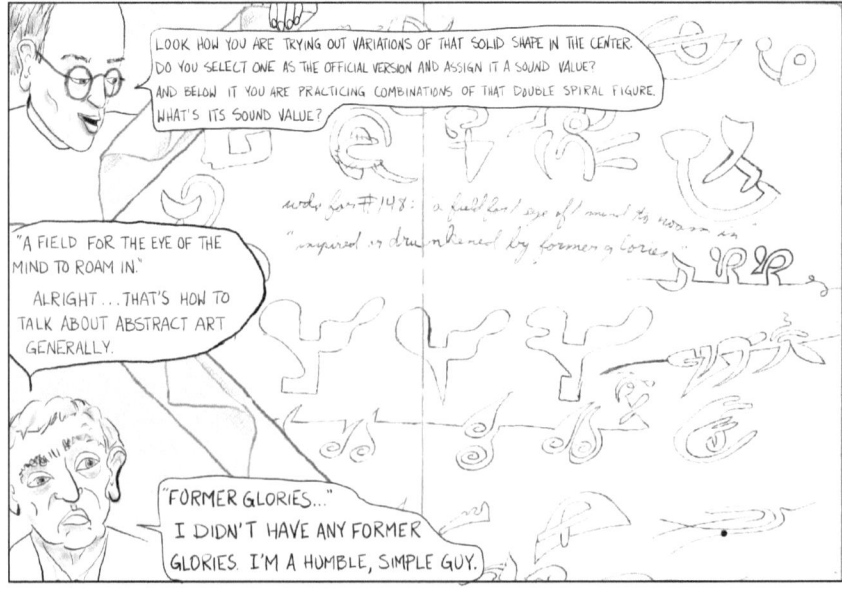

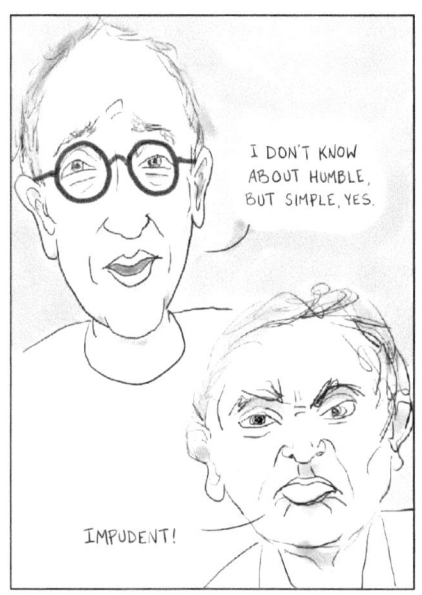
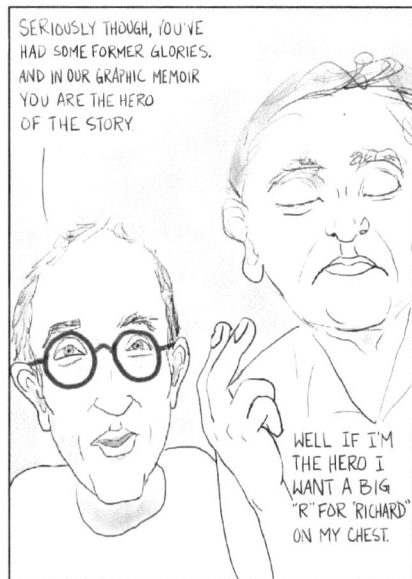
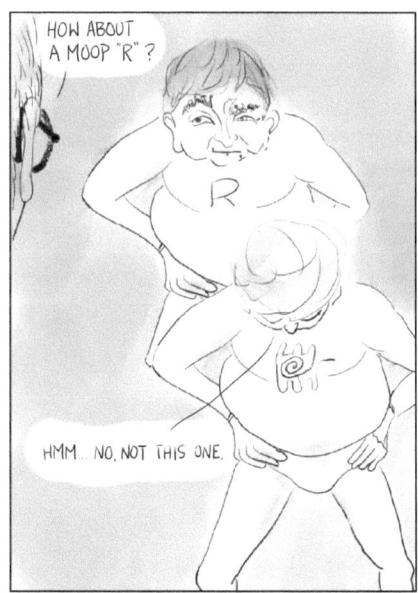
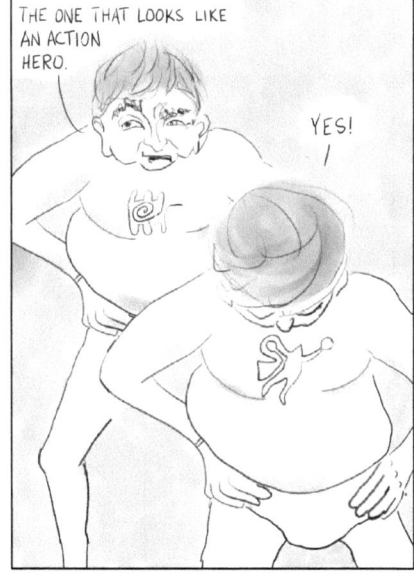

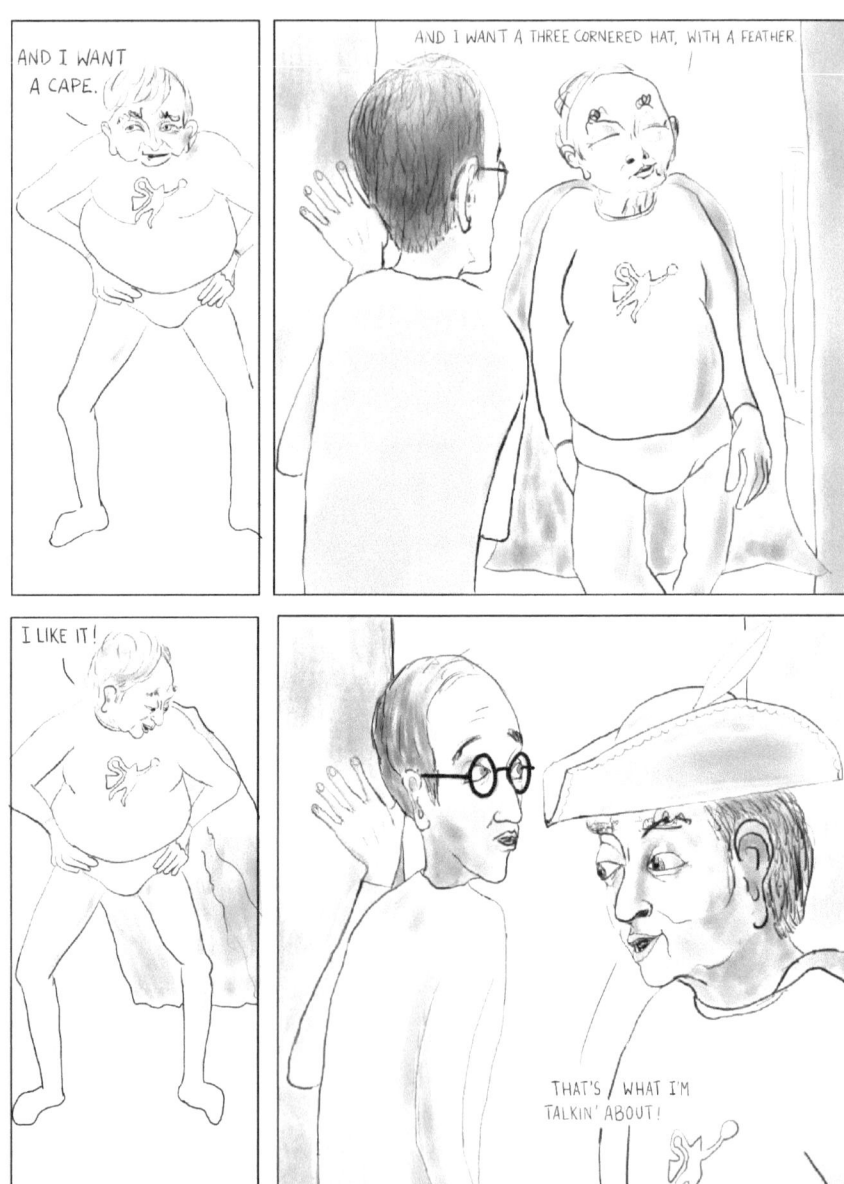

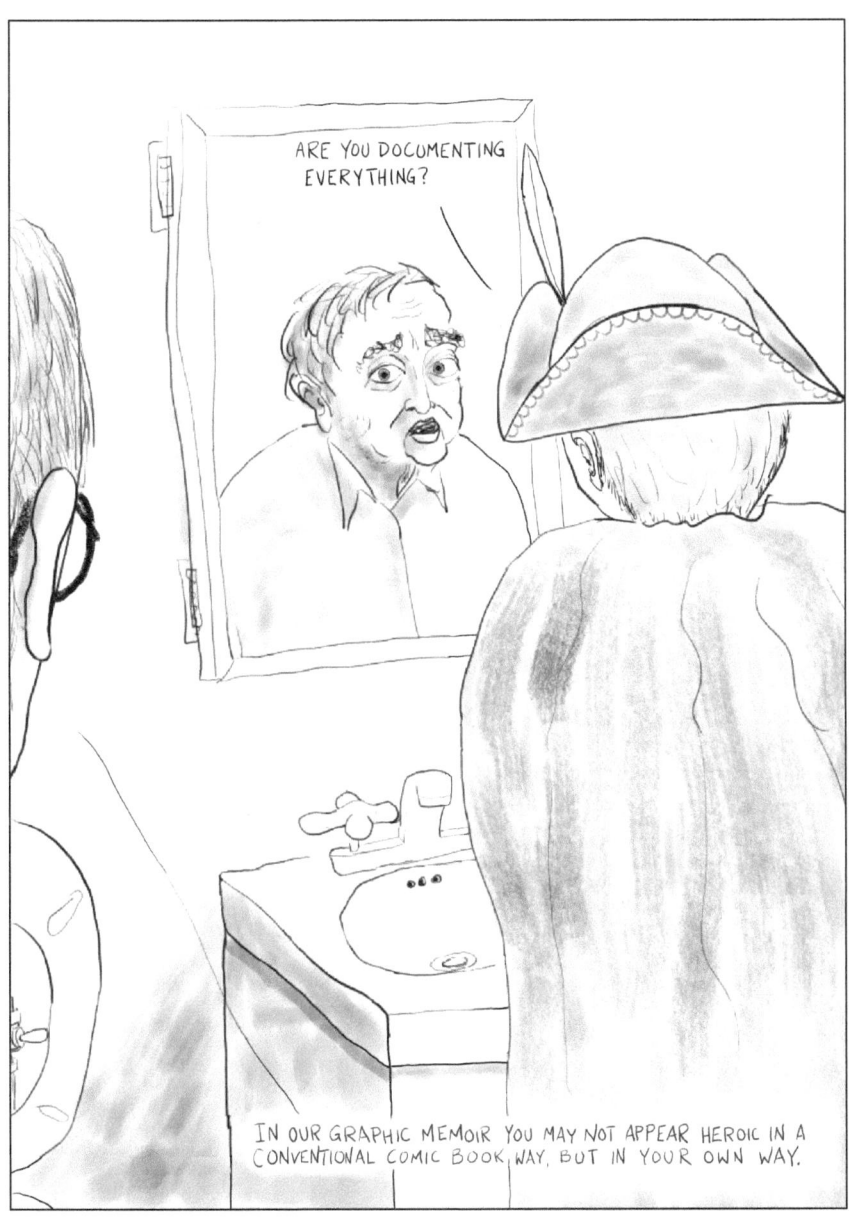

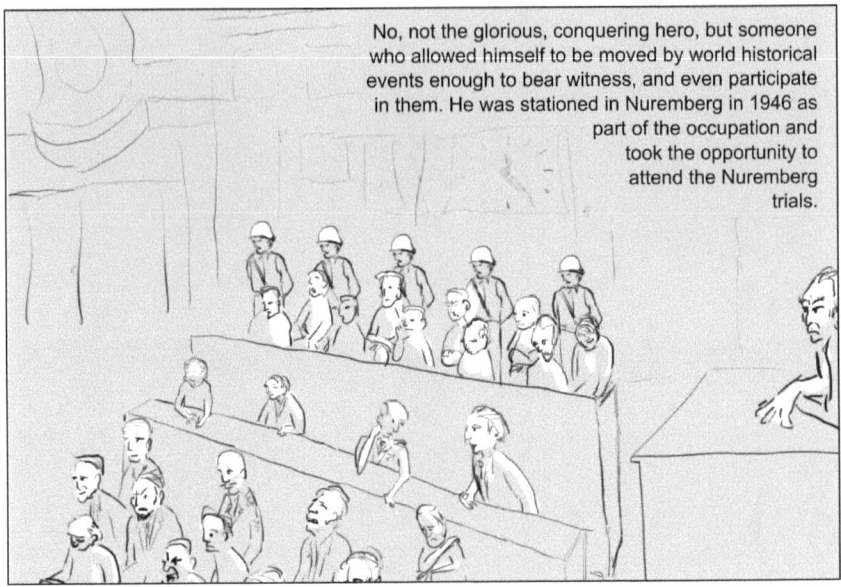

No, not the glorious, conquering hero, but someone who allowed himself to be moved by world historical events enough to bear witness, and even participate in them. He was stationed in Nuremberg in 1946 as part of the occupation and took the opportunity to attend the Nuremberg trials.

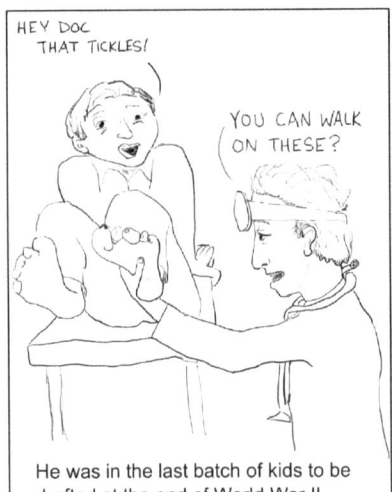

He was in the last batch of kids to be drafted at the end of World War II, and he didn't even have to go, having received a 4F diagnosis that he was unfit because of his club feet.

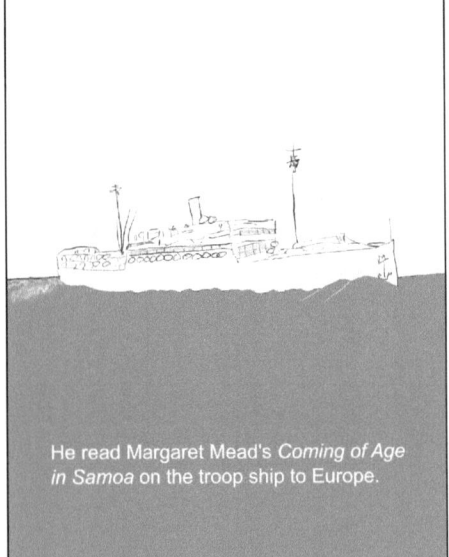

He read Margaret Mead's *Coming of Age in Samoa* on the troop ship to Europe.

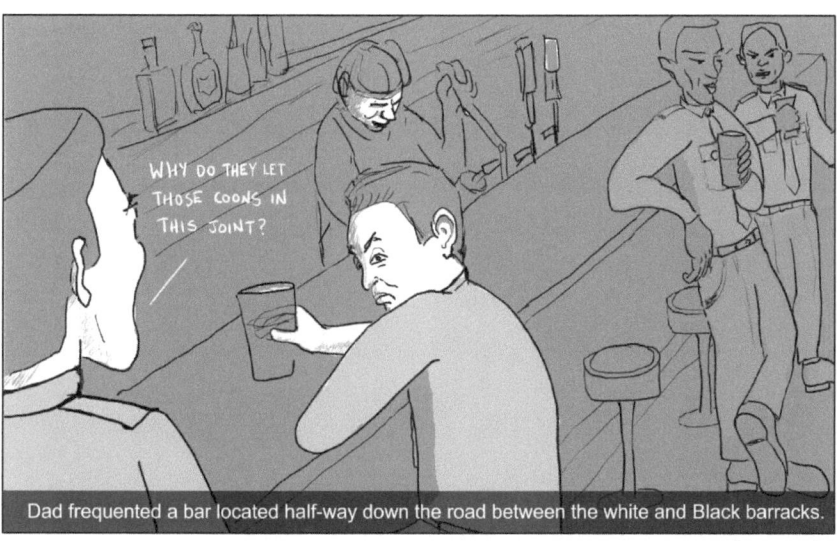

Dad frequented a bar located half-way down the road between the white and Black barracks.

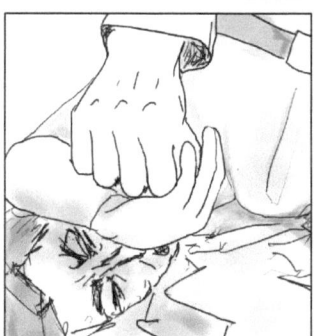

He got beat up once when he objected to the racial epithets cast by some of the white soldiers. He found himself transferred soon thereafter to a post in Munich.

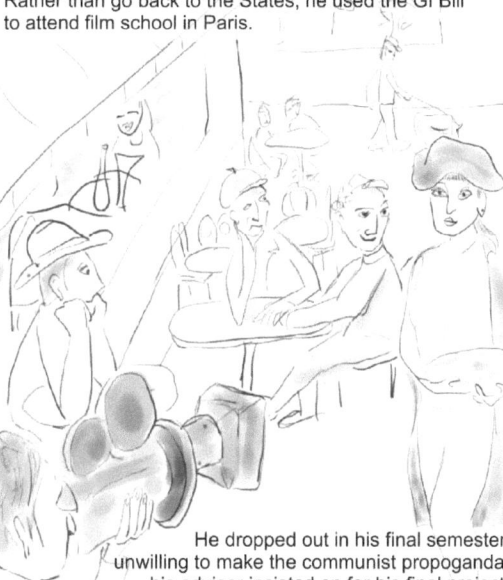

After a year, Dad received an honorable discharge. Rather than go back to the States, he used the GI Bill to attend film school in Paris.

He dropped out in his final semester, unwilling to make the communist propoganda his advisor insisted on for his final project.

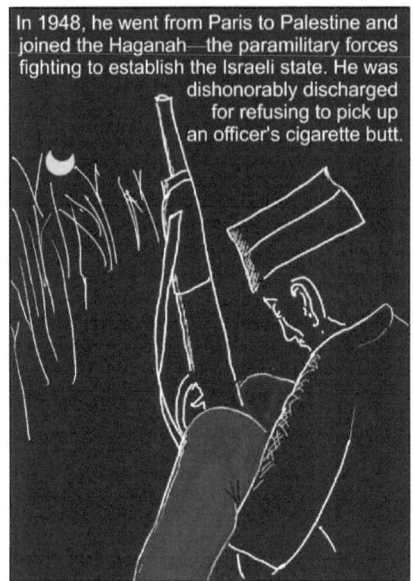
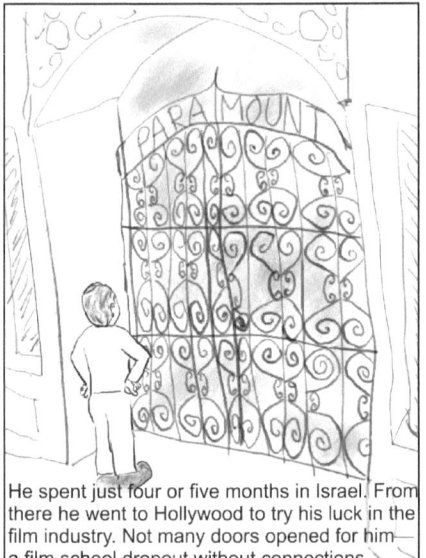

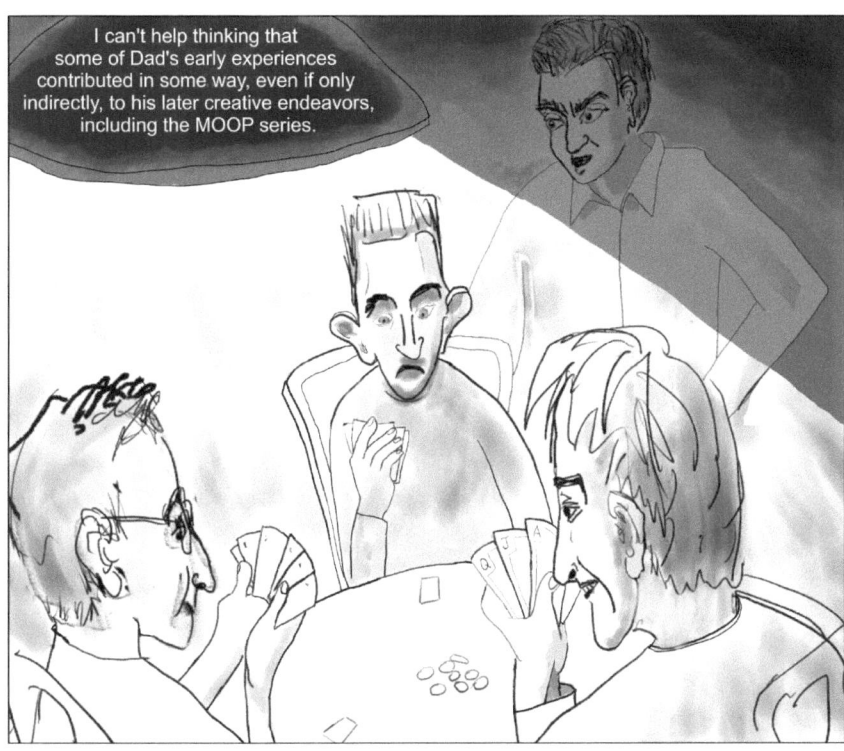

Kluwital

Chapter 5

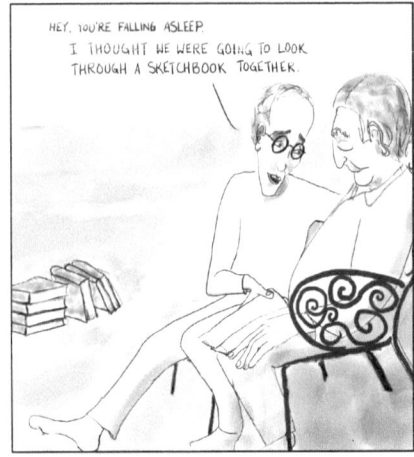

In the 1980-84 sketchbook, he started using a fine tipped dark black pen. He draws the same shape several times in sequence with minor variation of individual shapes.

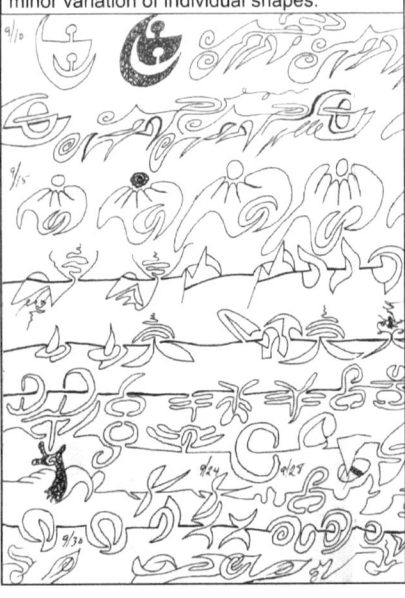

Page after page of the linearly connected script appears in this notebook.

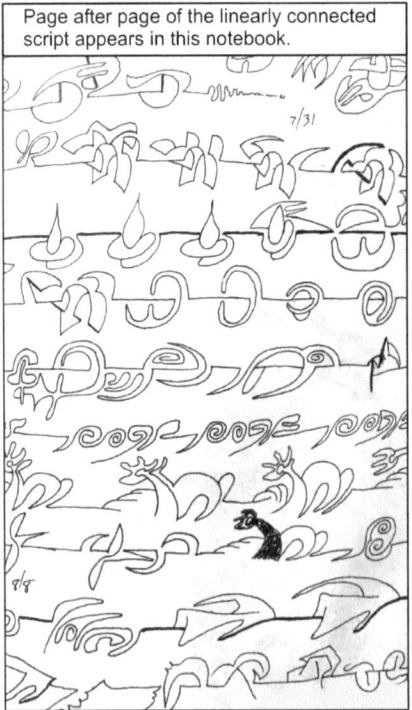

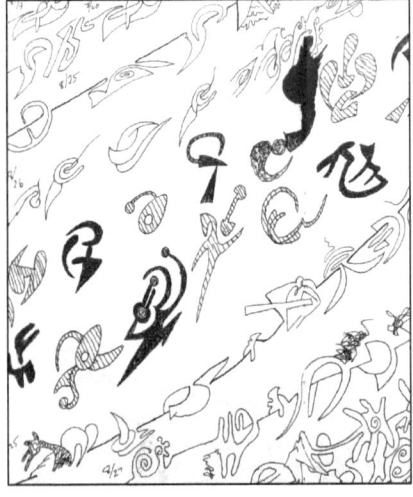

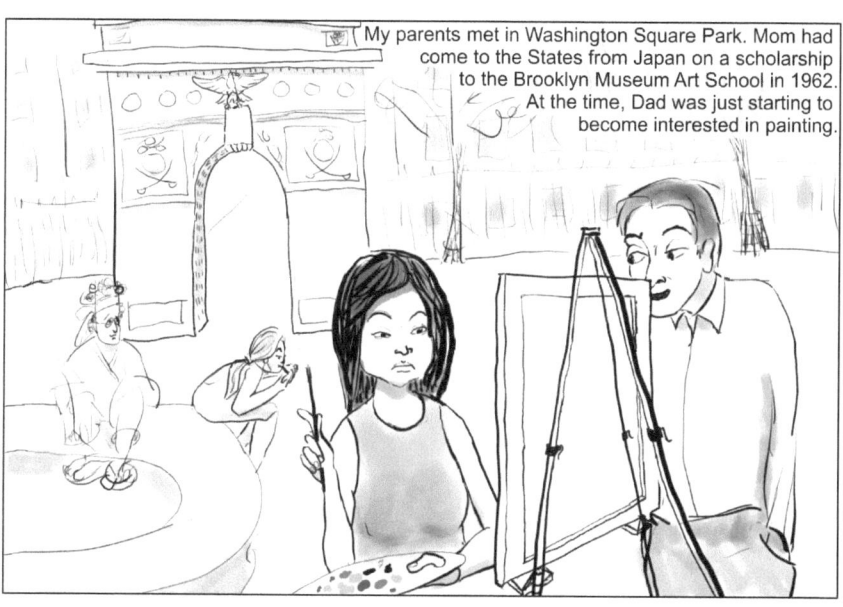
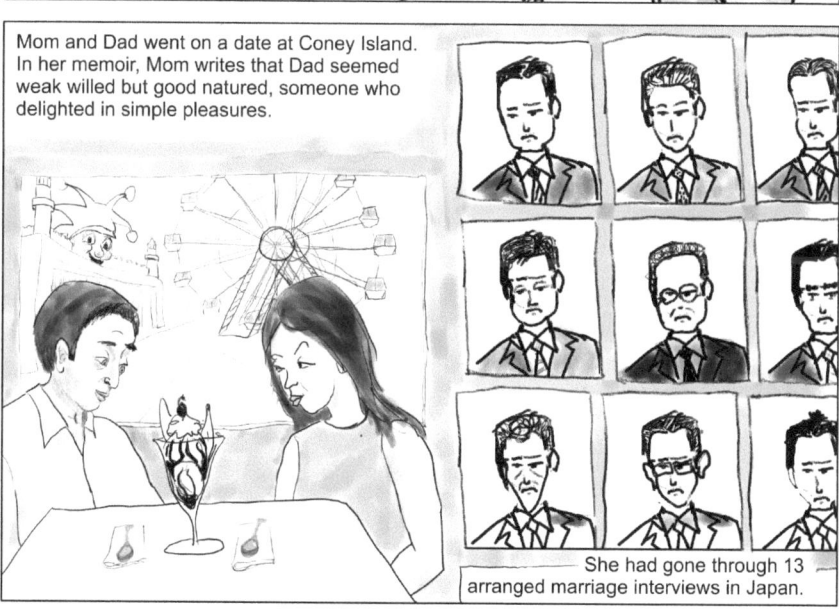

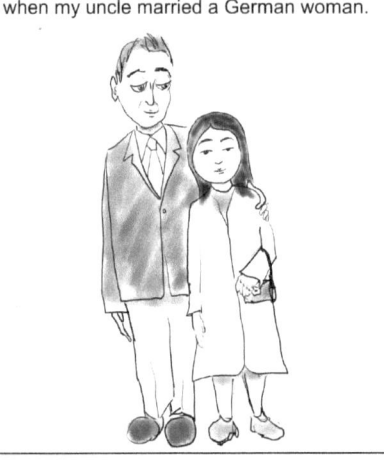

Mom and Dad got married at City Hall with only a few friends in attendance. My Jewish American grandparents could not accept the idea that Dad would marry a Japanese woman. There was no similar objection when my uncle married a German woman.

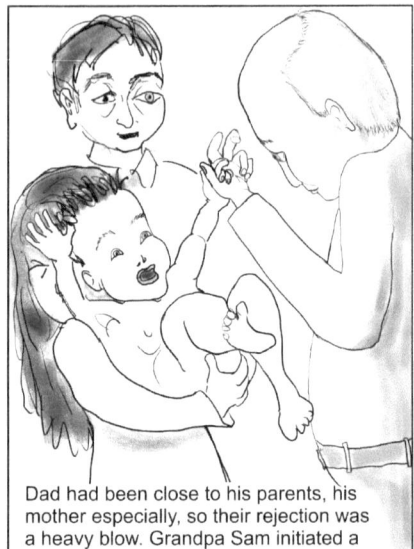

Dad had been close to his parents, his mother especially, so their rejection was a heavy blow. Grandpa Sam initiated a reconciliation when my brother was born.

I was born a year and five days after Abe. Photos suggest an idyllic time even though Grandma Ethel still refused to see us.

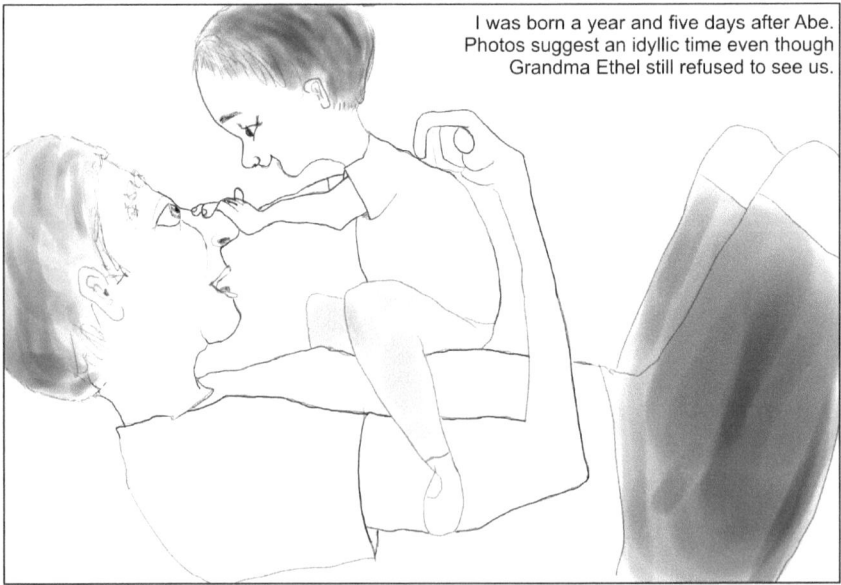

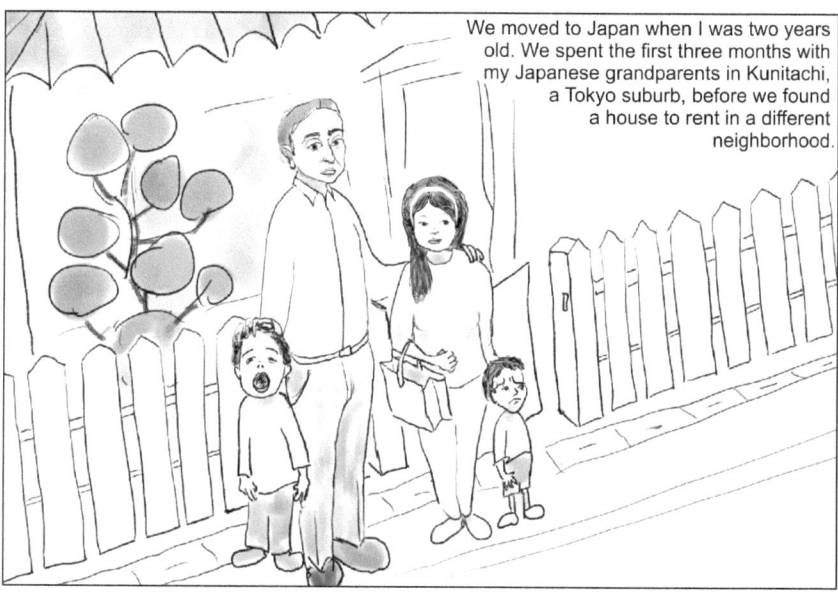

We moved to Japan when I was two years old. We spent the first three months with my Japanese grandparents in Kunitachi, a Tokyo suburb, before we found a house to rent in a different neighborhood.

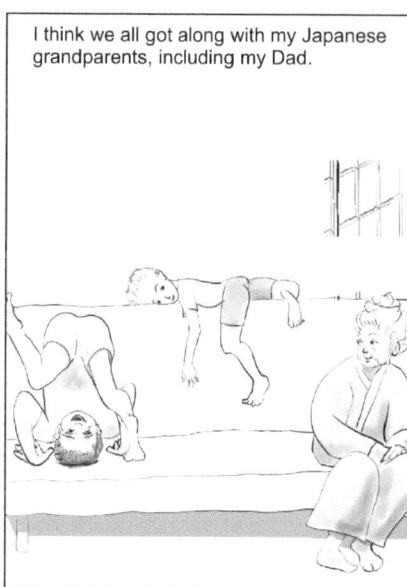

I think we all got along with my Japanese grandparents, including my Dad.

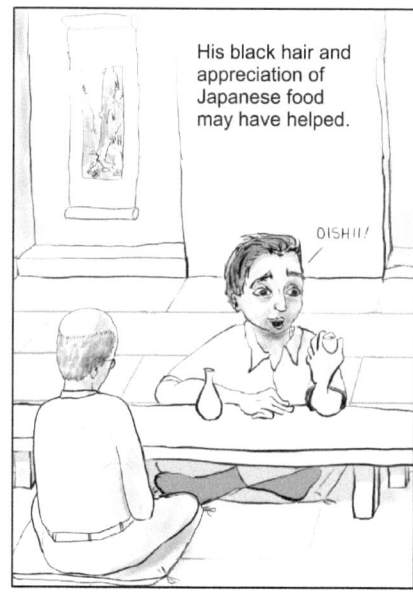

His black hair and appreciation of Japanese food may have helped.

OISHII!

We spent two years in Japan. Eventually, Dad decided he wanted to pursue art back in the States. The long separation must have softened Grandma Ethel, and we stayed with them for a month upon return. Abe was five and I was four. Reconciliation facilitated by peak cuteness.

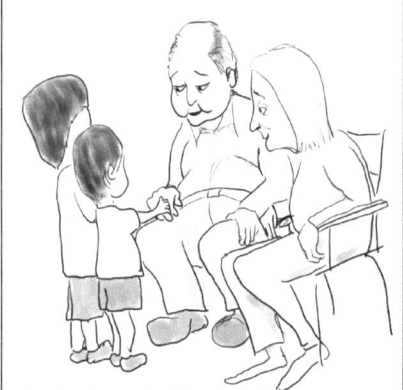

I visited Grandma by myself shortly after I finished college, when she was 88. She confided in me that Dad had never really forgiven her.

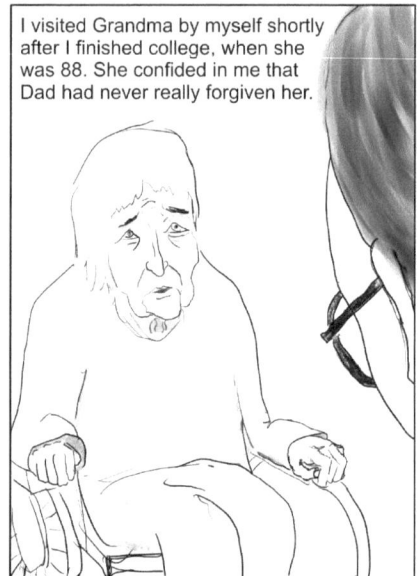

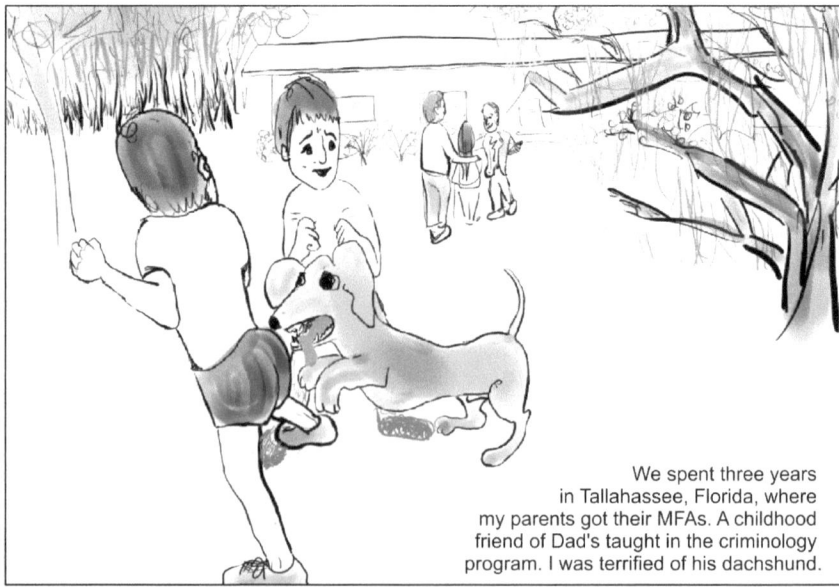

We spent three years in Tallahassee, Florida, where my parents got their MFAs. A childhood friend of Dad's taught in the criminology program. I was terrified of his dachshund.

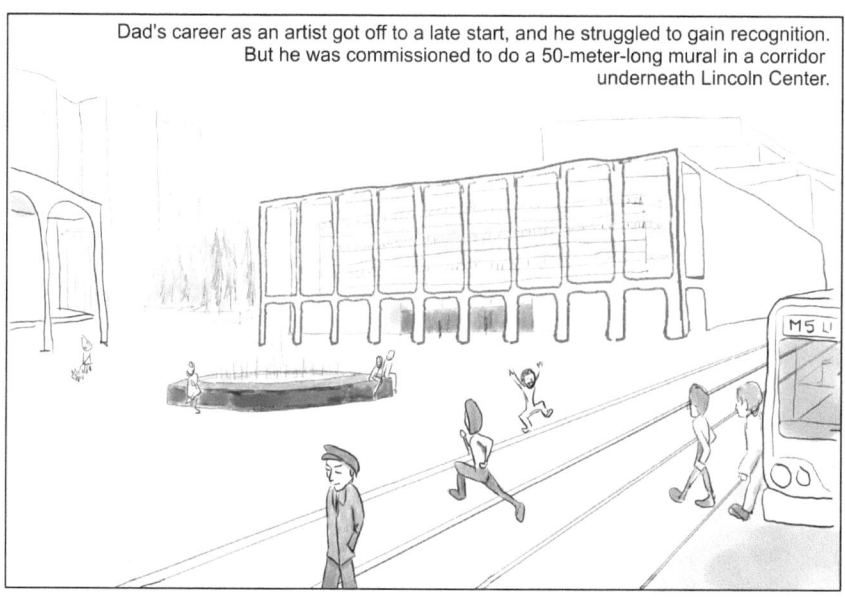

Dad's career as an artist got off to a late start, and he struggled to gain recognition. But he was commissioned to do a 50-meter-long mural in a corridor underneath Lincoln Center.

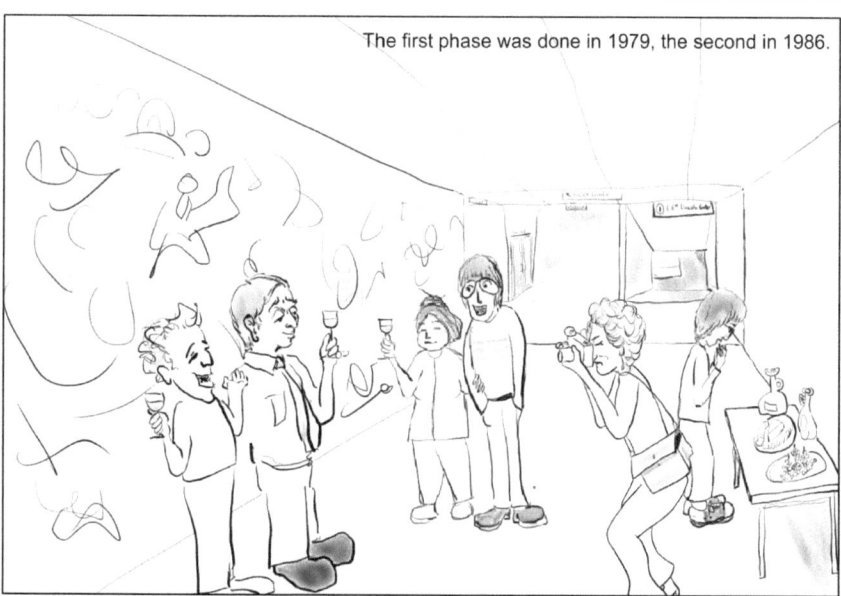

The first phase was done in 1979, the second in 1986.

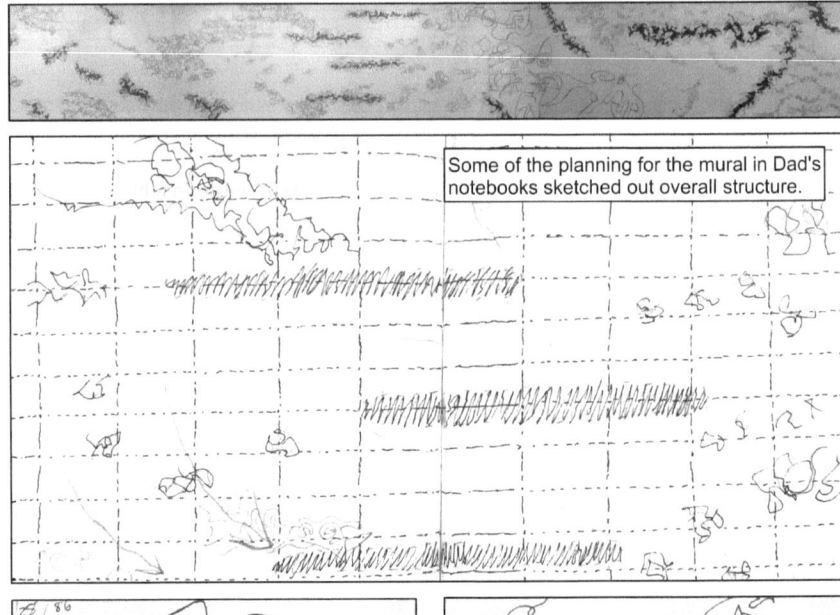

Some of the planning for the mural in Dad's notebooks sketched out overall structure.

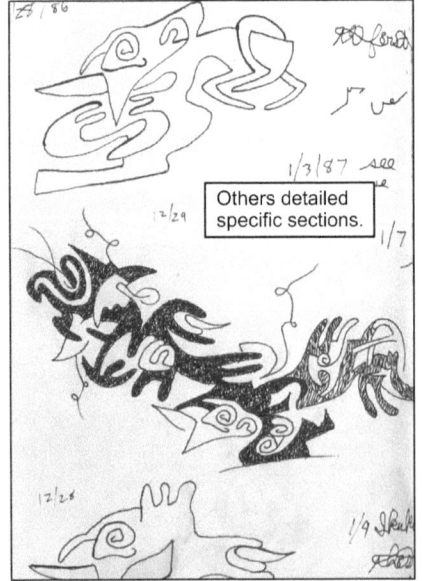

Others detailed specific sections.

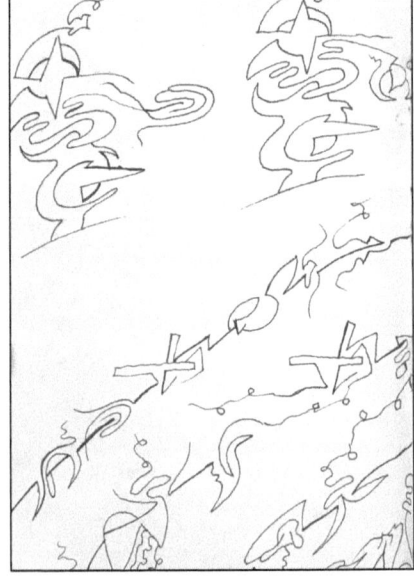

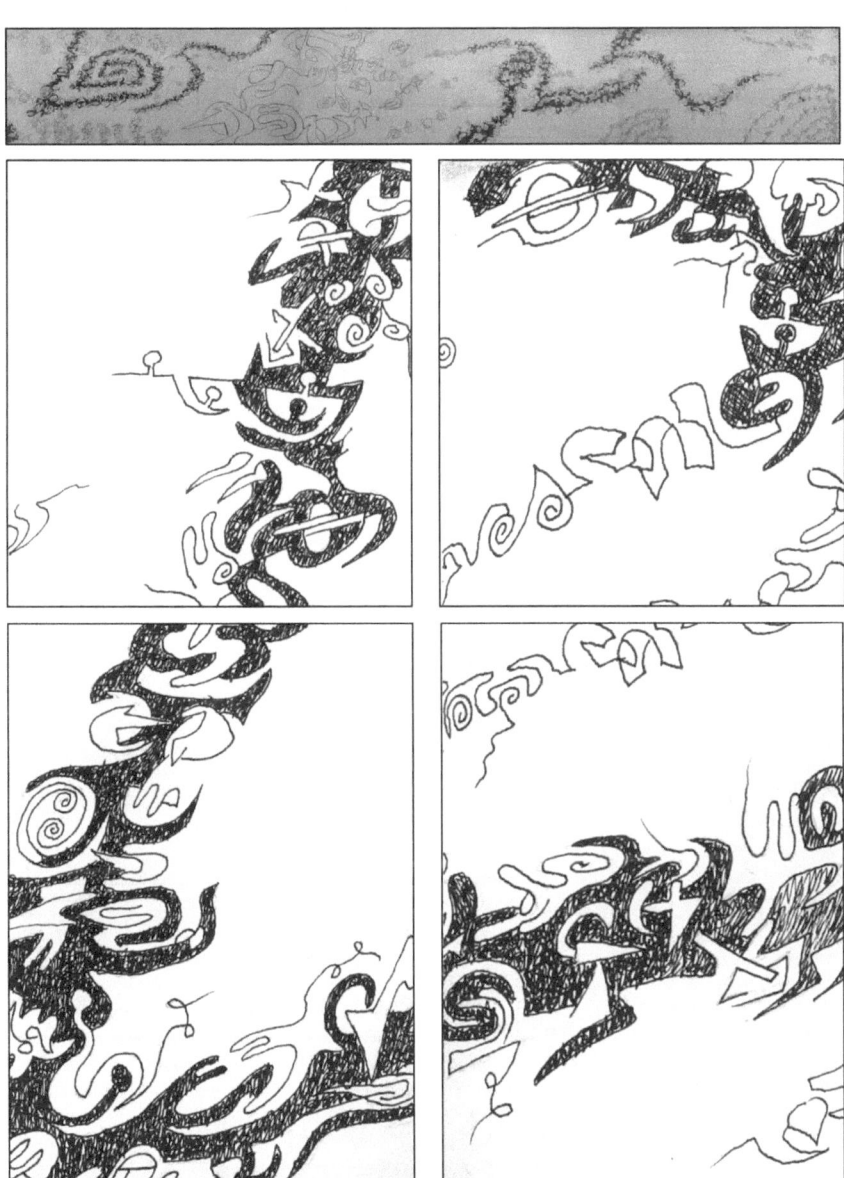

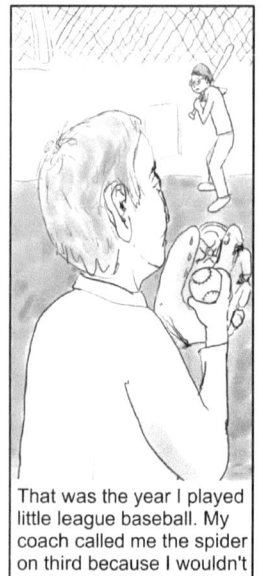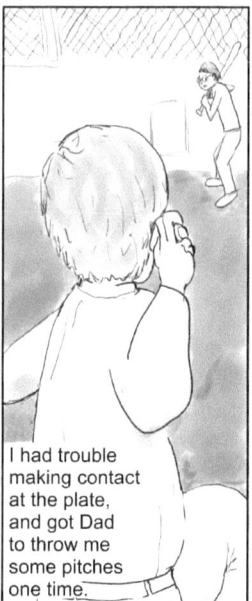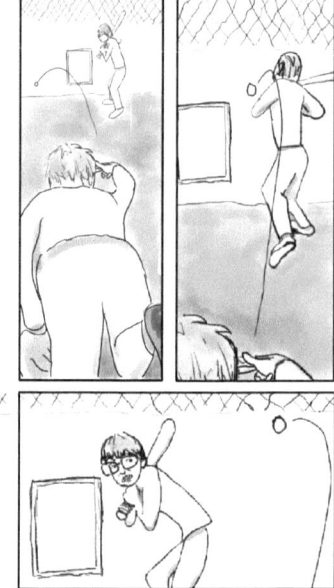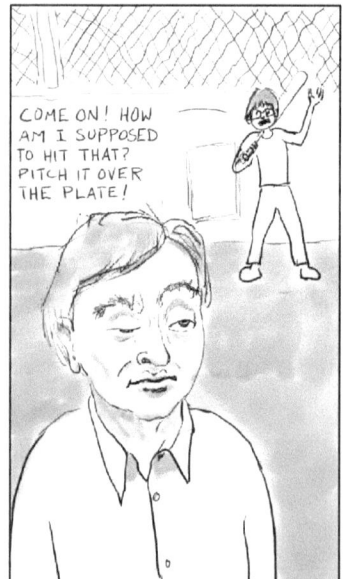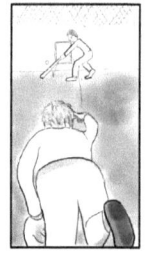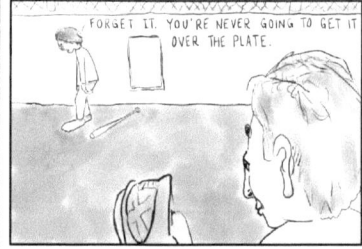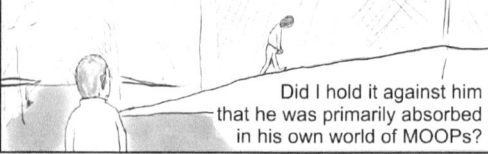

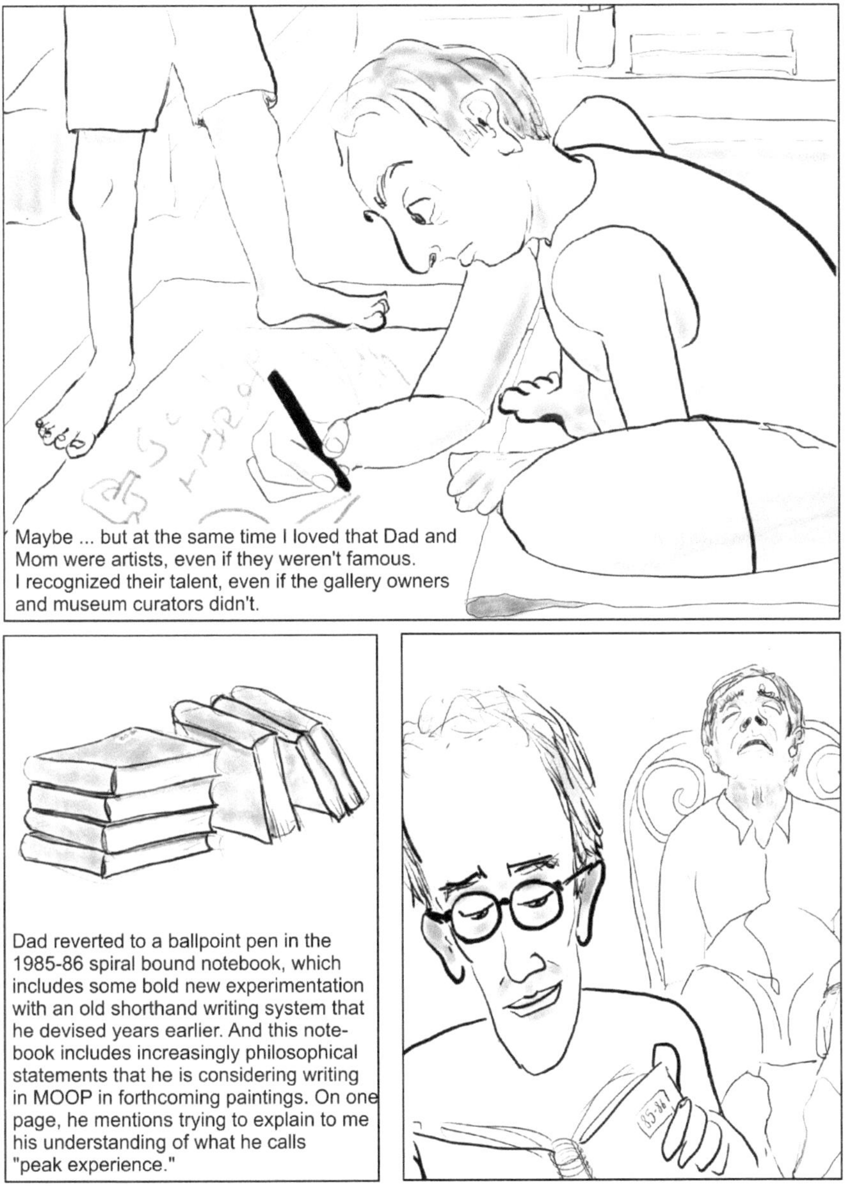

Maybe ... but at the same time I loved that Dad and Mom were artists, even if they weren't famous. I recognized their talent, even if the gallery owners and museum curators didn't.

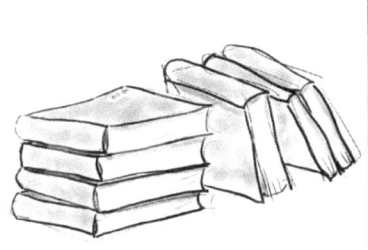

Dad reverted to a ballpoint pen in the 1985-86 spiral bound notebook, which includes some bold new experimentation with an old shorthand writing system that he devised years earlier. And this notebook includes increasingly philosophical statements that he is considering writing in MOOP in forthcoming paintings. On one page, he mentions trying to explain to me his understanding of what he calls "peak experience."

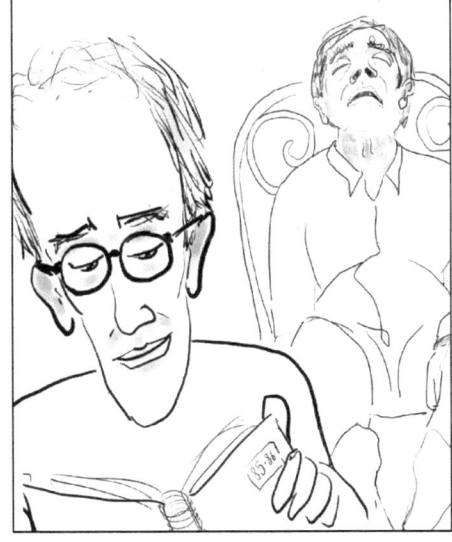

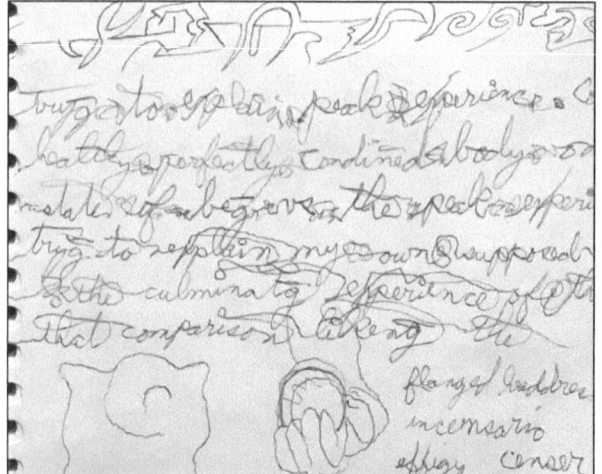

He writes, "How did I say it to Joshua? In trying to explain peak experience, comparing the ailing body v. the perfectly conditioned body on the one hand, with the everyday state of being v. the peak experience state of being on the other."

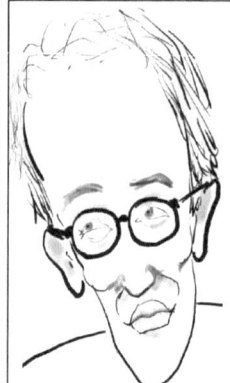

I'm surprised that Dad mentioned discussing this idea with me, for I don't remember being much of an interlocutor for Dad about his thought method. Abe engaged with him more on such matters.

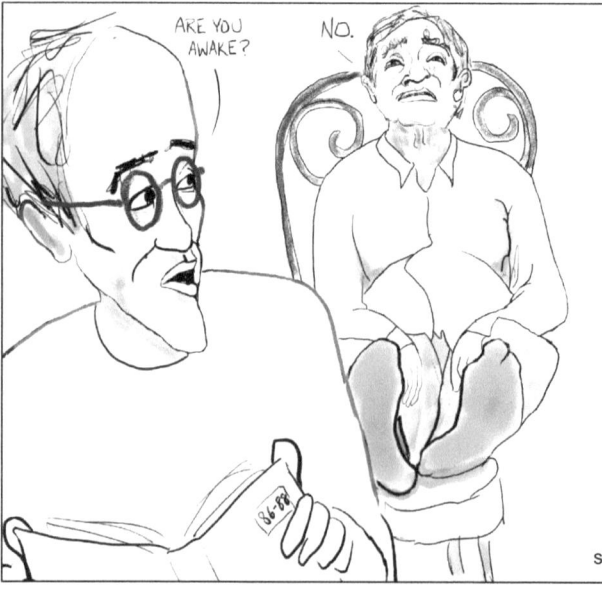

The 1986-88 notebook might be the highpoint of all of the MOOP notebooks. While continuing to develop his MOOPs, Dad was experimenting with different non-MOOP patterns inspired by a variety of sources, including German expressionist Paul Klee, the geometric patterns of Sol Lewitt, and Kuba textiles. He referred to these influences as "Kluwital," short for Klee, Lewitt, et al.

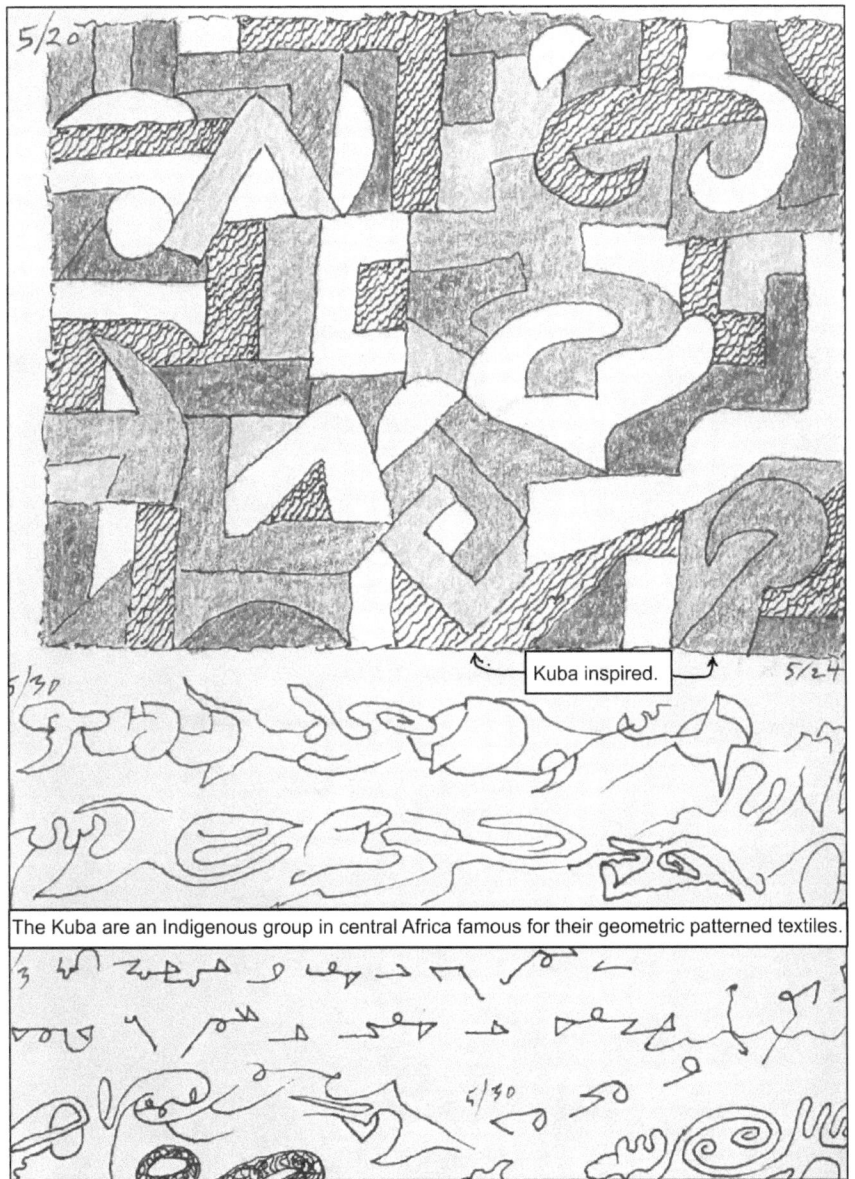

Kuba inspired.

The Kuba are an Indigenous group in central Africa famous for their geometric patterned textiles.

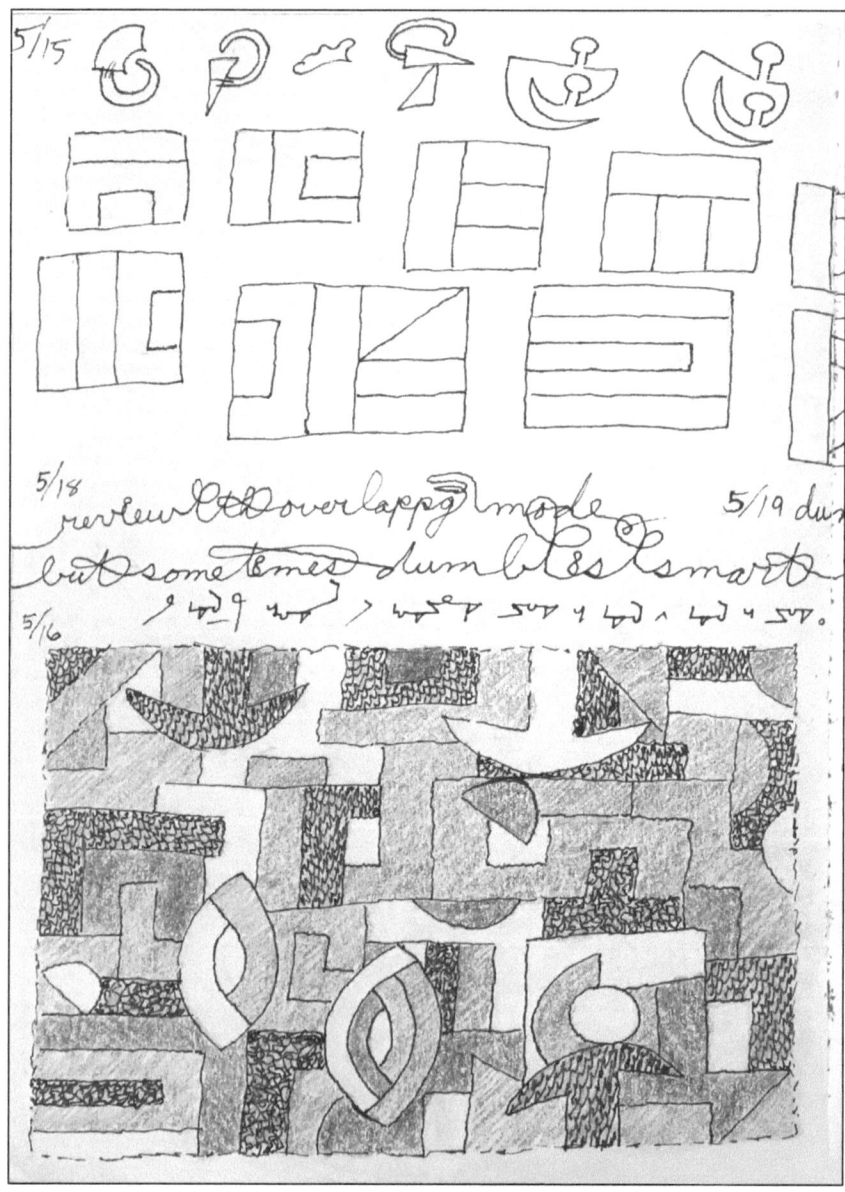

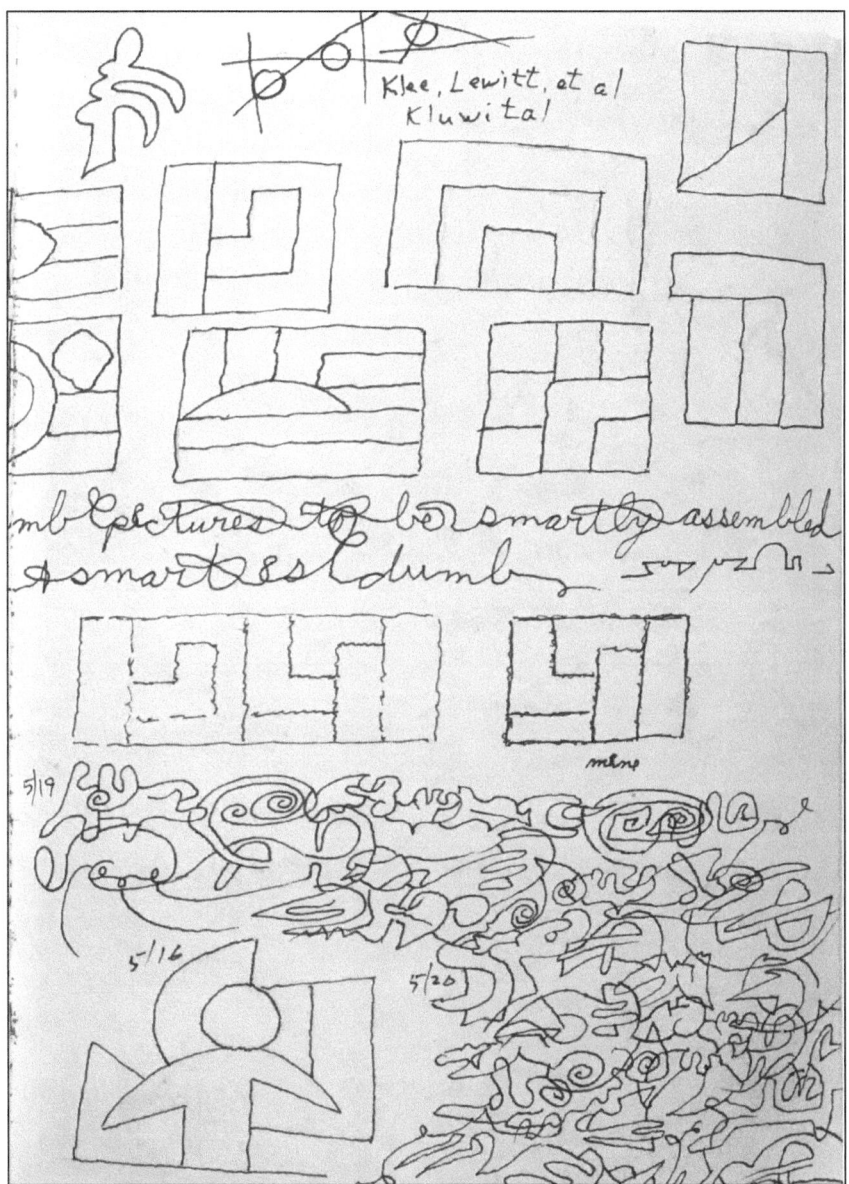

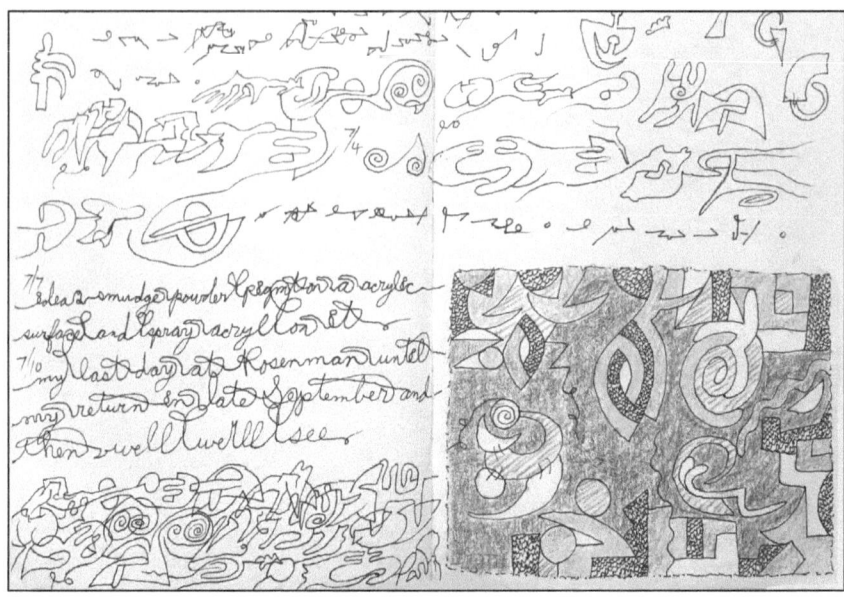

Here Dad was developing his system of circles and segments, which involved combinations of intersecting, non-intersecting, and tangential arrangements.

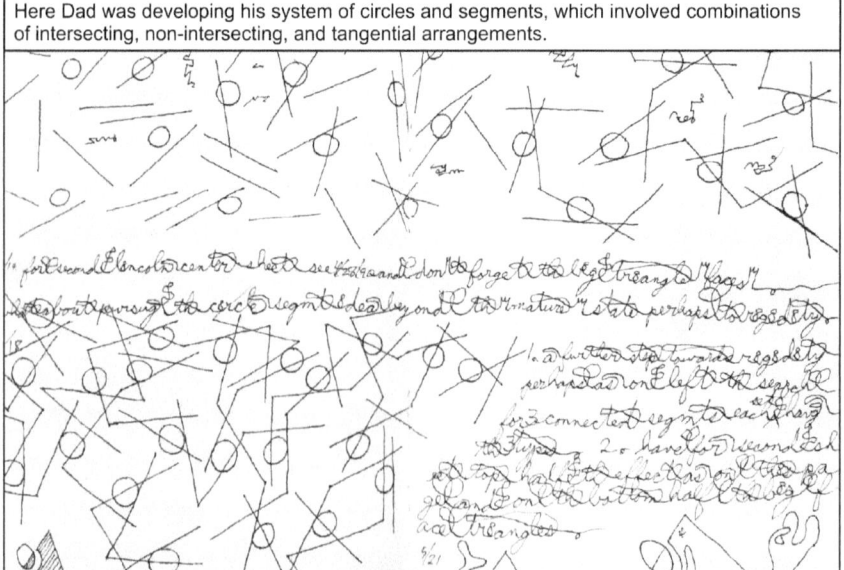

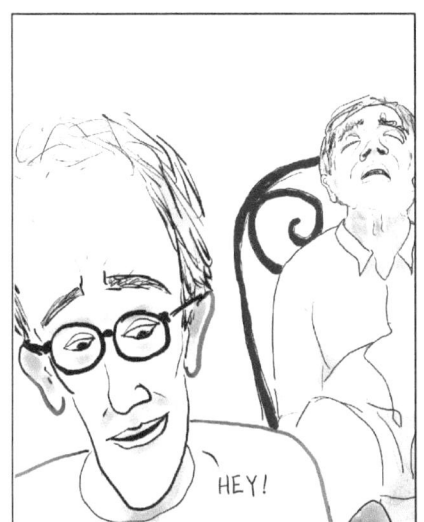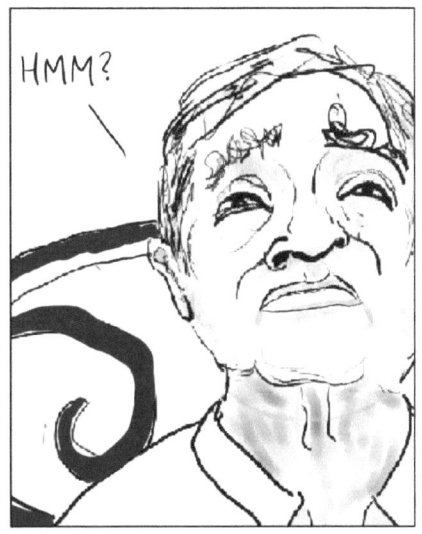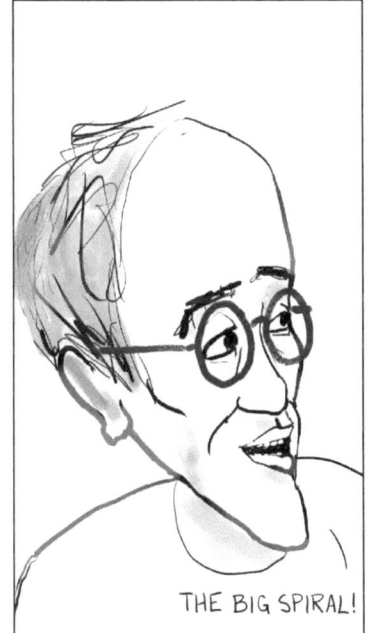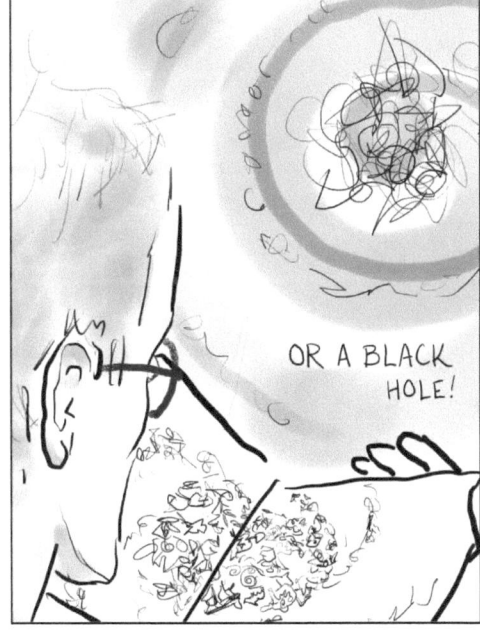

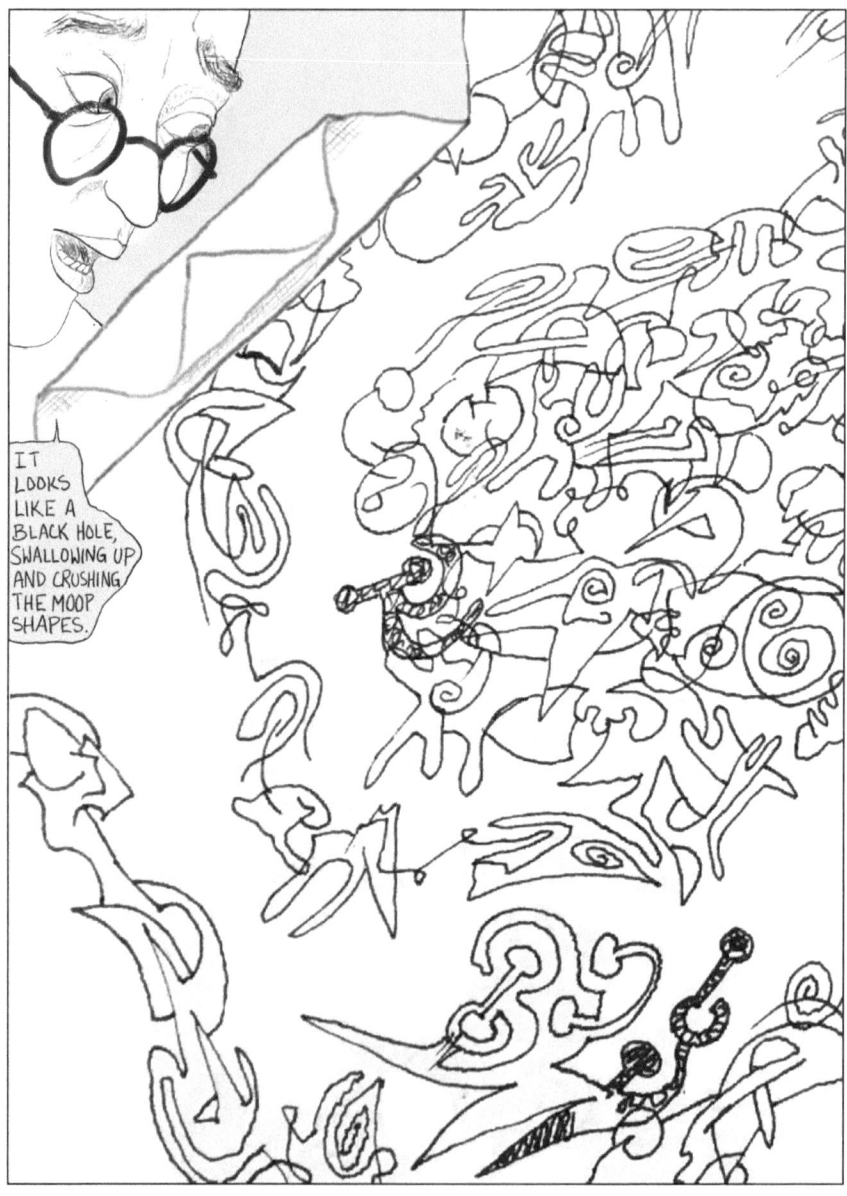

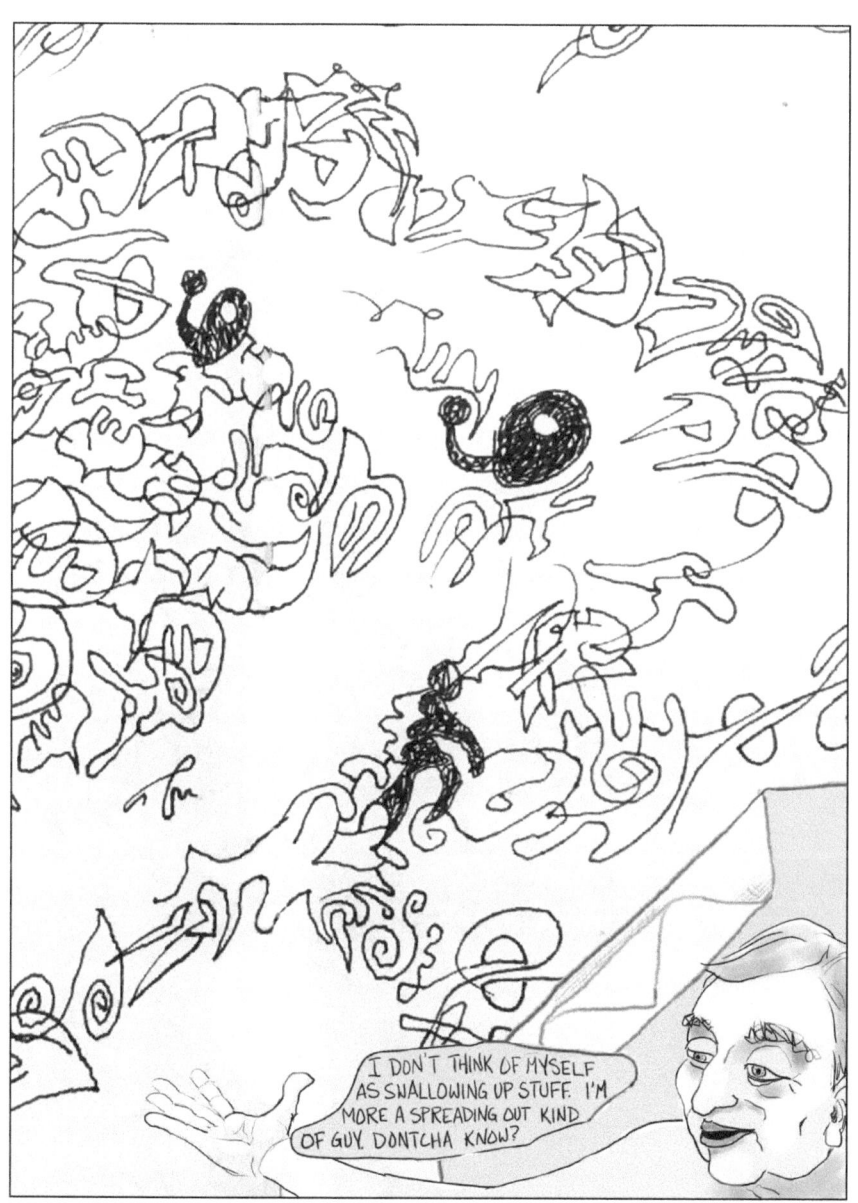

Everyday Rituals

Chapter 6

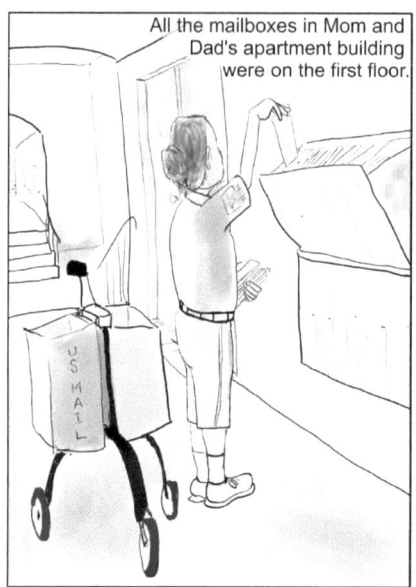
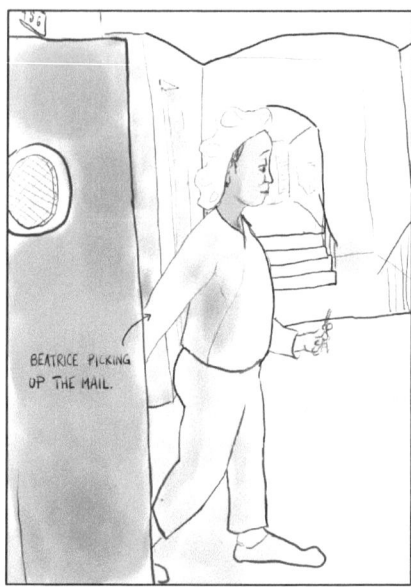
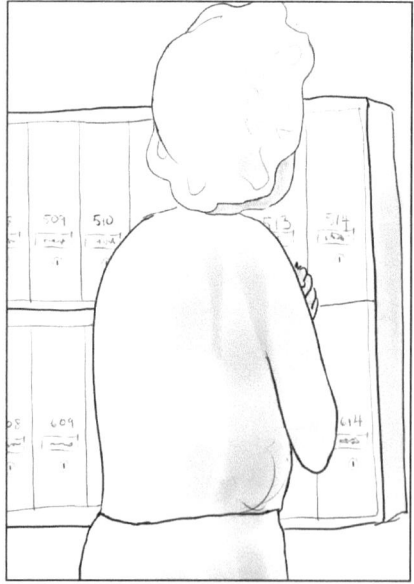
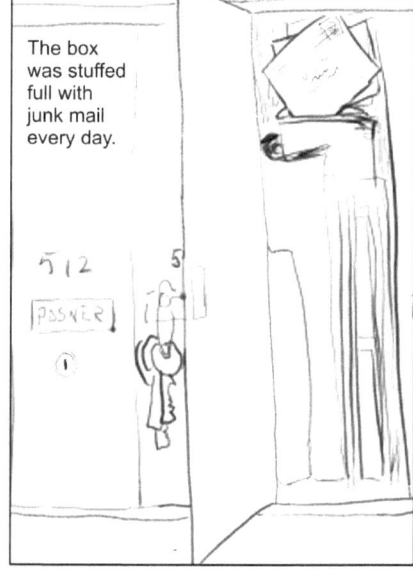

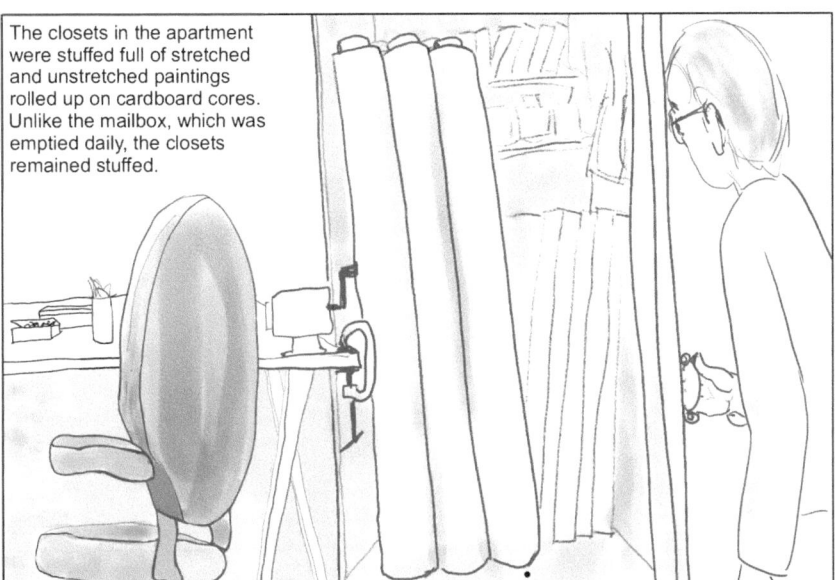

The closets in the apartment were stuffed full of stretched and unstretched paintings rolled up on cardboard cores. Unlike the mailbox, which was emptied daily, the closets remained stuffed.

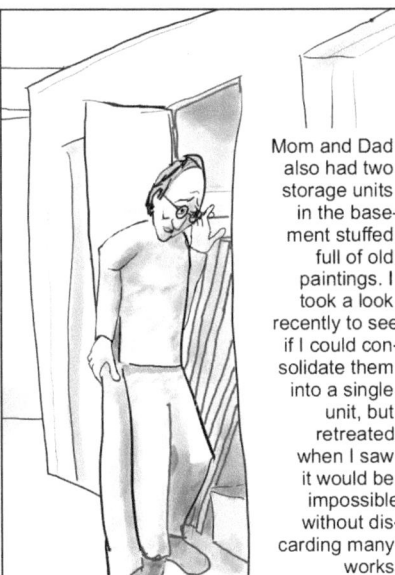

Mom and Dad also had two storage units in the basement stuffed full of old paintings. I took a look recently to see if I could consolidate them into a single unit, but retreated when I saw it would be impossible without discarding many works.

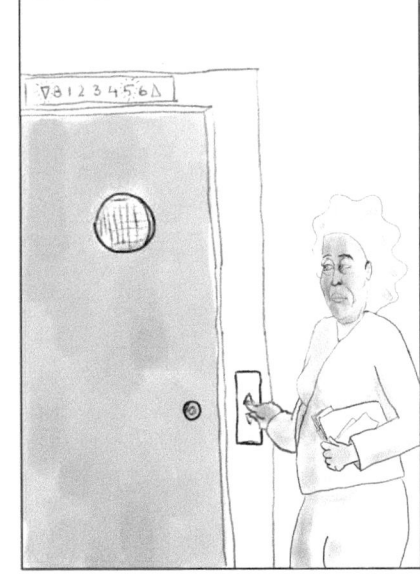

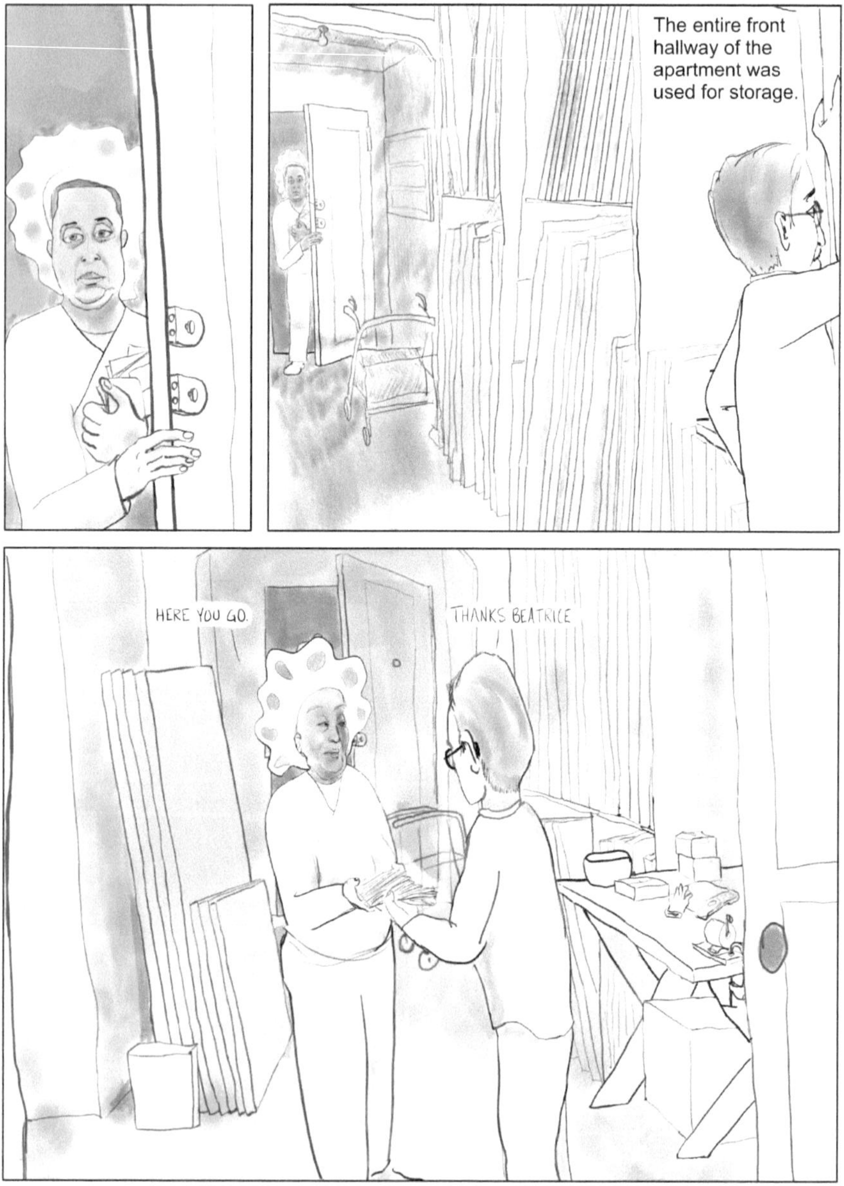

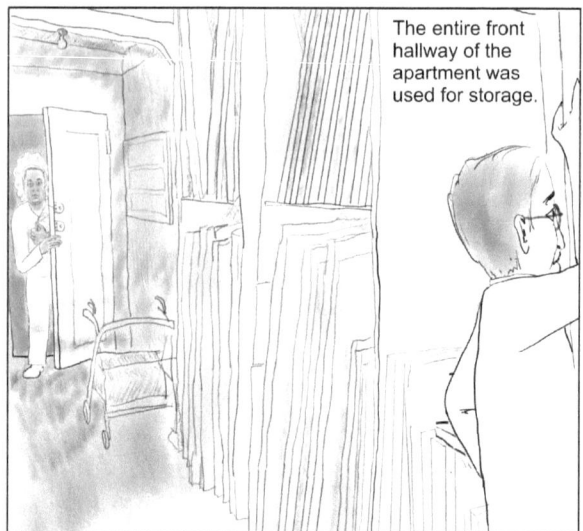

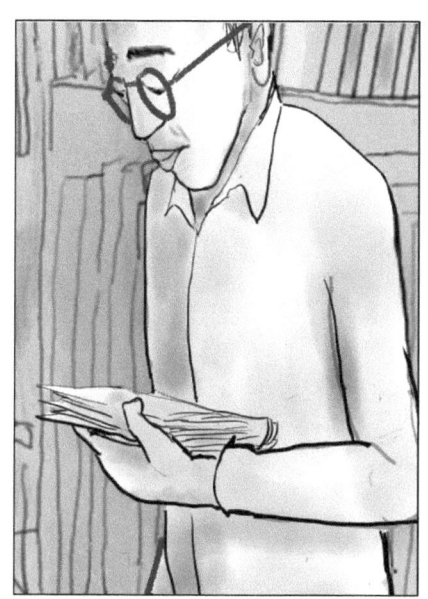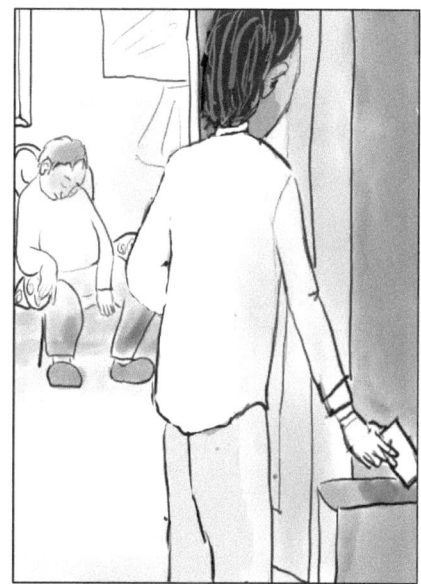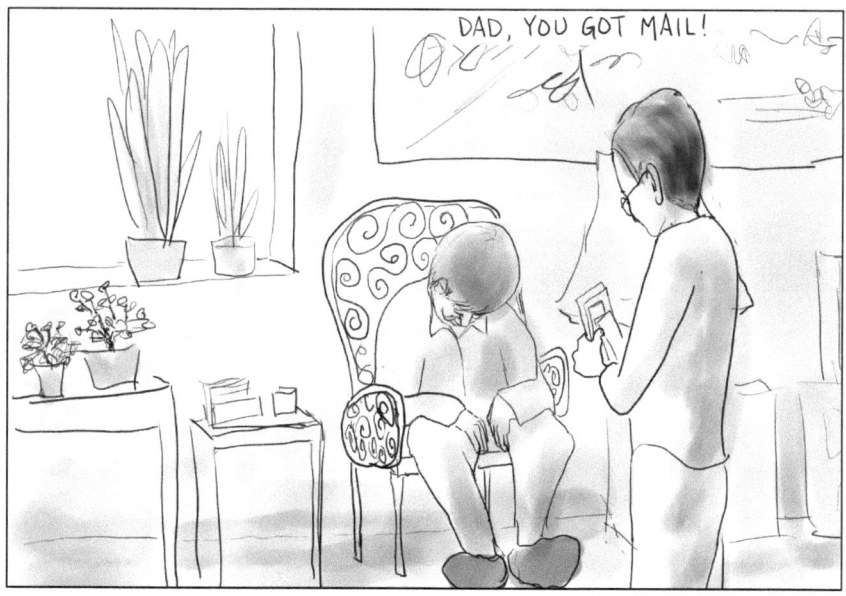

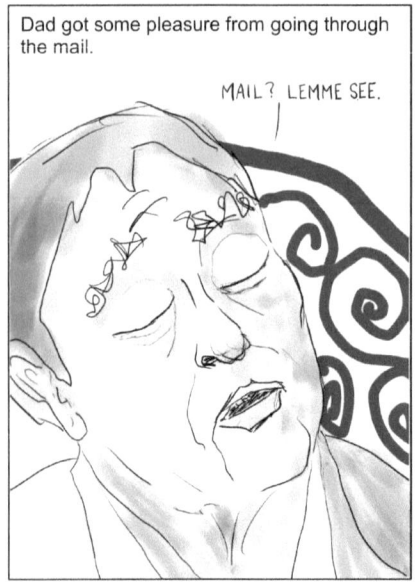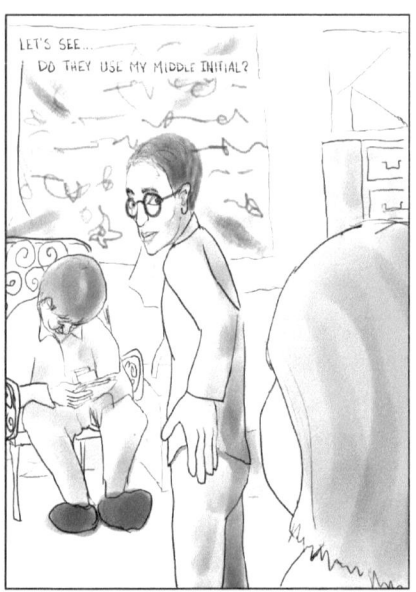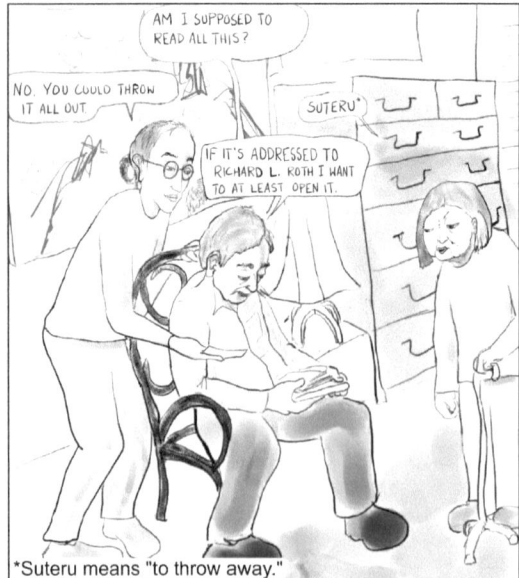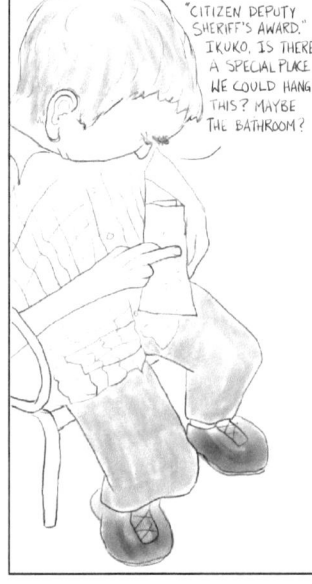

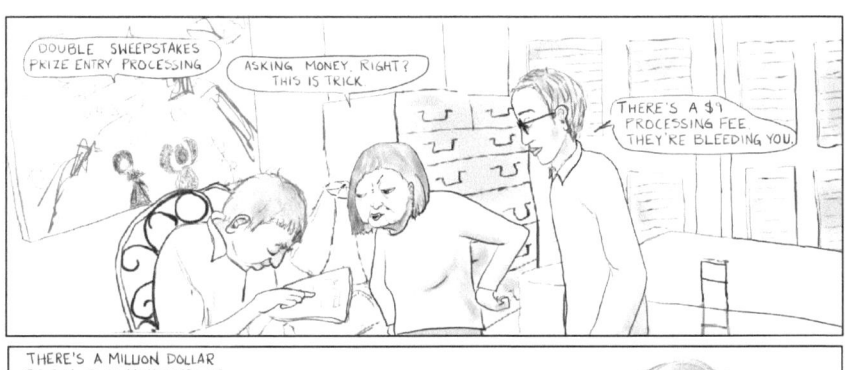
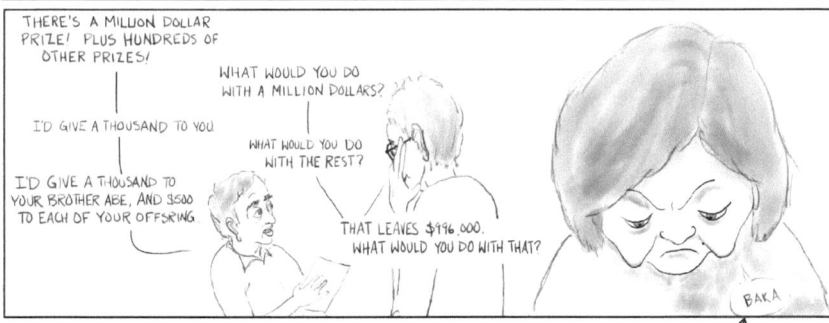
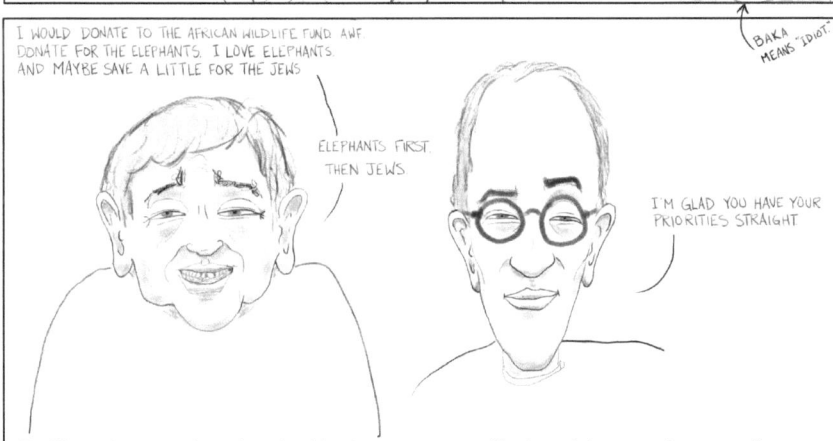

Dad has given to quite a few charities in recent years. He doesn't keep track very well and gave multiple times to some organizations and made single contributions to well over 40 others, mostly in the $20 to $50 range. While this makes my mom anxious about money, my brother and I have been more concerned about sweepstakes scams.

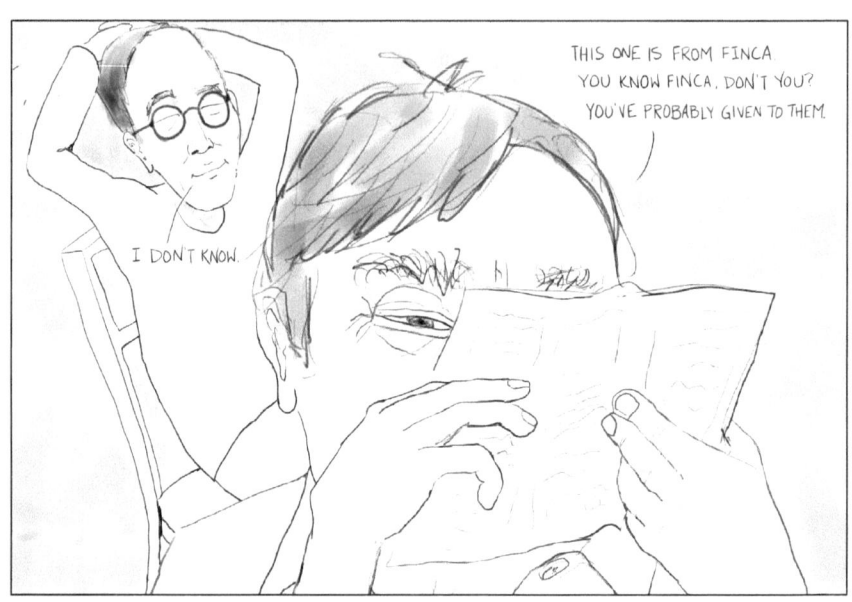

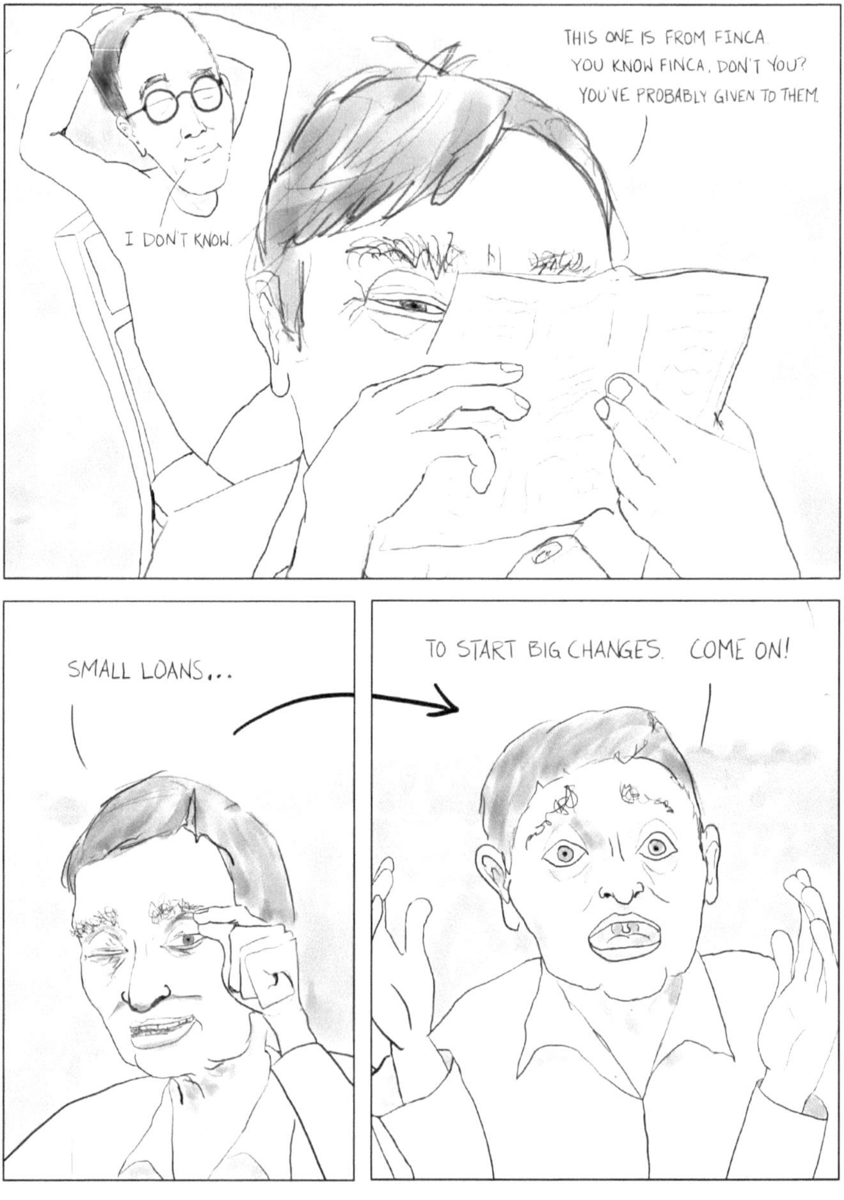

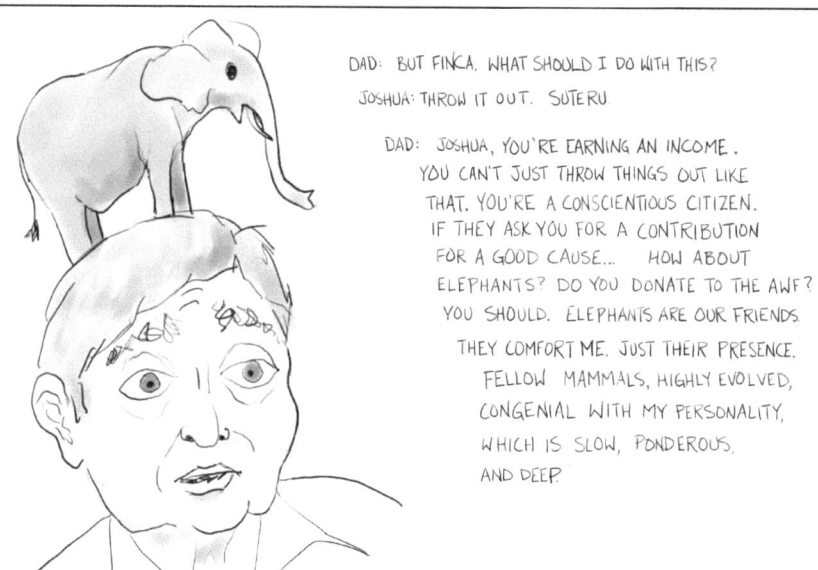

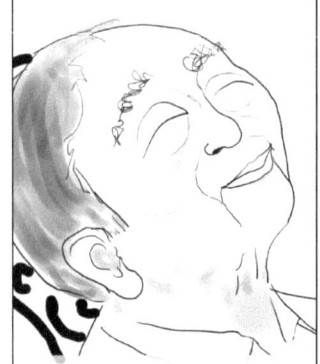

We were improvising a ritual around opening the mail, one that made it a light-hearted activity. This was just one of many such routines—repeated actions as well as formulaic speech—with which Dad filled his days.

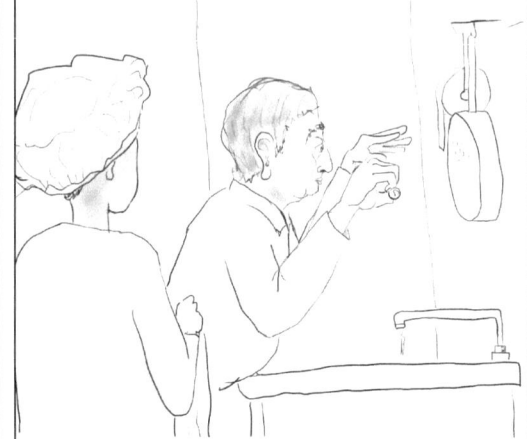

Every time Dad washed his hands before eating, he'd end by flicking his fingers at a pan hanging over the kitchen sink, listening for the tinkling sound created as the droplets hit the metal surface. Only then would he wipe his hands on the towel offered to him.

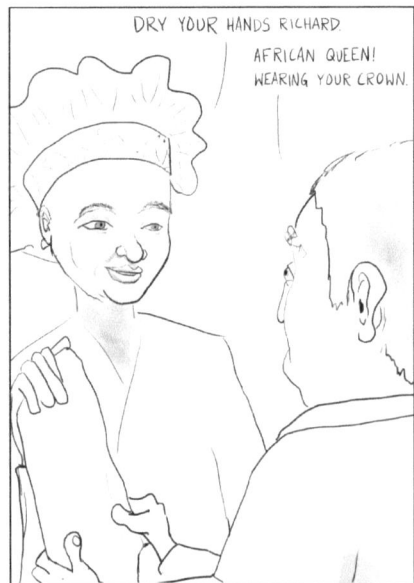

DRY YOUR HANDS RICHARD. AFRICAN QUEEN! WEARING YOUR CROWN.

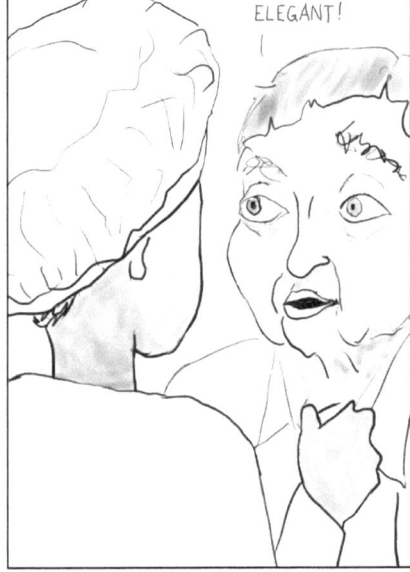

ELEGANT!

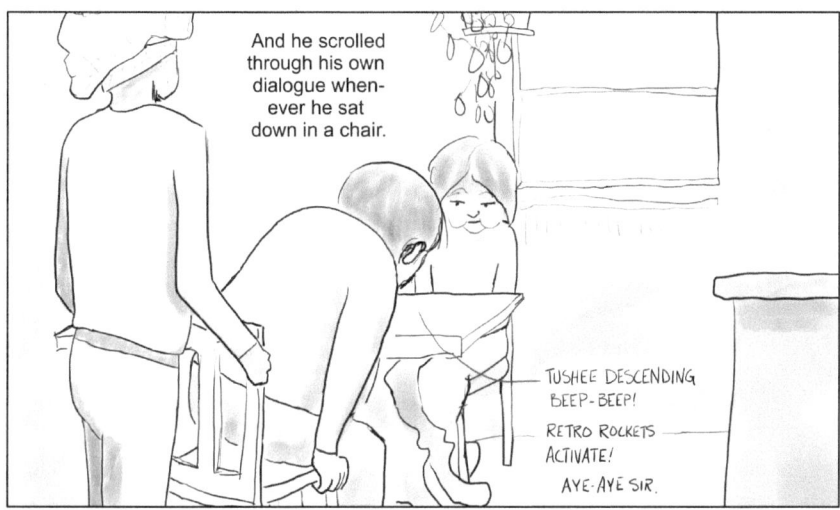

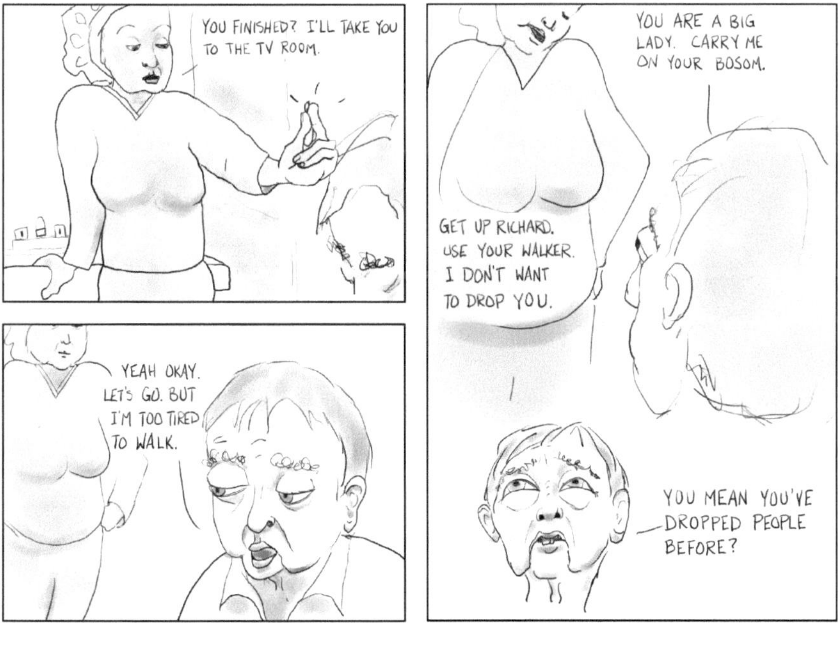

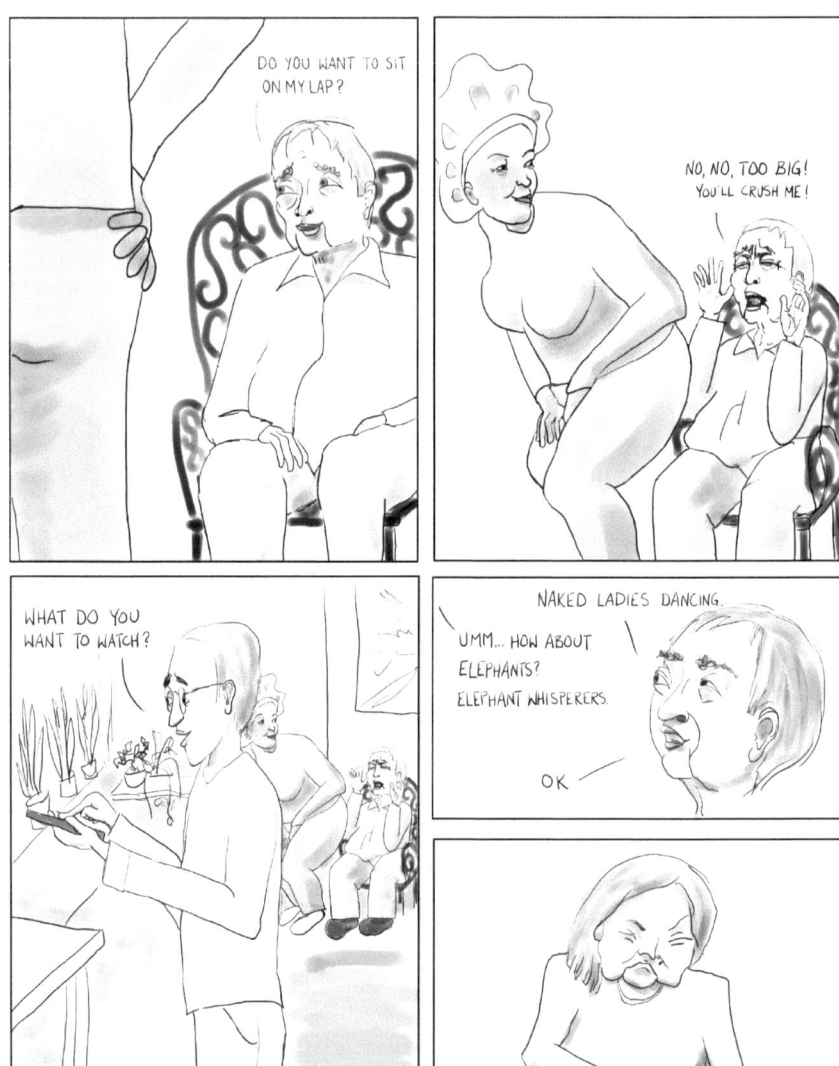

Look at me, pretending not to notice Dad's indiscretions. Was I too forgiving, allowing his bad behavior to become another kind of ritual? Maybe I was deferring to the care workers who easily rebuffed Dad, or contained the interactions in the frame of play. But what if he became harder to handle? And Mom wasn't pleased the times she picked up on these interactions.

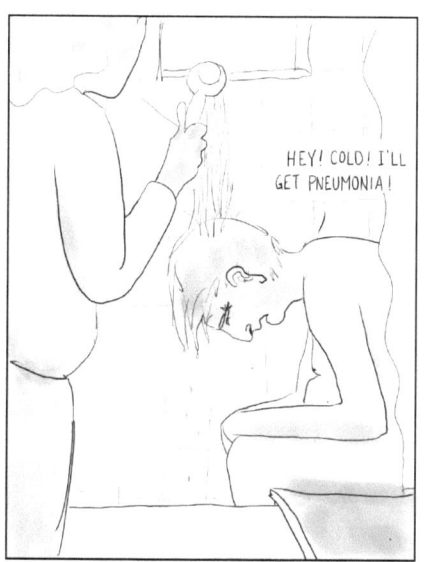
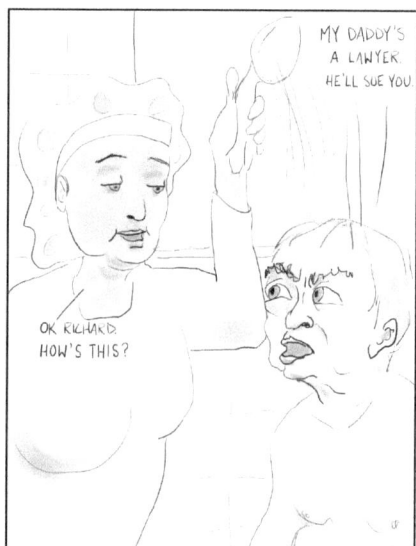
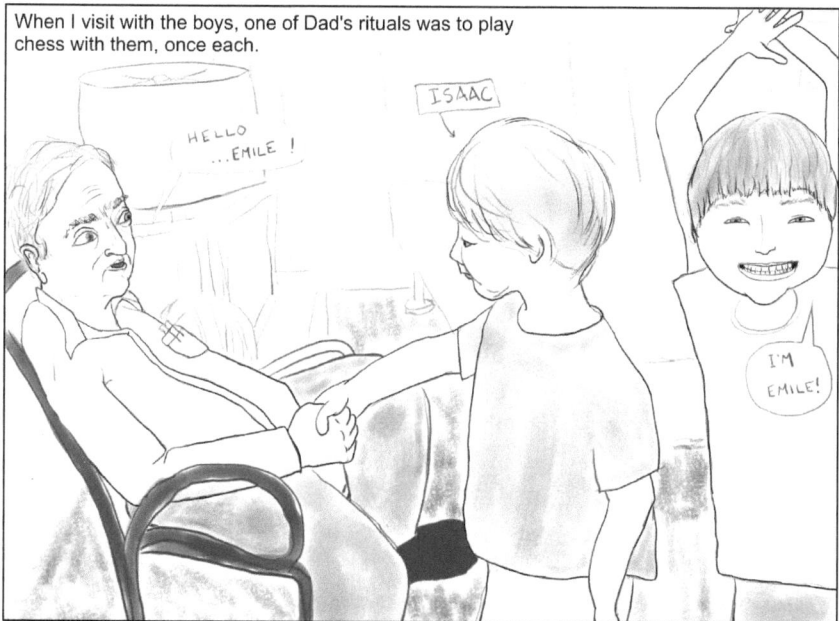

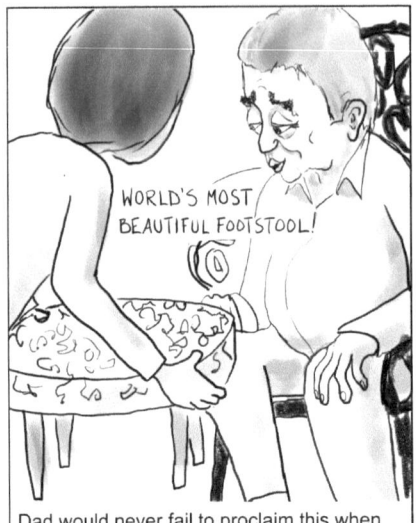

Dad would never fail to proclaim this when we set the chess board on our footstool that had been upholstered with an old MOOP.

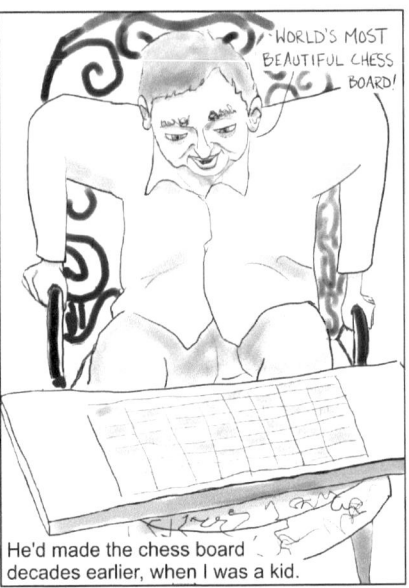

He'd made the chess board decades earlier, when I was a kid.

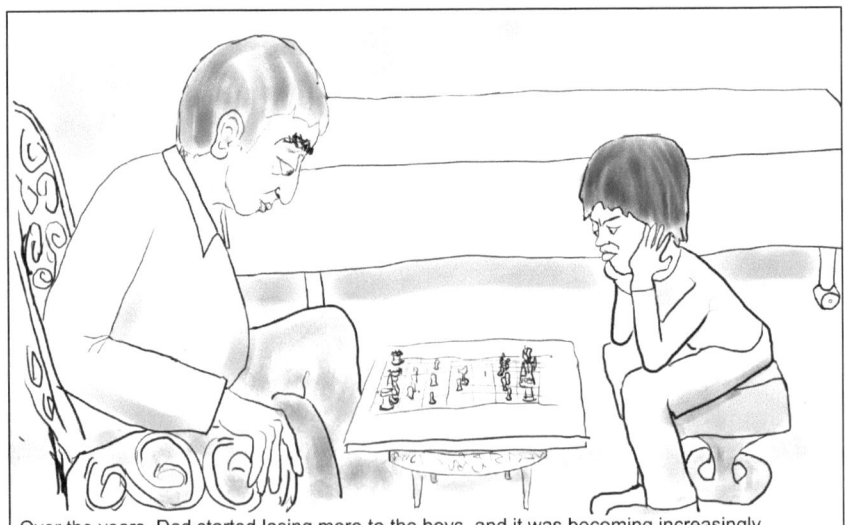

Over the years, Dad started losing more to the boys, and it was becoming increasingly apparent that his memory was failing. I'm sure it was disturbing for him, but he brushed it off. "I'm 90 years old!" became a common refrain in the house, every time he missed something.

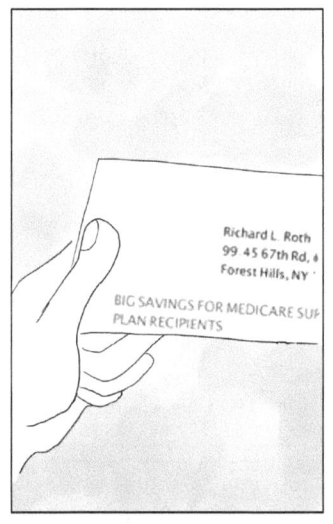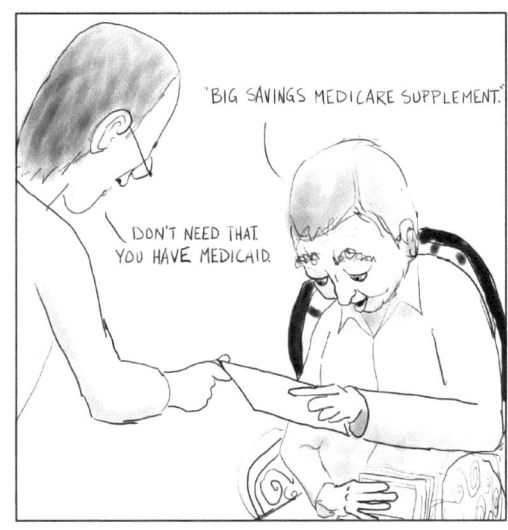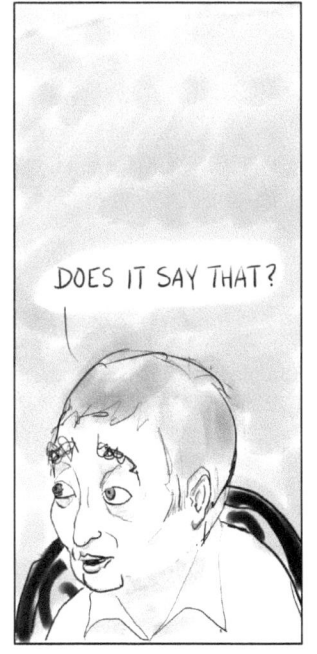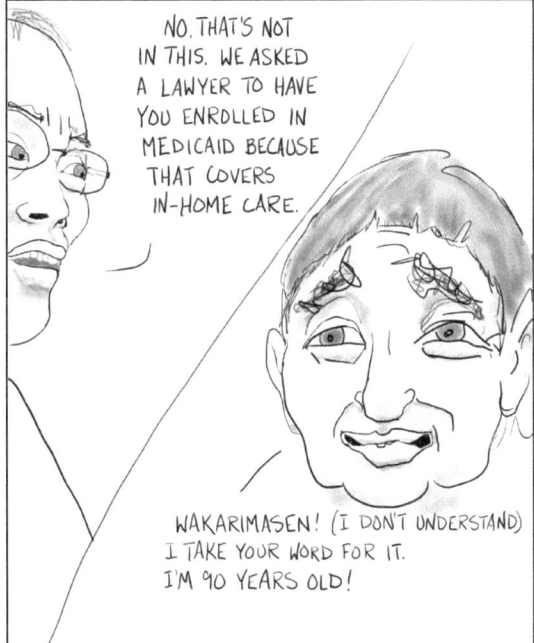

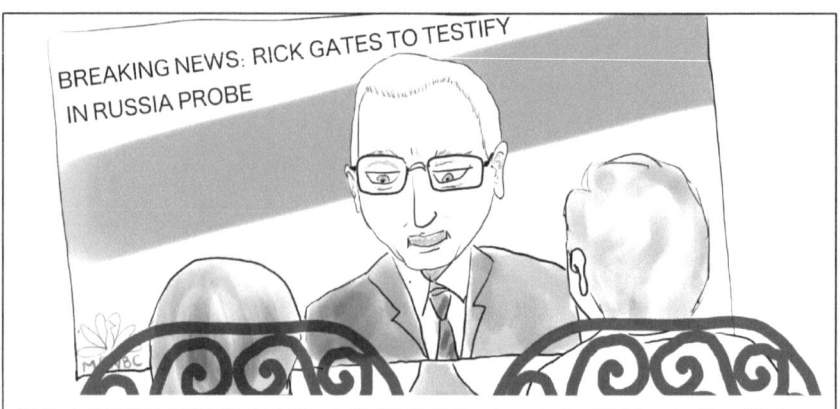

As my parents' eyesight dimmed, they pulled their chairs closer to the TV. They continued to do so even after I finally discarded their old 19" Sony Trinitron in favor of a 36" Samsung flat panel.

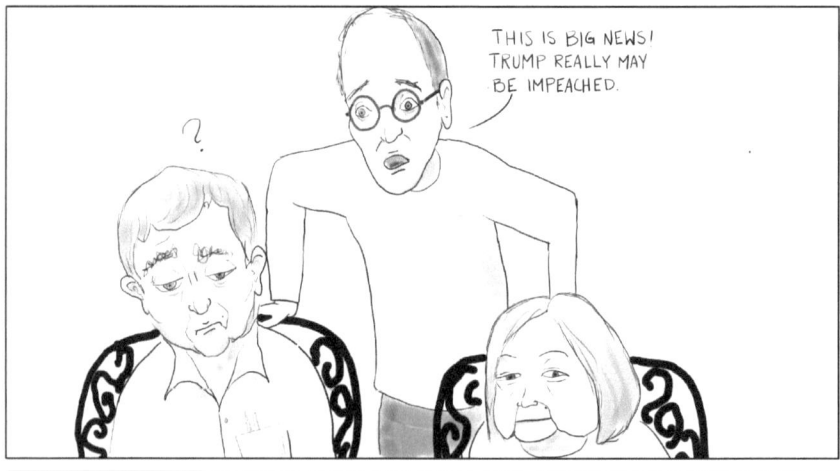

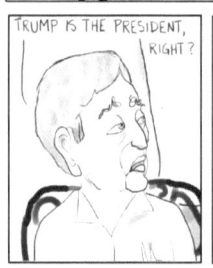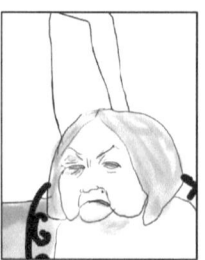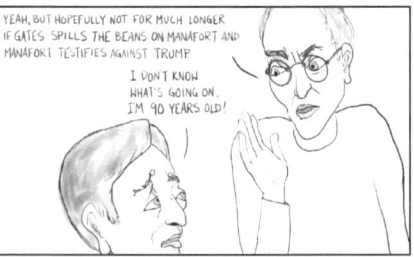

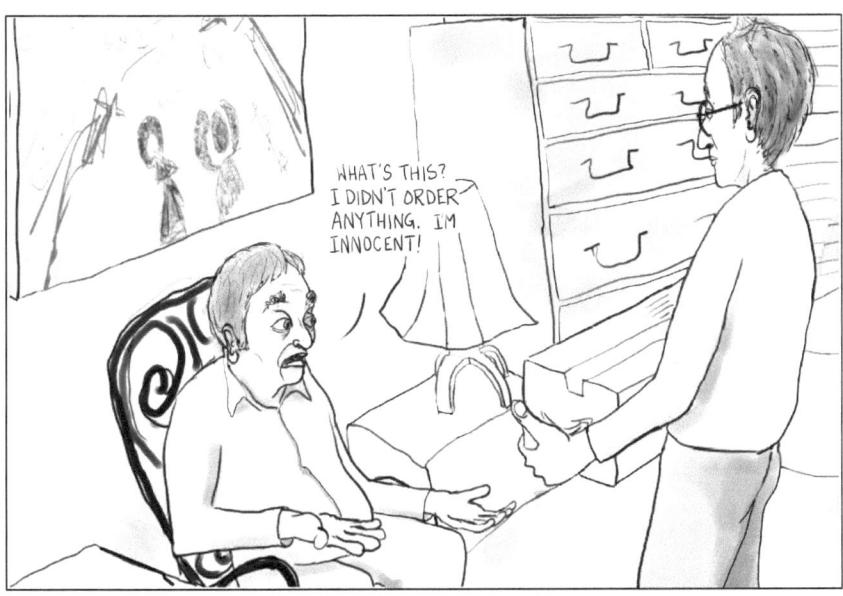

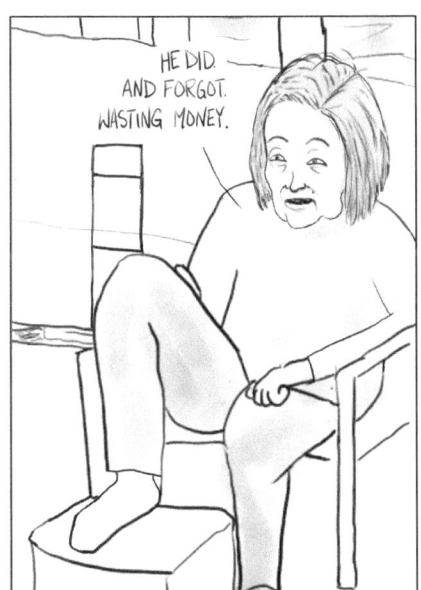

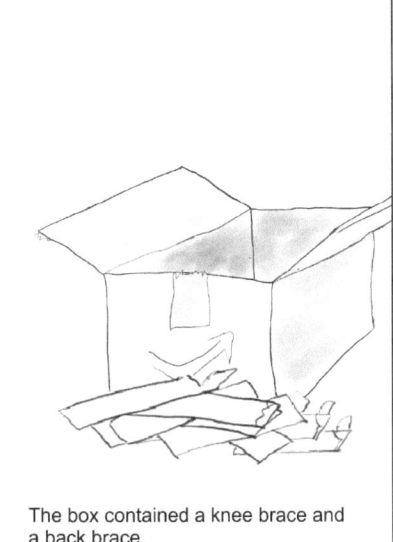

The box contained a knee brace and a back brace.

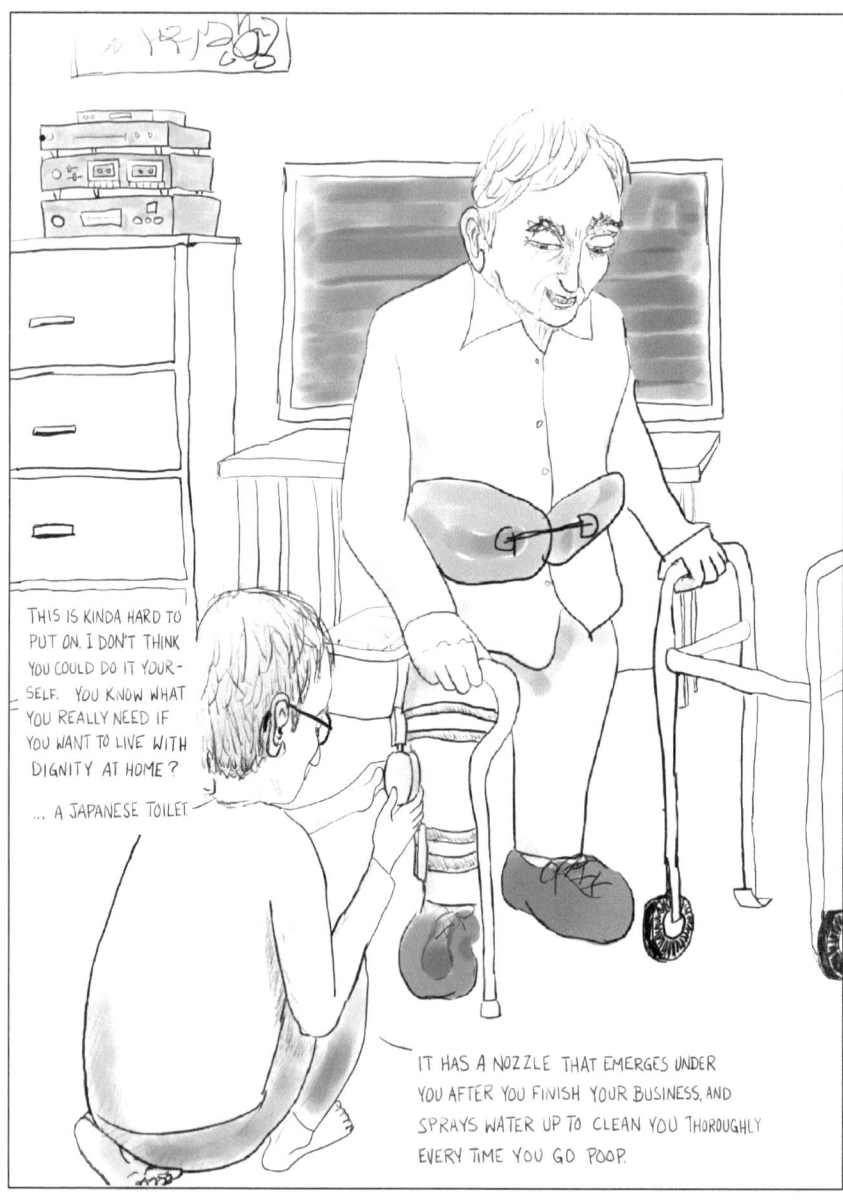

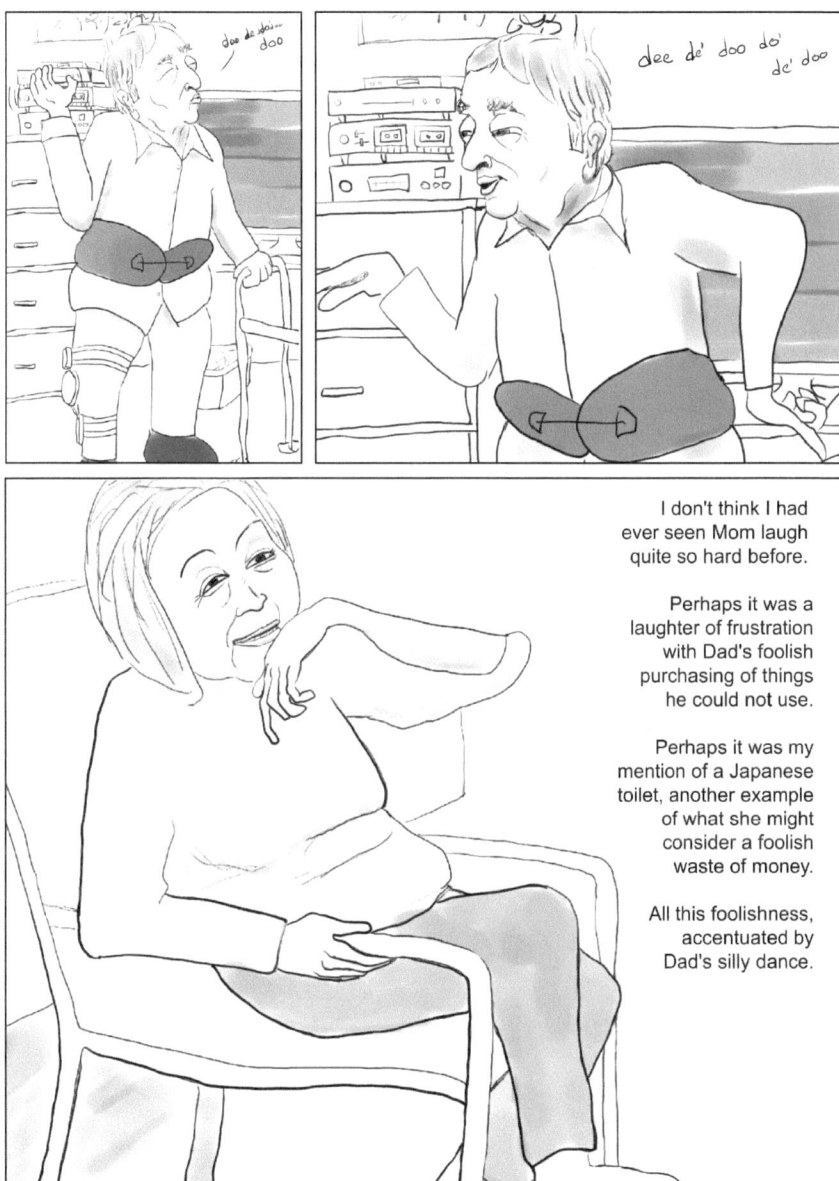

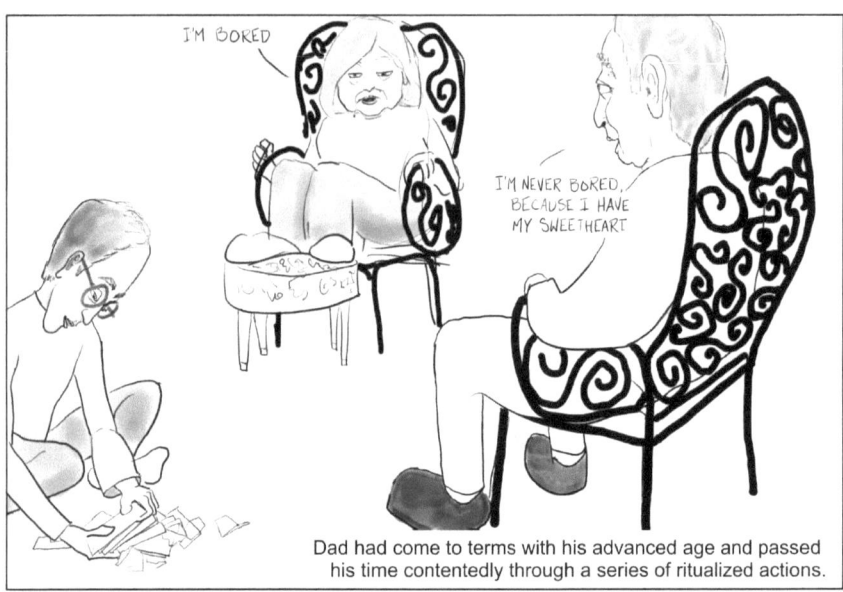
Dad had come to terms with his advanced age and passed his time contentedly through a series of ritualized actions.

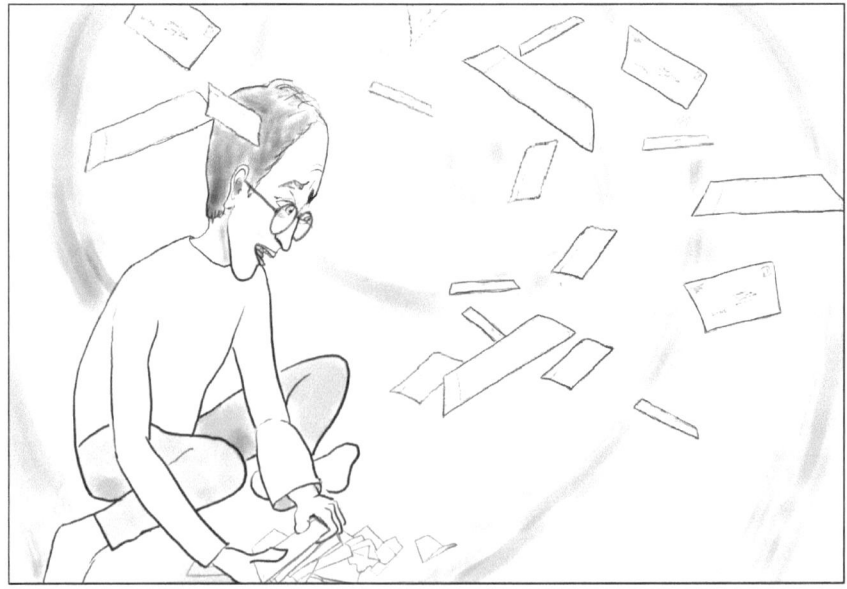

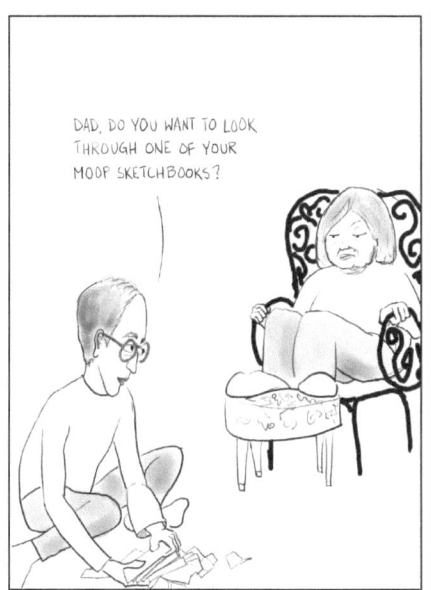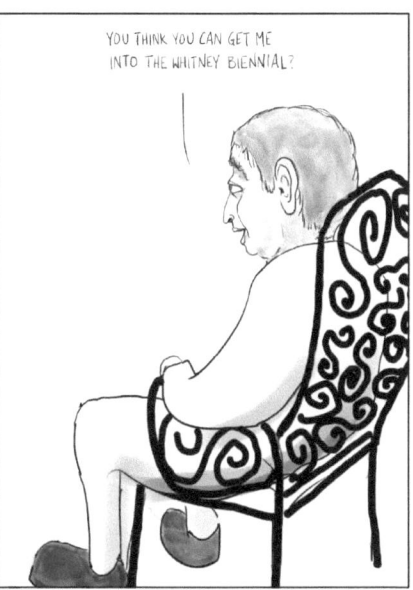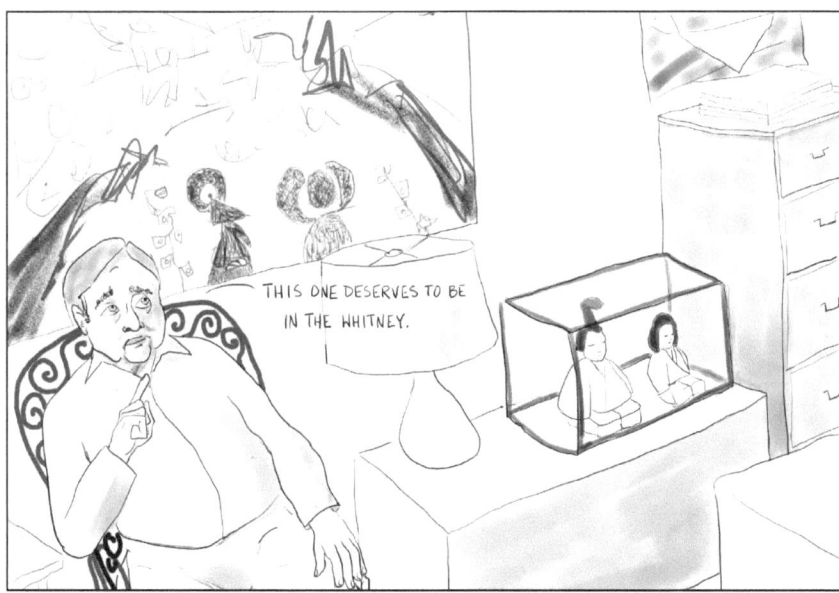

Text and Image

Chapter 7

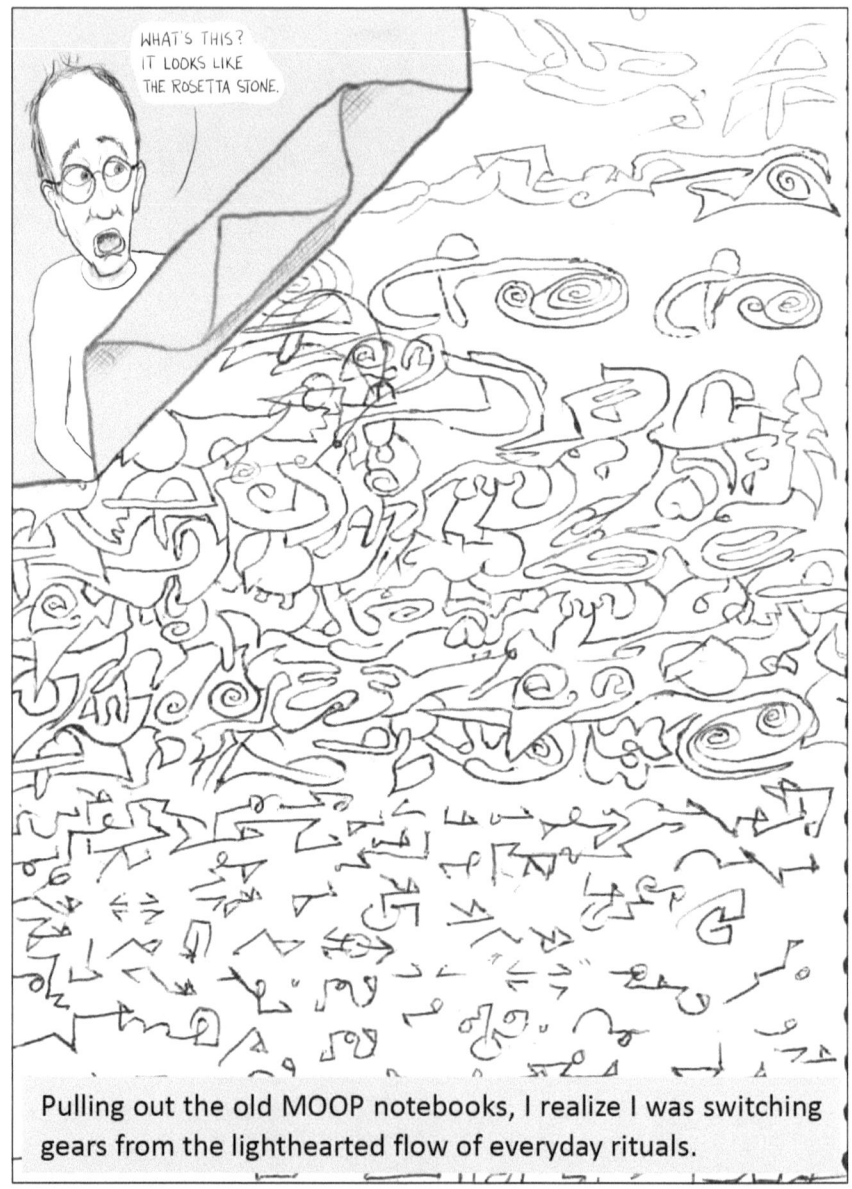

Pulling out the old MOOP notebooks, I realize I was switching gears from the lighthearted flow of everyday rituals.

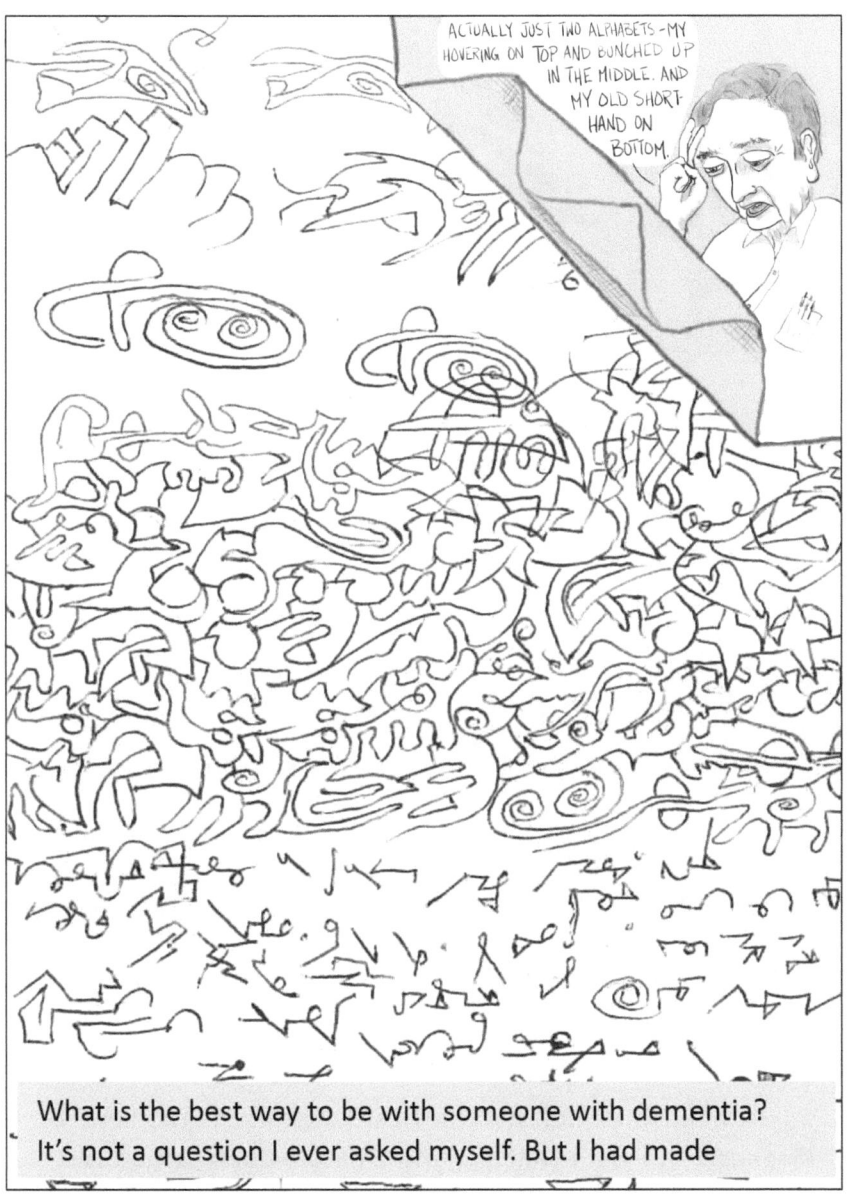

What is the best way to be with someone with dementia? It's not a question I ever asked myself. But I had made

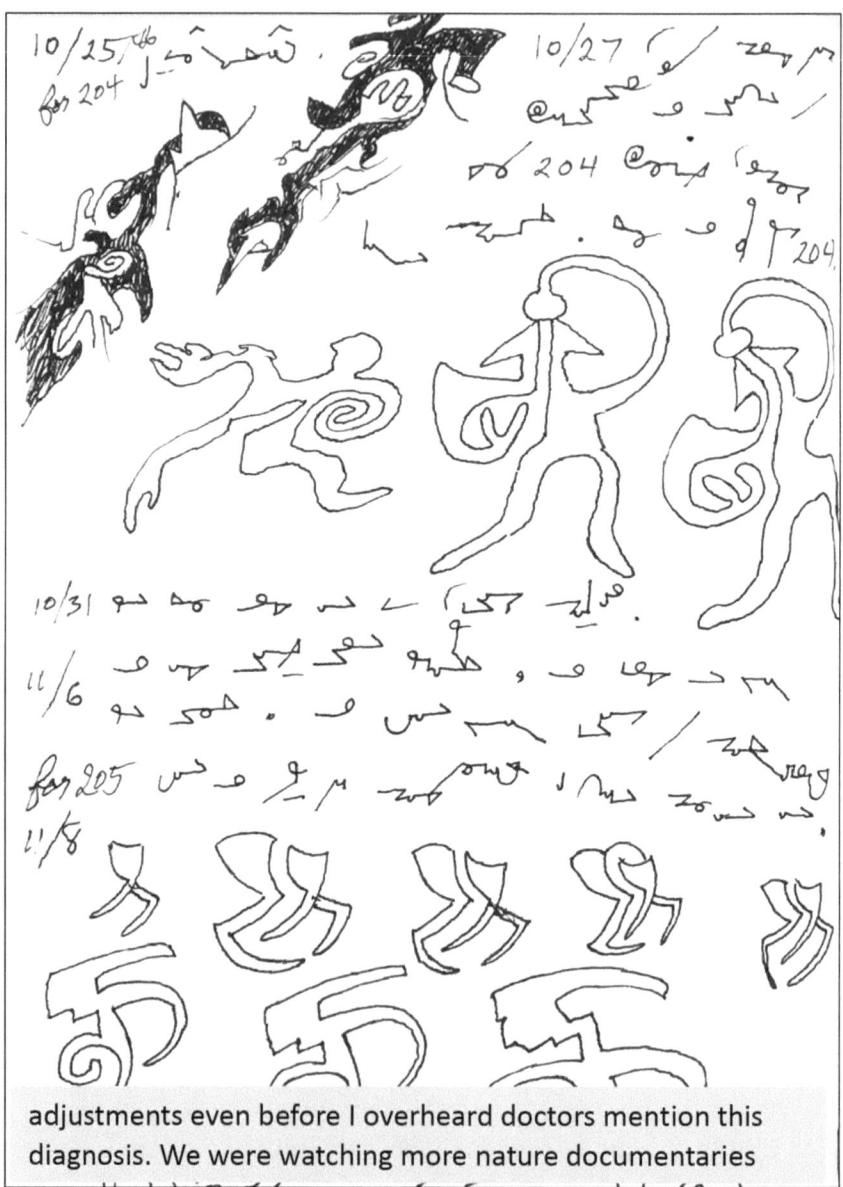

adjustments even before I overheard doctors mention this diagnosis. We were watching more nature documentaries

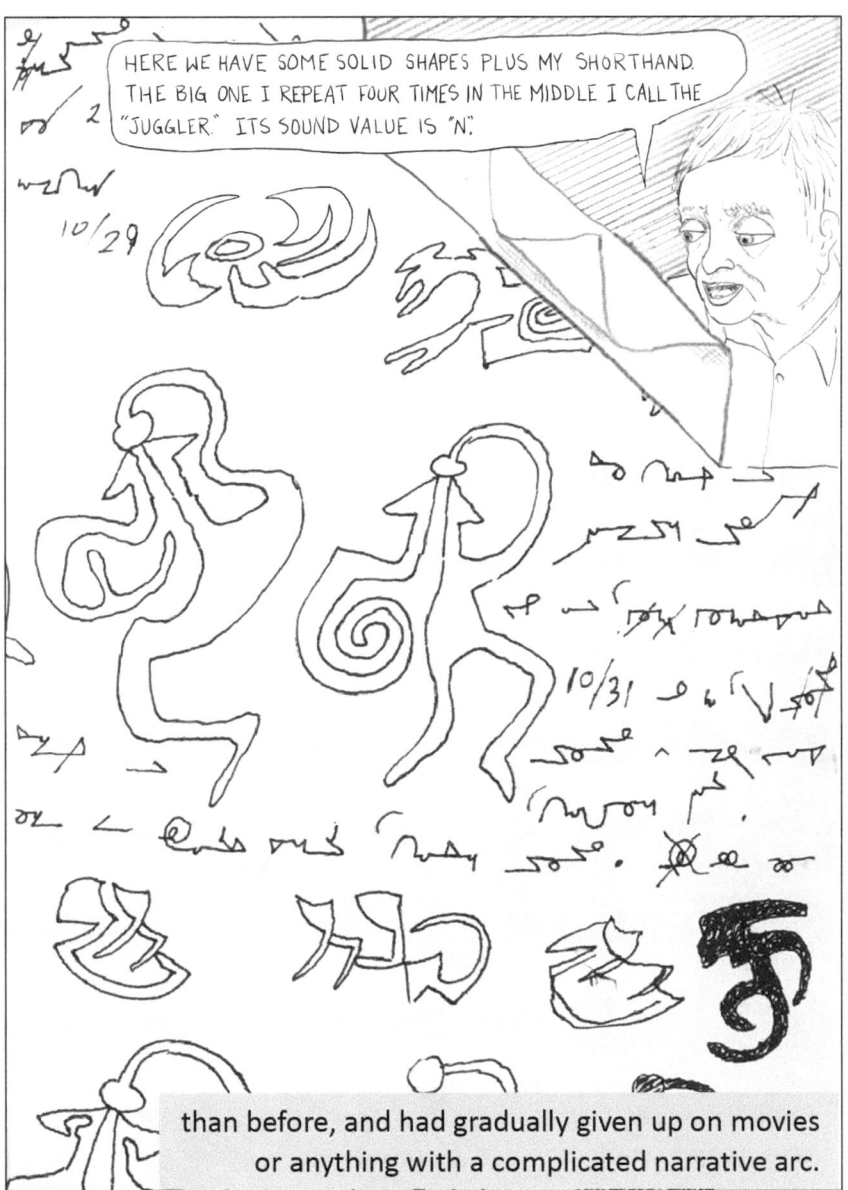

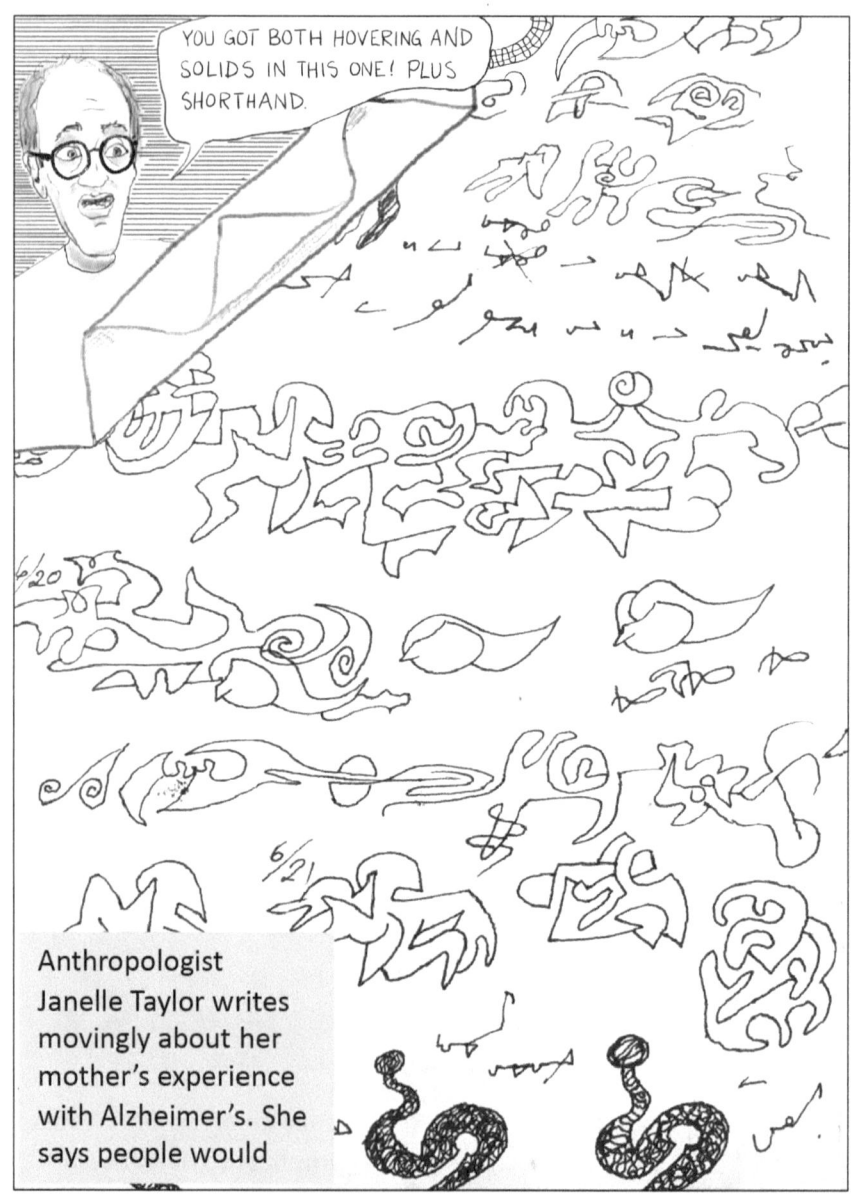

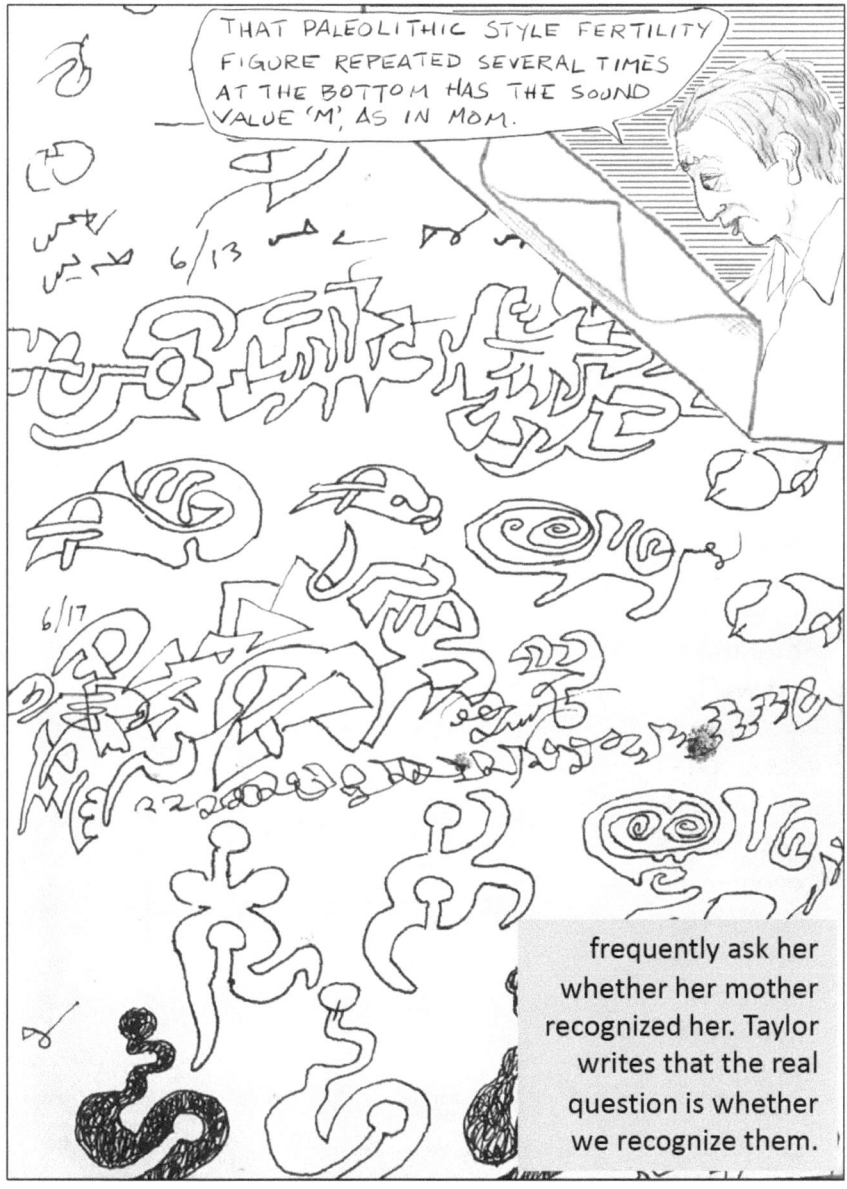

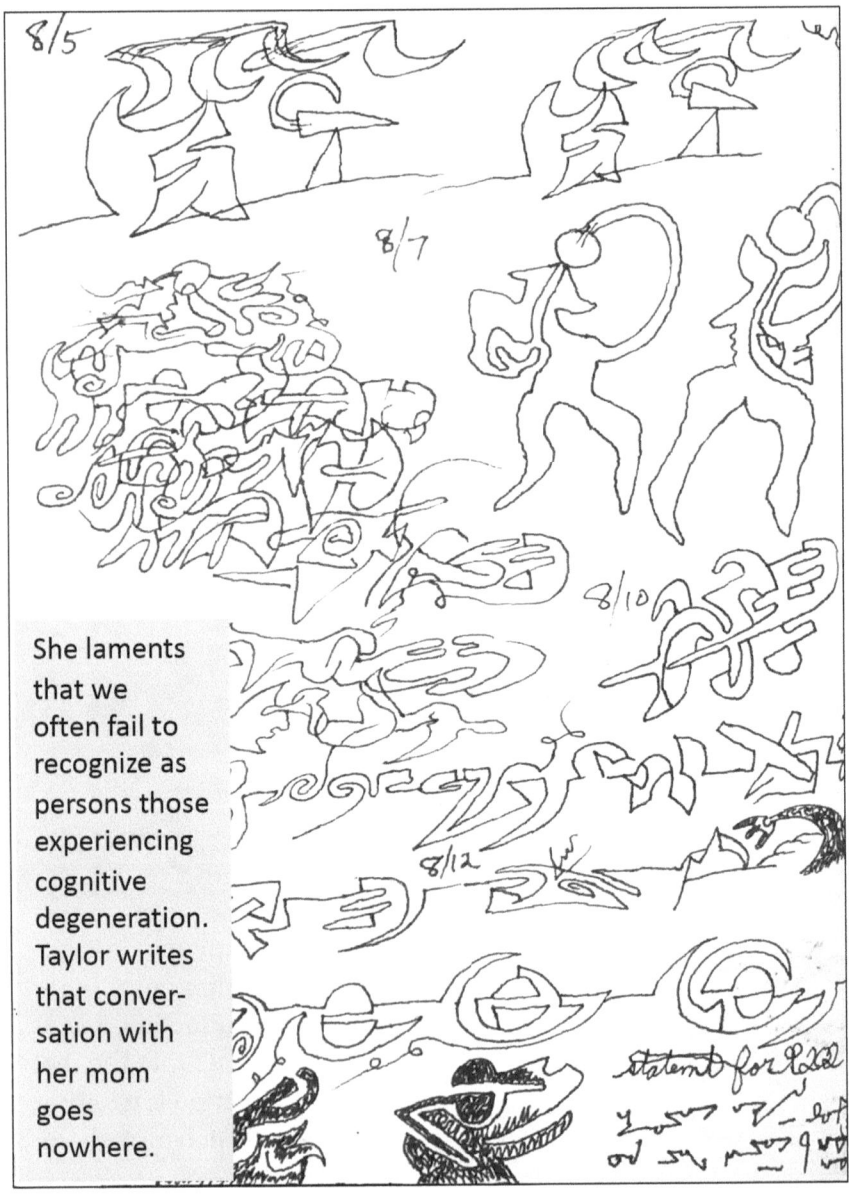

She laments that we often fail to recognize as persons those experiencing cognitive degeneration. Taylor writes that conversation with her mom goes nowhere.

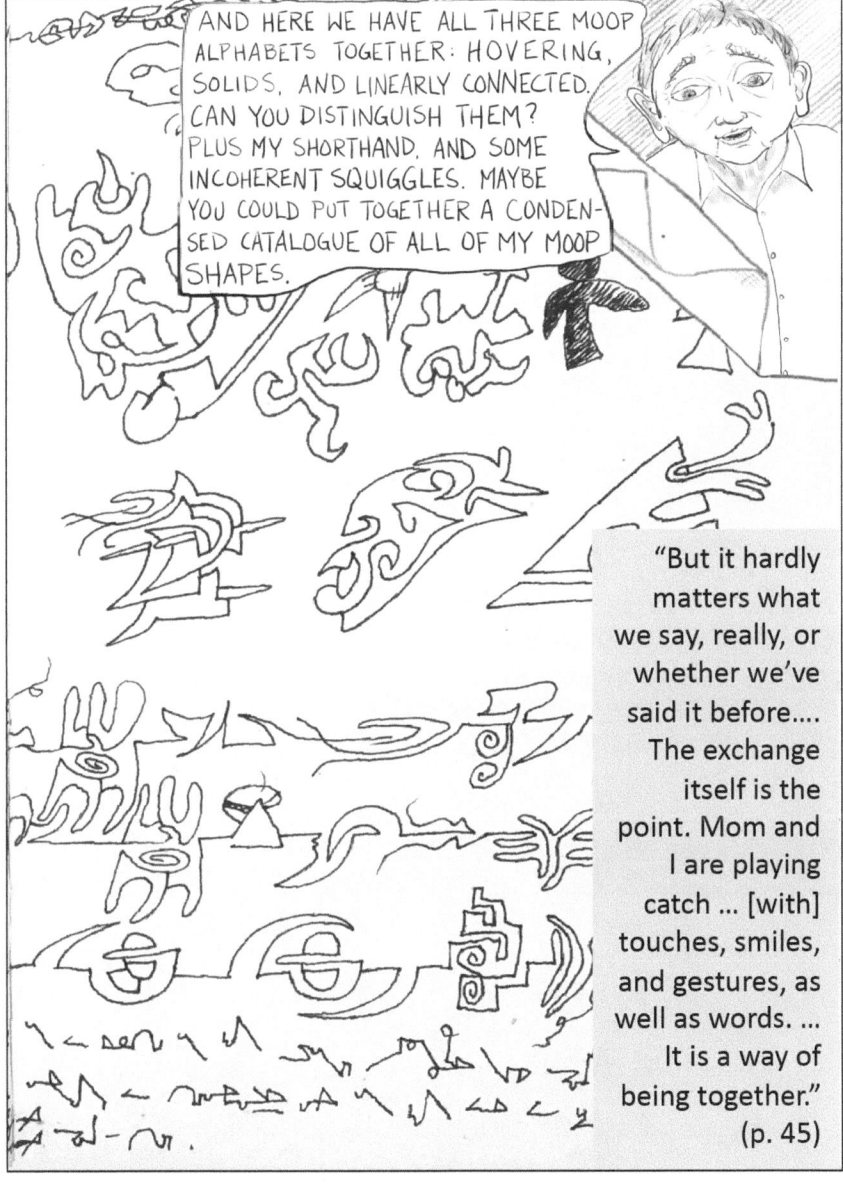

		1 GENERALIZED SHORT VOWELS A, E, I, O, U, AU	2 SHWA ə	3 ENDING "R" - SHORT VOWEL + R
	HOVERING			
	LINEARLY CONNECTED			
SOLID				

		6: "B" or "P"	7: "D" or "T"	8: "G" or "K"
	HOVERING			
	LINEARLY CONNECTED			
SOLID				

		11 TH	12 S or Z	13 SH or ZH	14 H	15 CH or J
	HOVERING					
	LINEARLY CONNECTED					
SOLID						

		18 NG	19: L or R (STARTING R)	20 W	21 Y	WORDS a the and of	END OF WO
	HOVERING						
	LINEARLY CONNECTED						
SOLID							

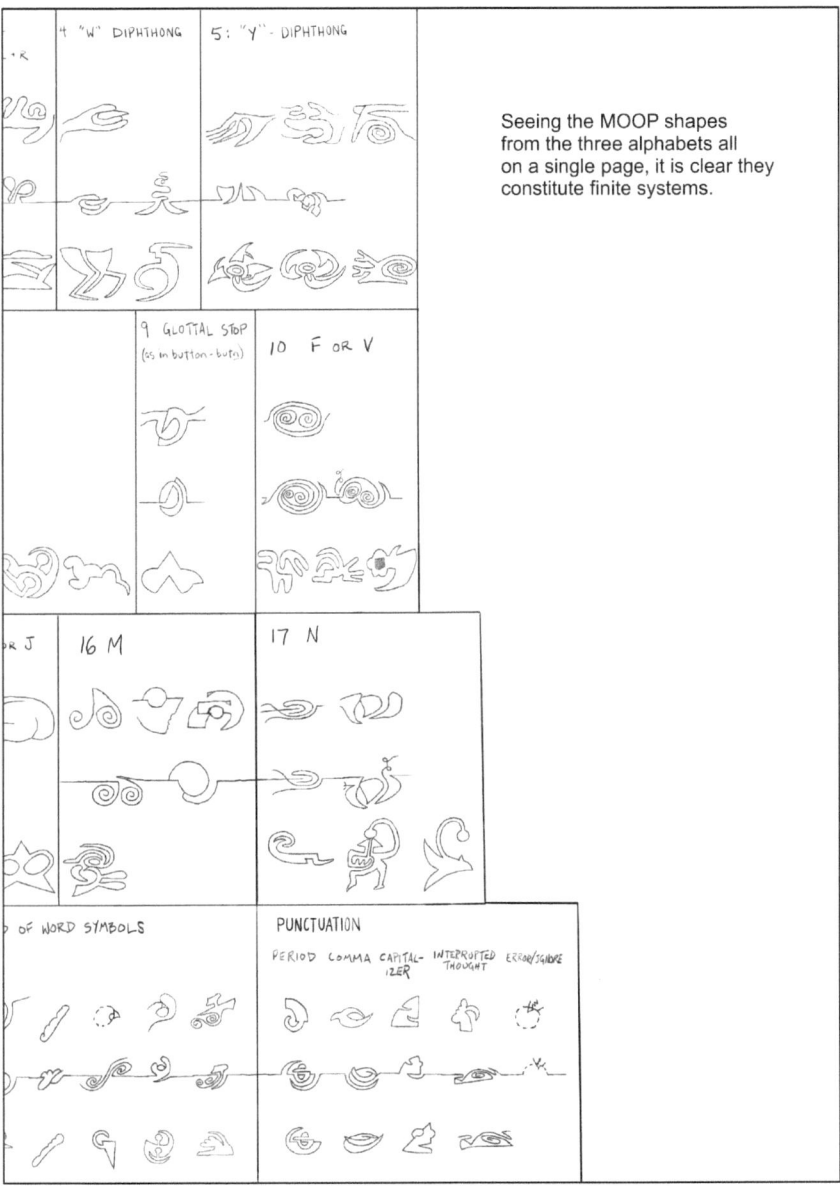

Seeing the MOOP shapes from the three alphabets all on a single page, it is clear they constitute finite systems.

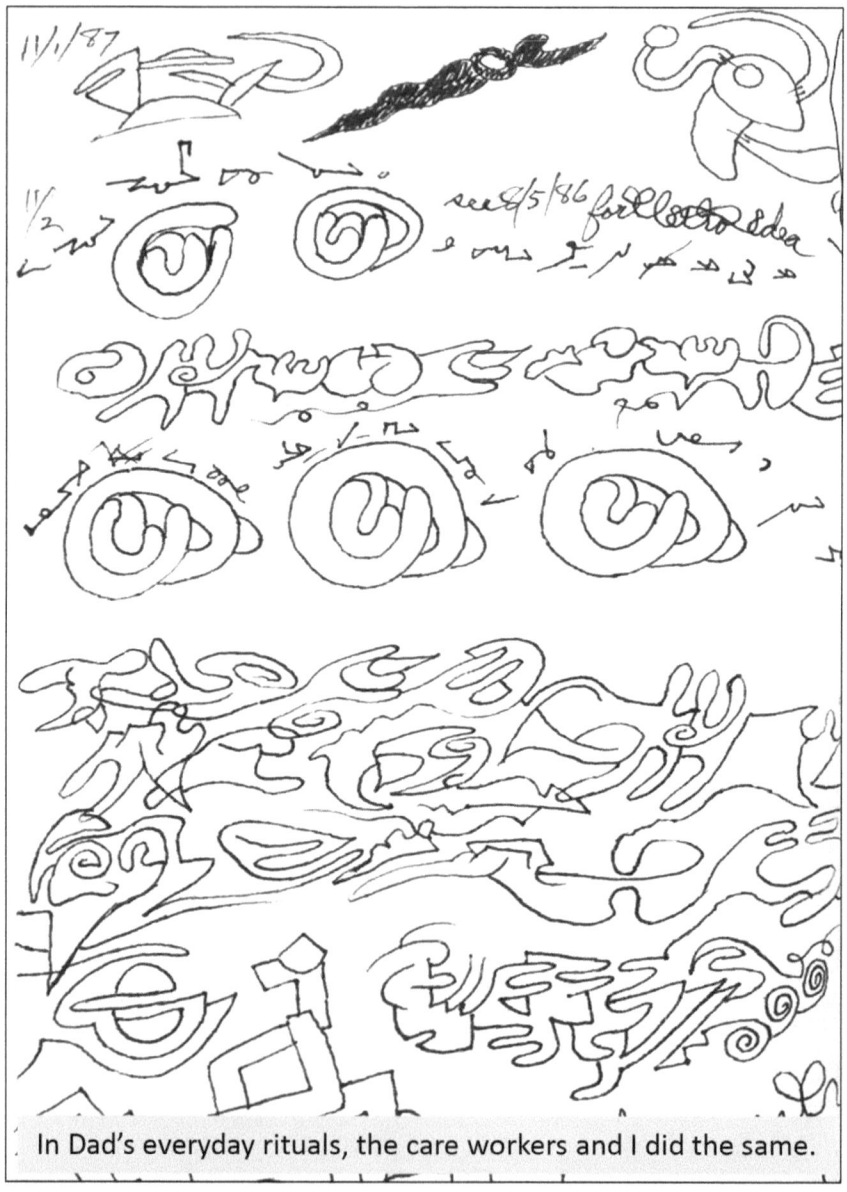

In Dad's everyday rituals, the care workers and I did the same.

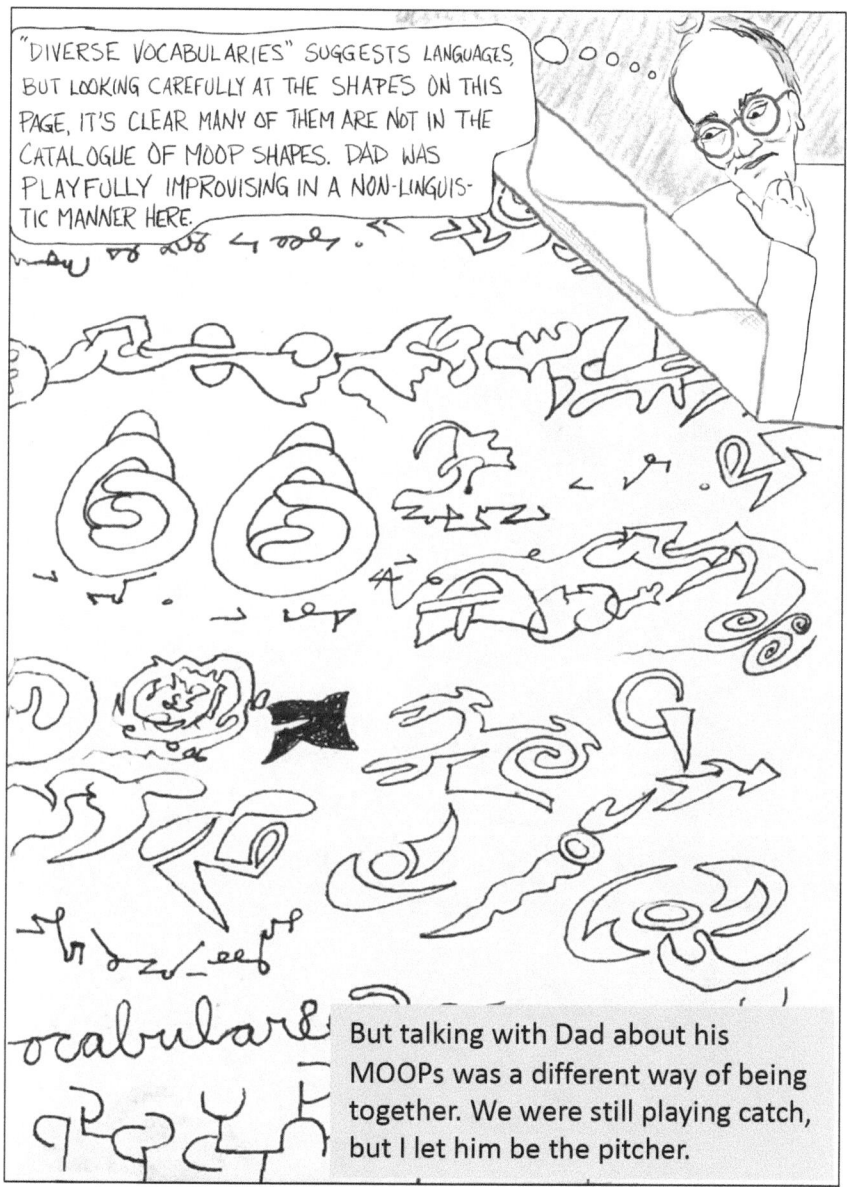

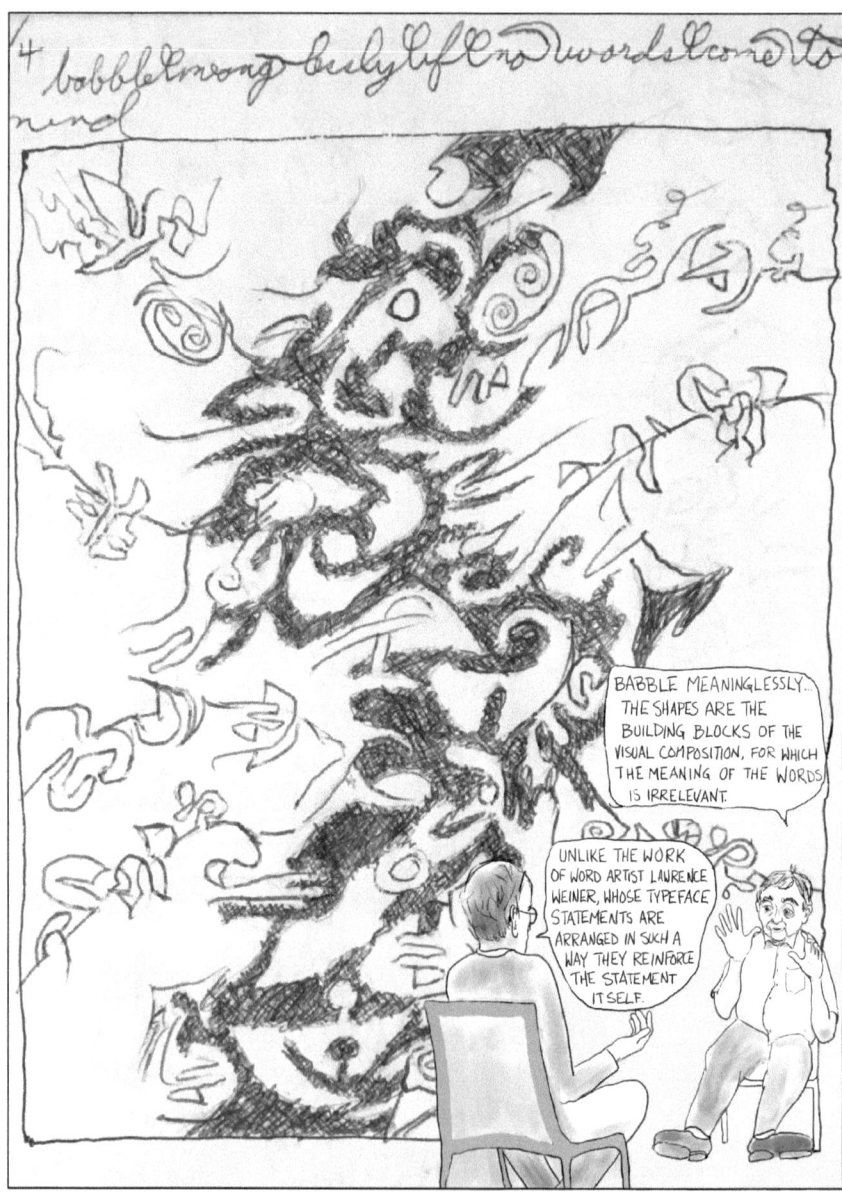

Dad communicated with word artist Lawrence Weiner, who sent him a postcard of one of his works, "Caught between Ships Passing in the Night." Dad taped it to the kitchen cupboard.

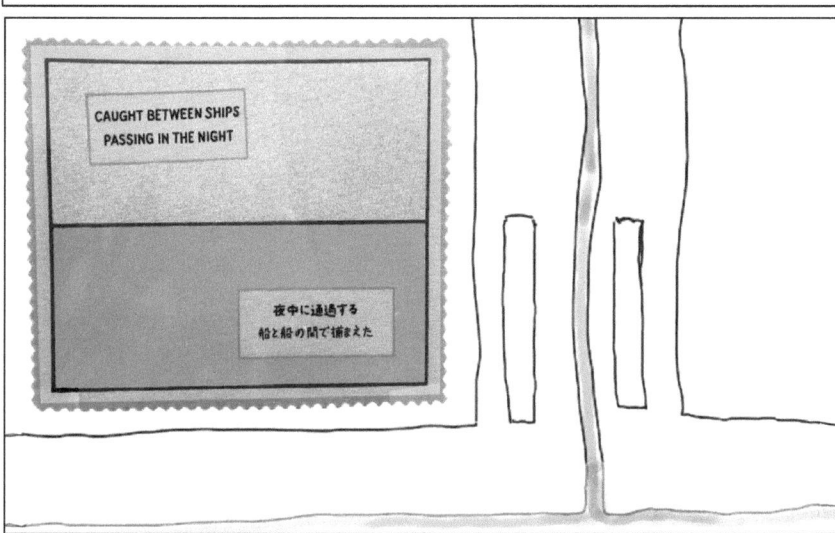

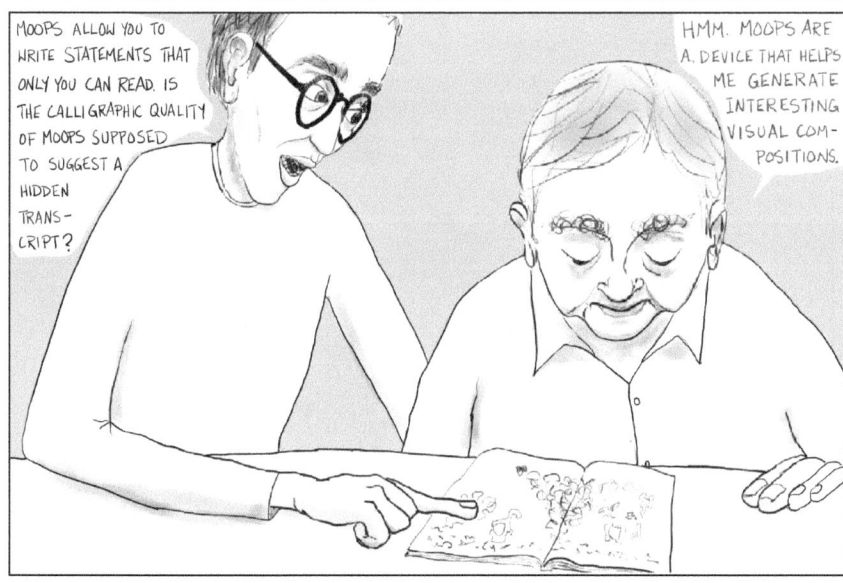

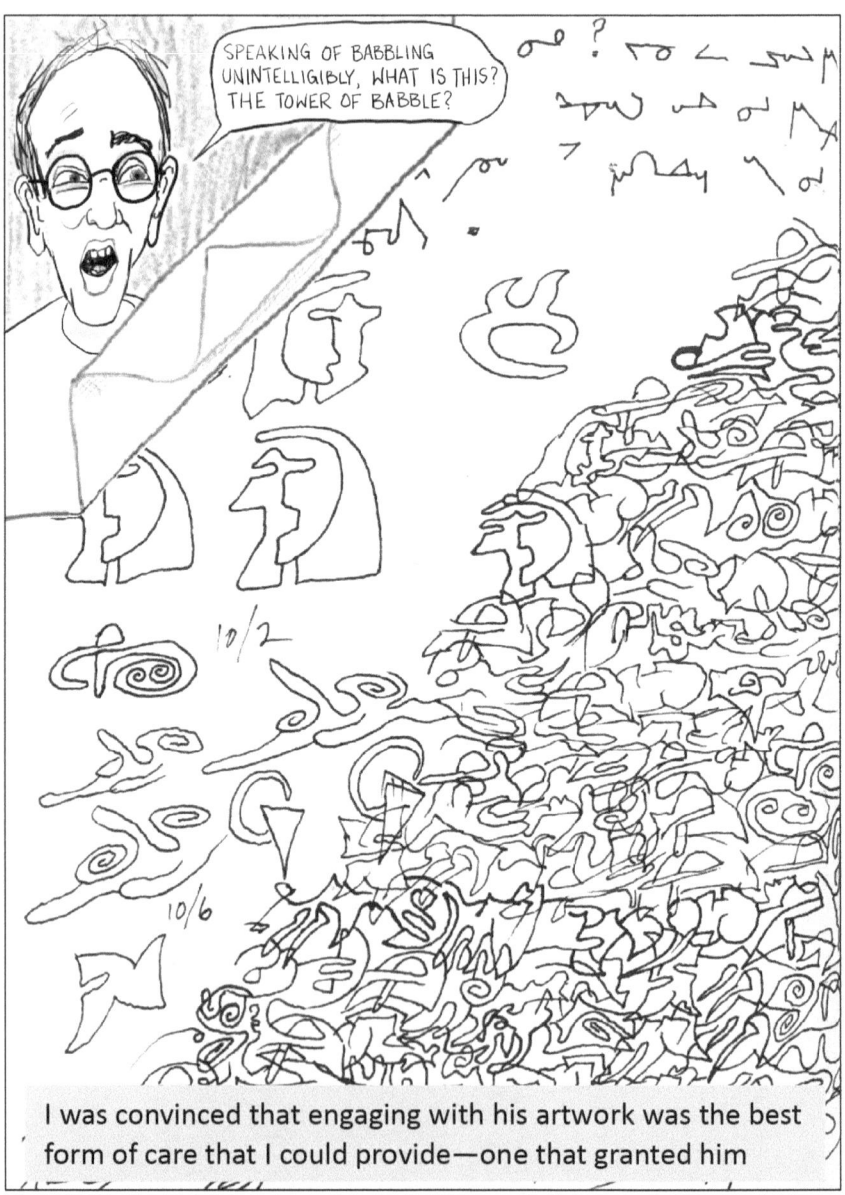

I was convinced that engaging with his artwork was the best form of care that I could provide—one that granted him

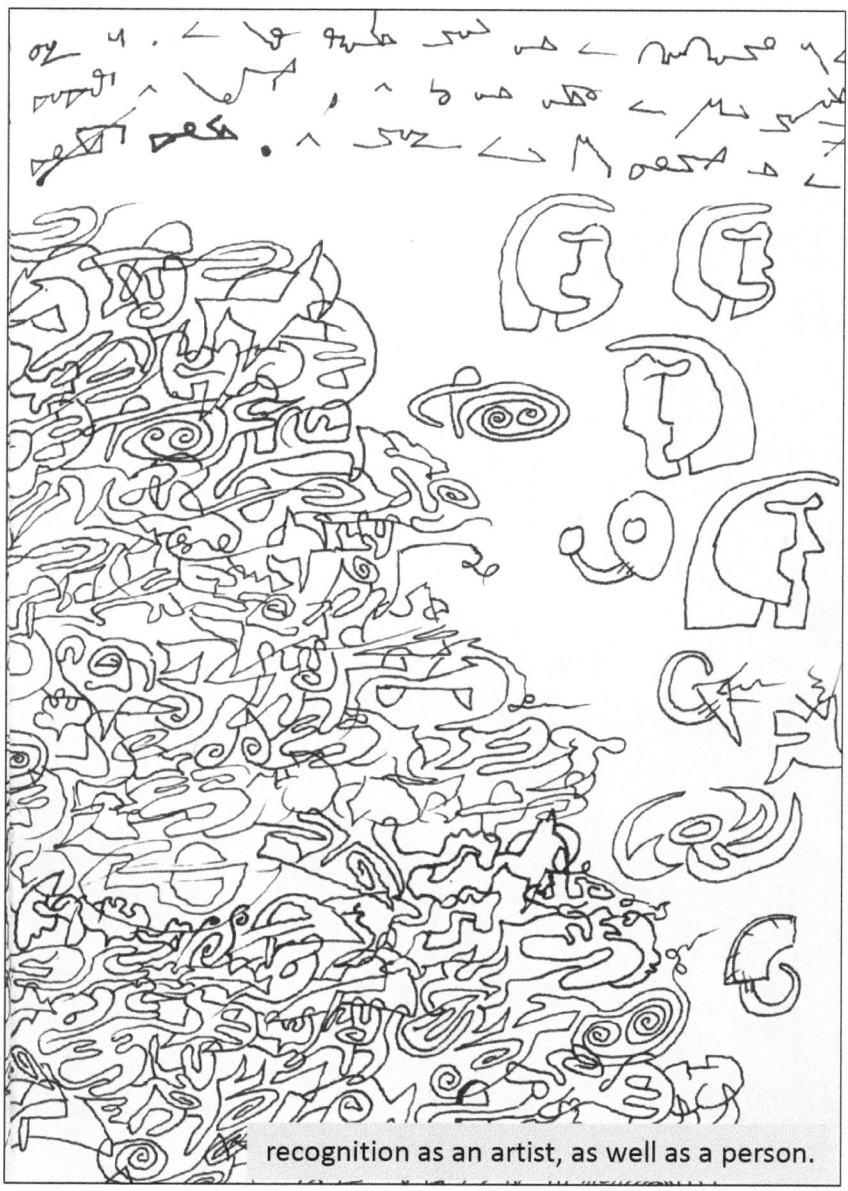

recognition as an artist, as well as a person.

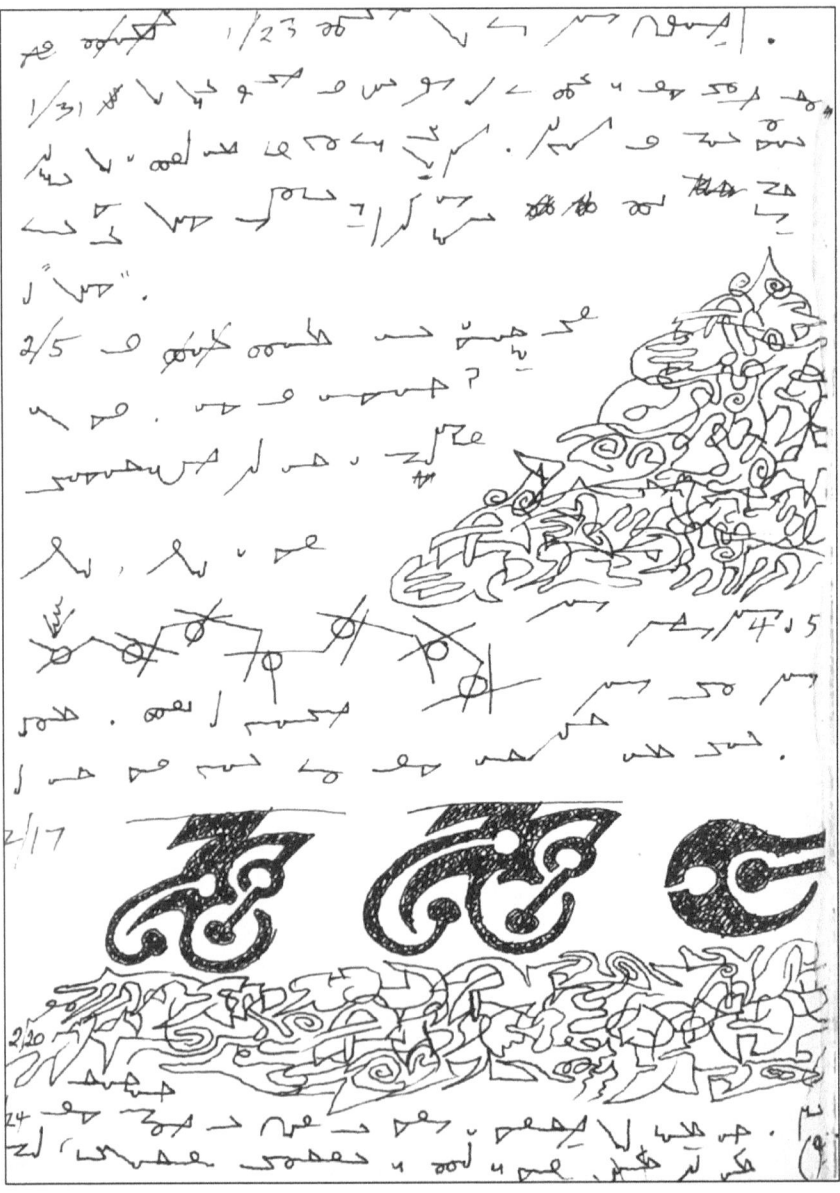

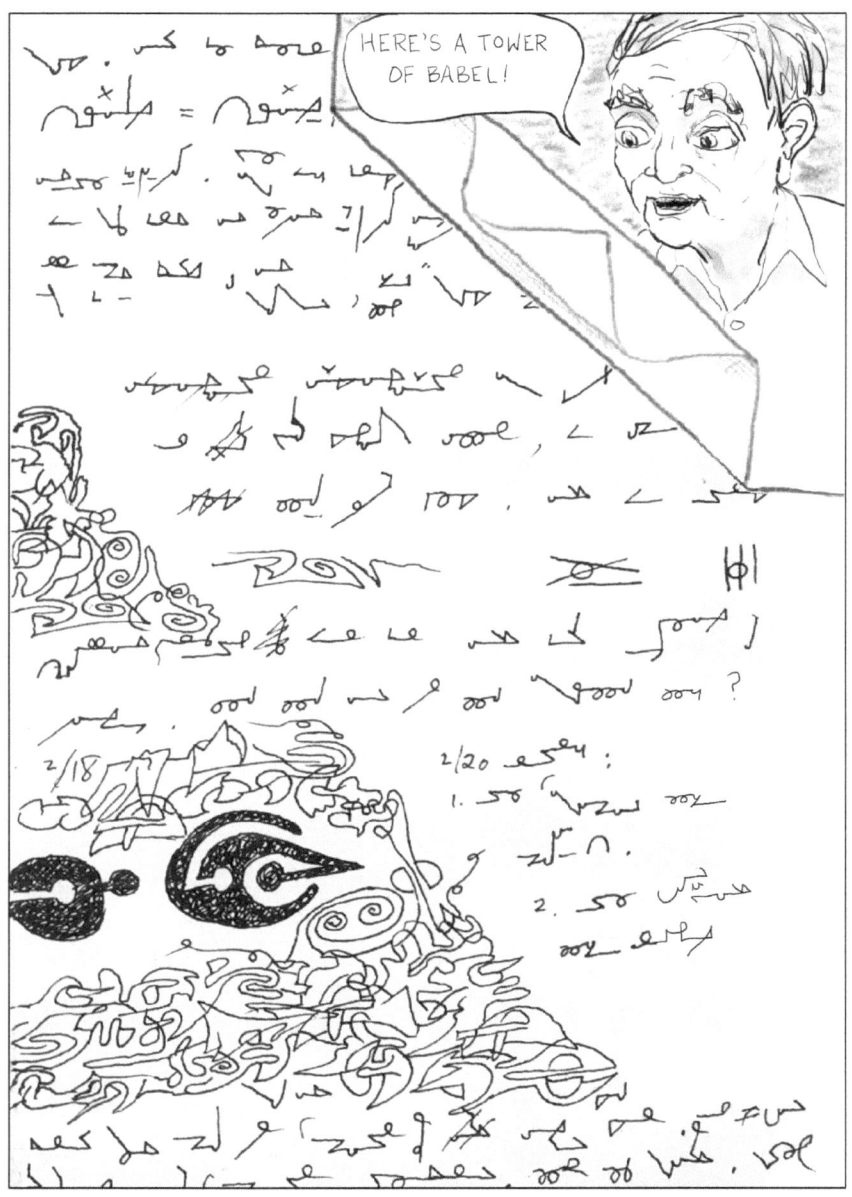

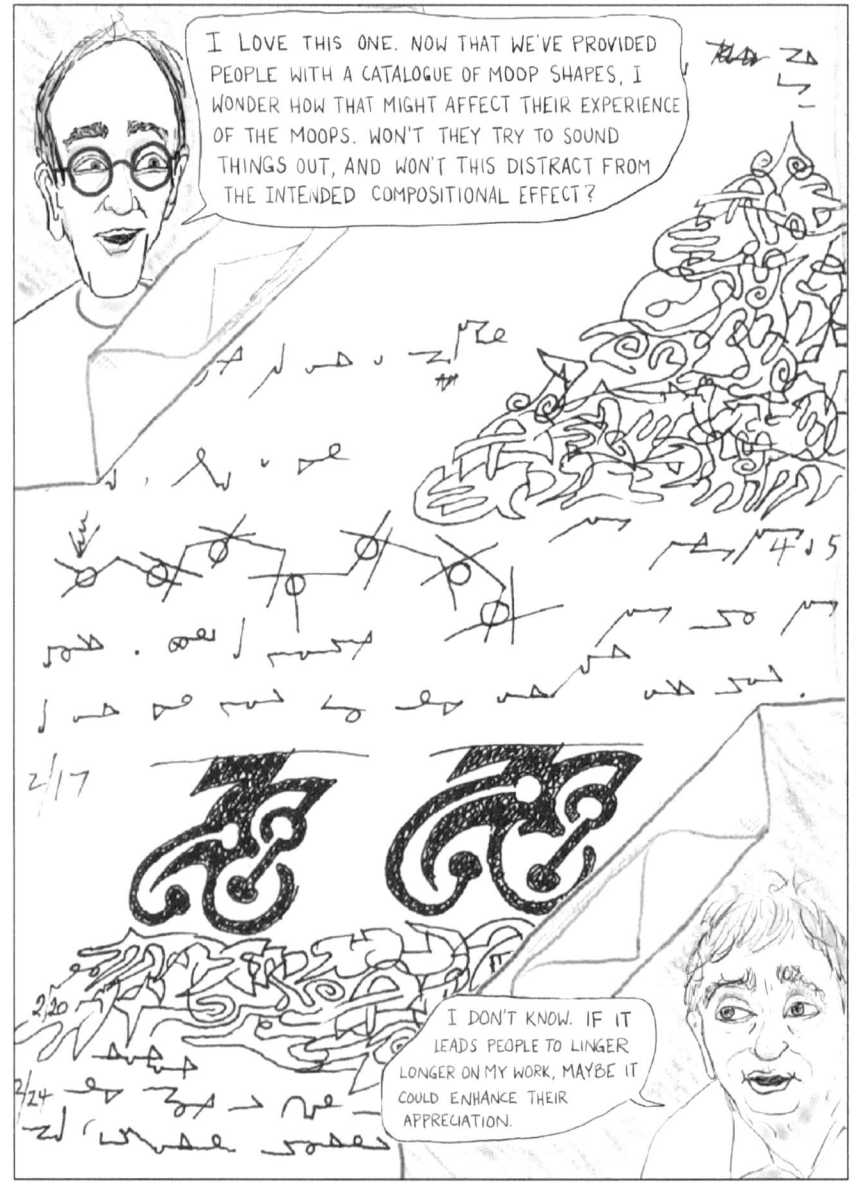

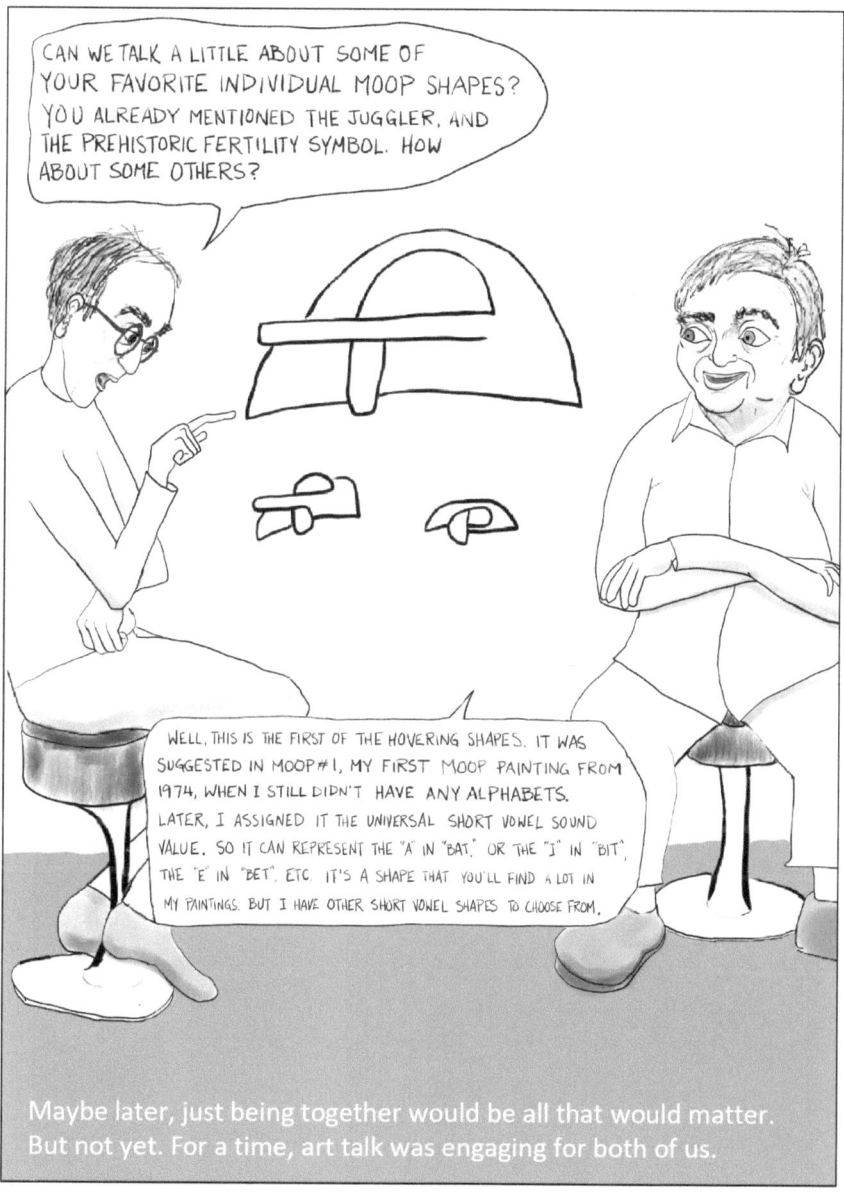

Maybe later, just being together would be all that would matter. But not yet. For a time, art talk was engaging for both of us.

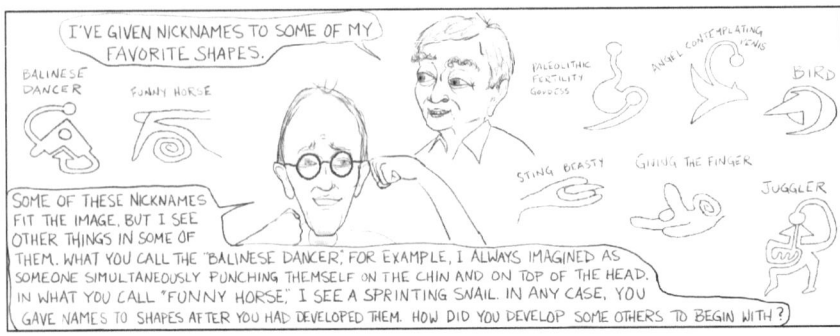

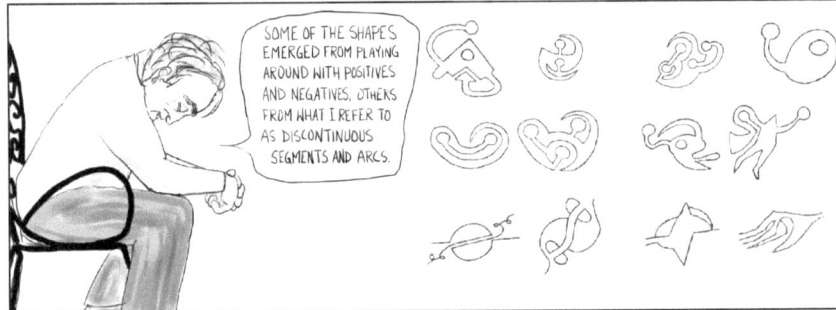

Eventually, Dad went pretty wild with the positive/negative figures. While these involved conceptual innovation, the influence of Indigenous art is clear.

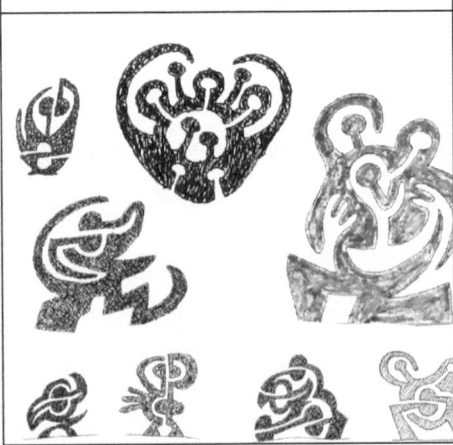

In one notebook, Dad jotted some shapes he saw at a MOMA exhibit of Rongo-rongo talking boards from Easter Island.

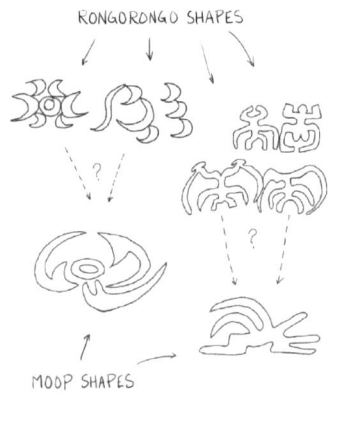

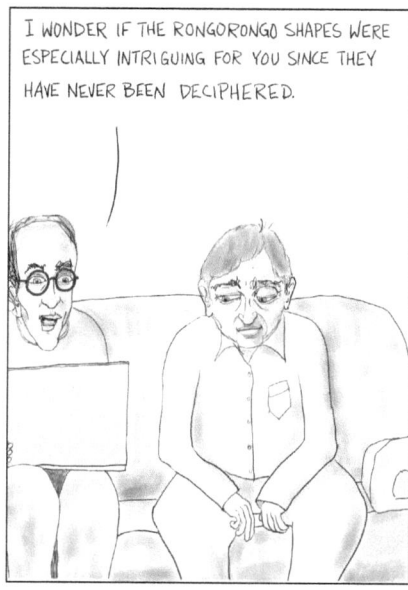
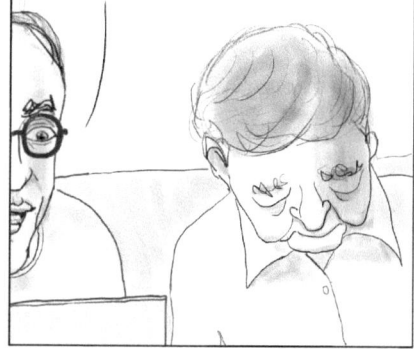
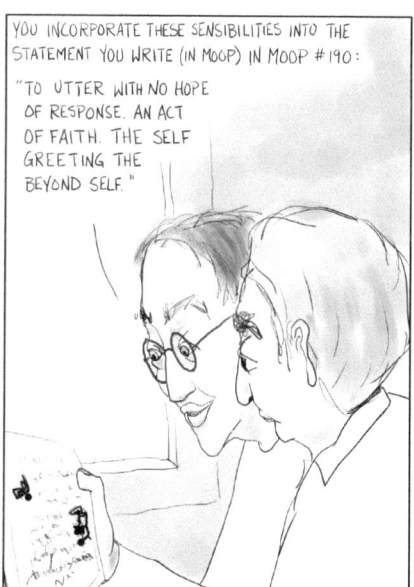
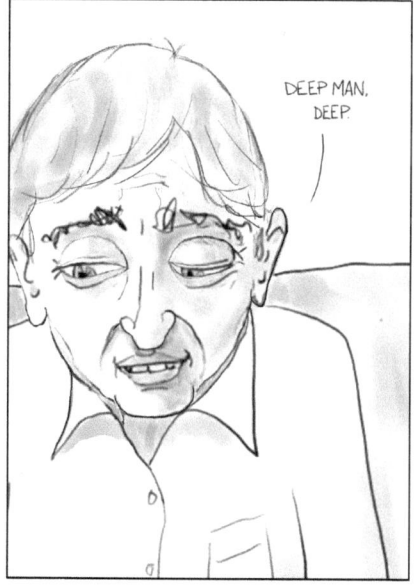

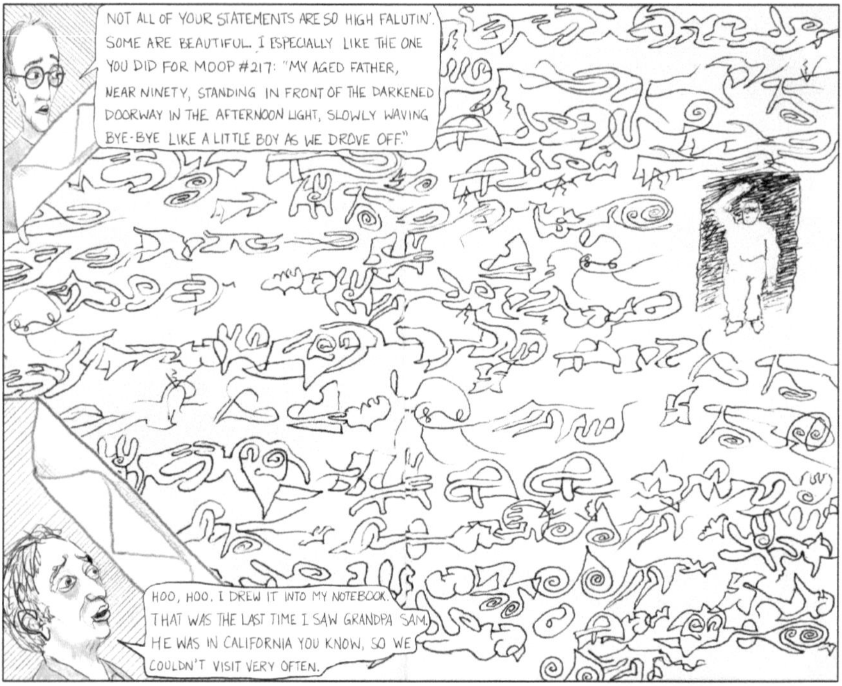

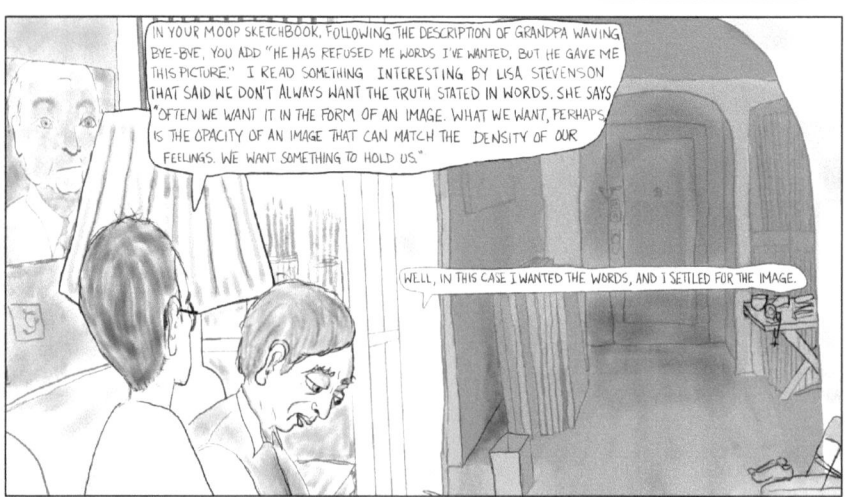

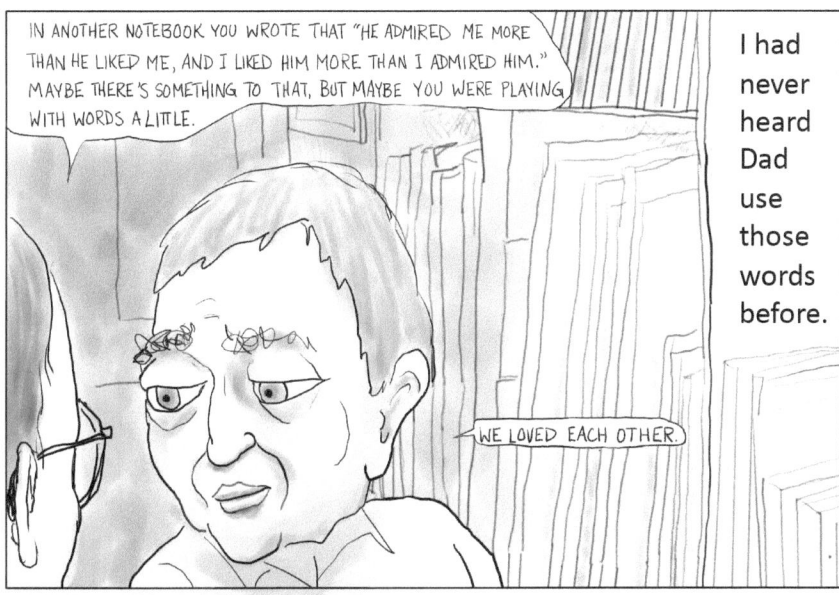

I had never heard Dad use those words before.

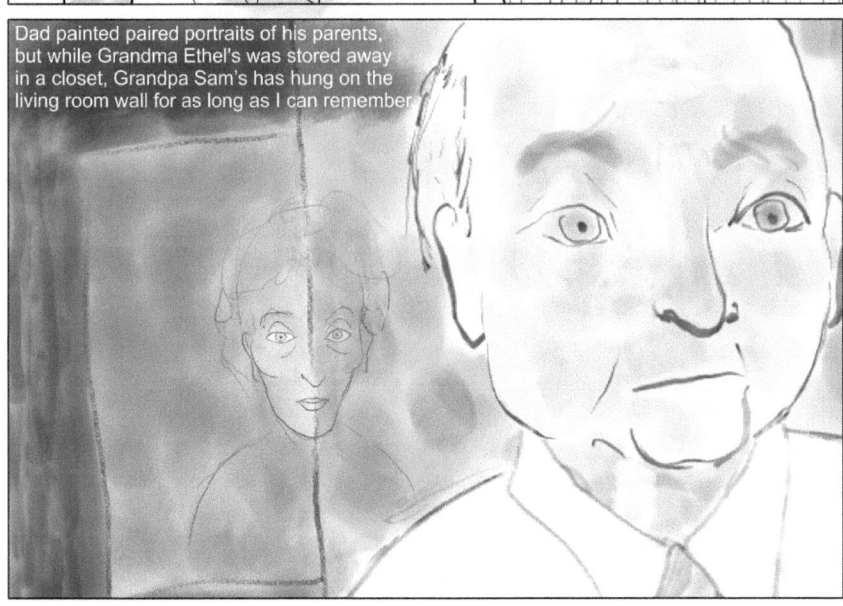

Documenting the Progress of My Decrepitude

Chapter 8

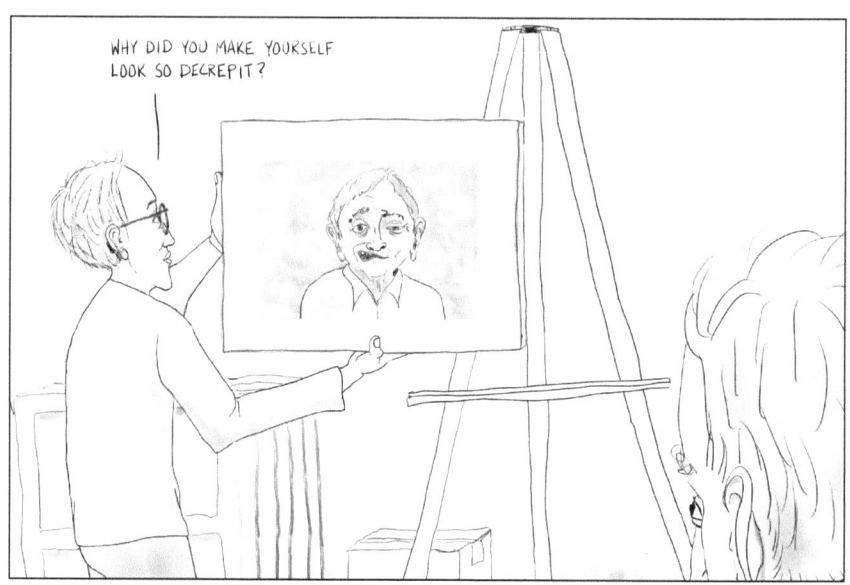
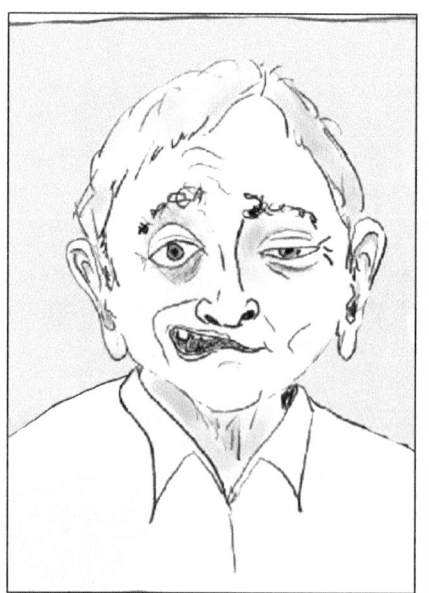
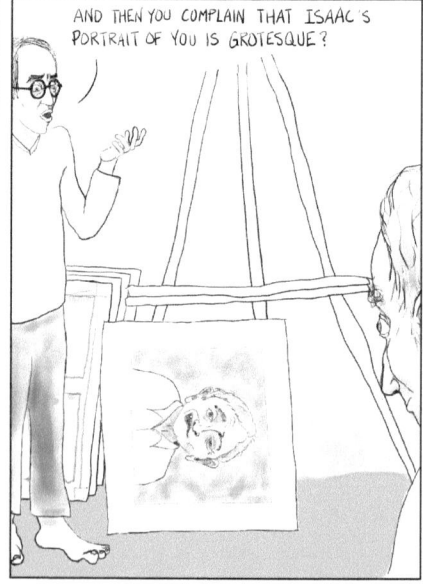

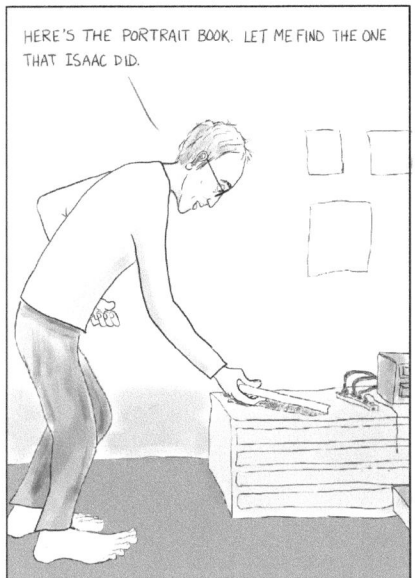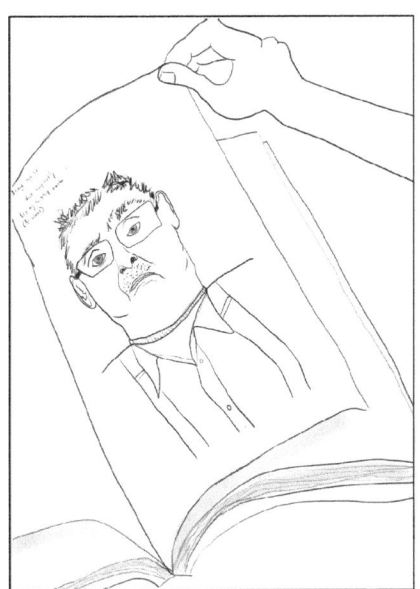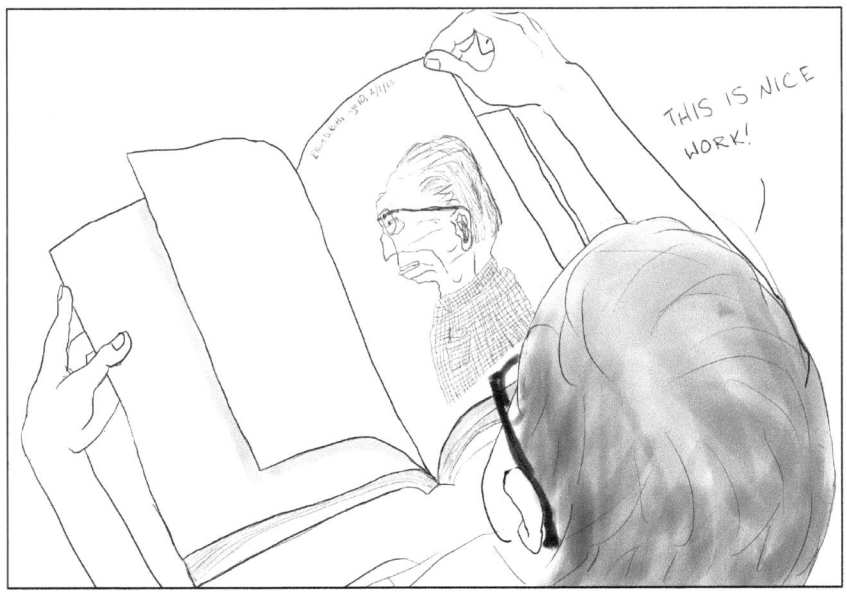

Dad would have Isaac and Emile do his portrait every time they visited. Little by little, they filled the sketchbook set aside for these portraits. The sessions only lasted about 20 minutes, but Dad would often end up falling asleep.

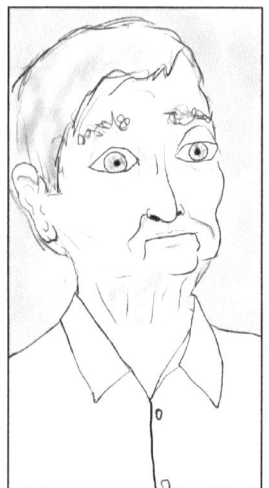
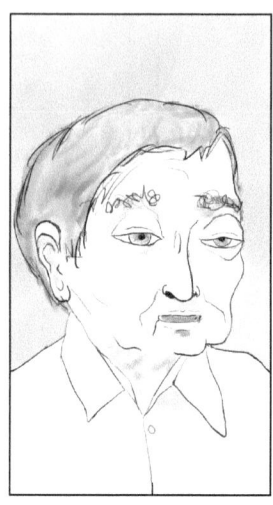
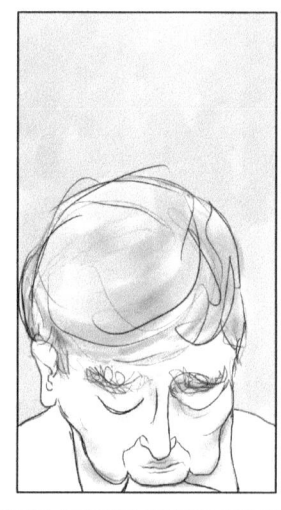

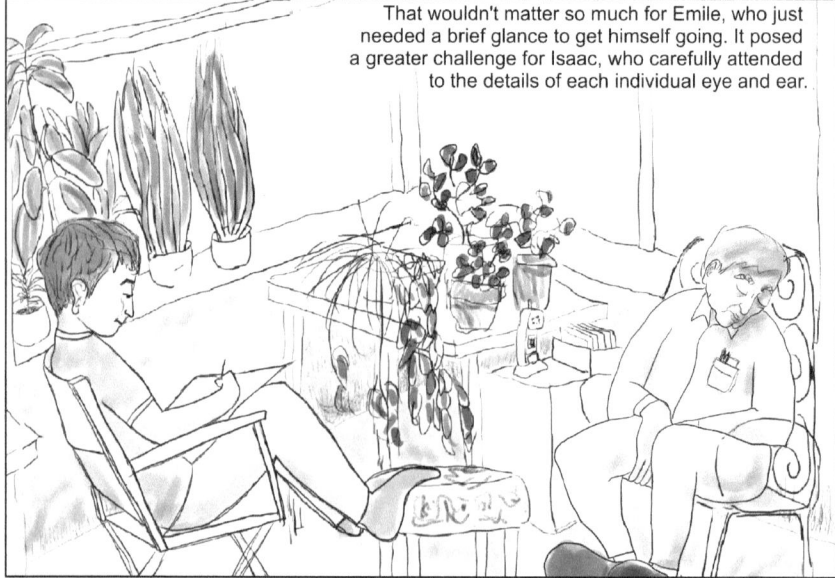

That wouldn't matter so much for Emile, who just needed a brief glance to get himself going. It posed a greater challenge for Isaac, who carefully attended to the details of each individual eye and ear.

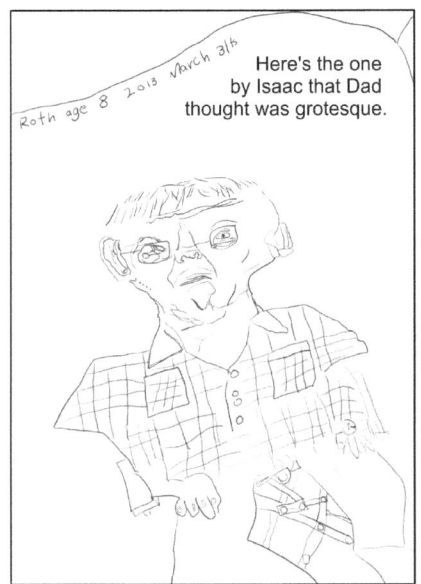

Here's the one by Isaac that Dad thought was grotesque.

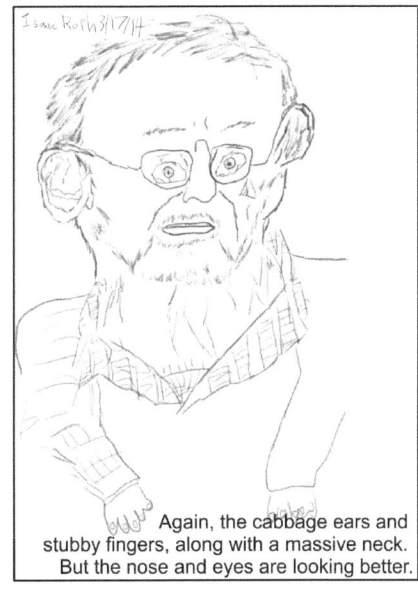

Again, the cabbage ears and stubby fingers, along with a massive neck. But the nose and eyes are looking better.

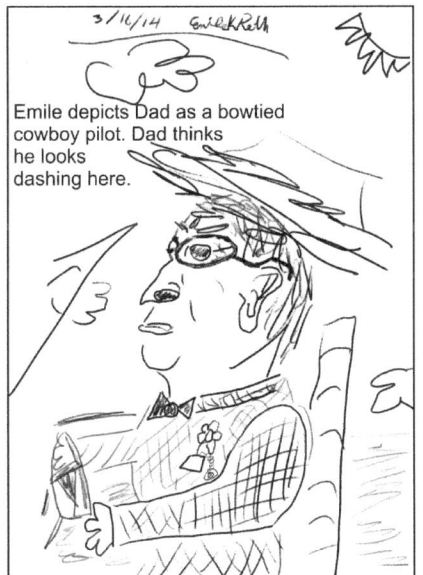

Emile depicts Dad as a bowtied cowboy pilot. Dad thinks he looks dashing here.

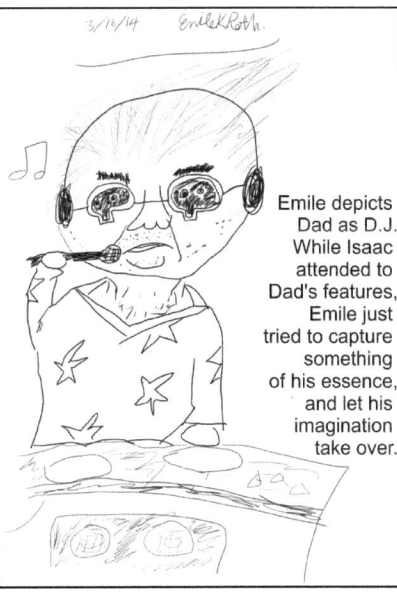

Emile depicts Dad as D.J. While Isaac attended to Dad's features, Emile just tried to capture something of his essence, and let his imagination take over.

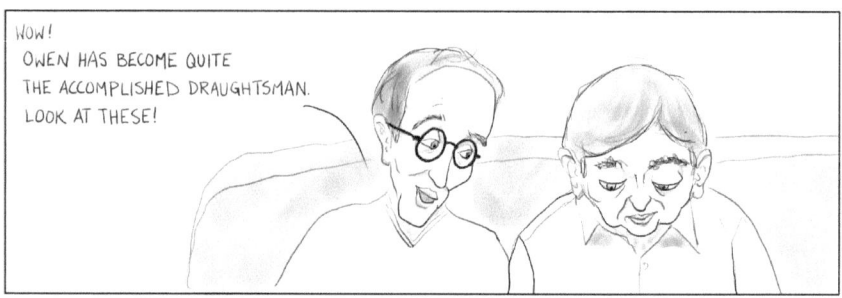

WOW! OWEN HAS BECOME QUITE THE ACCOMPLISHED DRAUGHTSMAN. LOOK AT THESE!

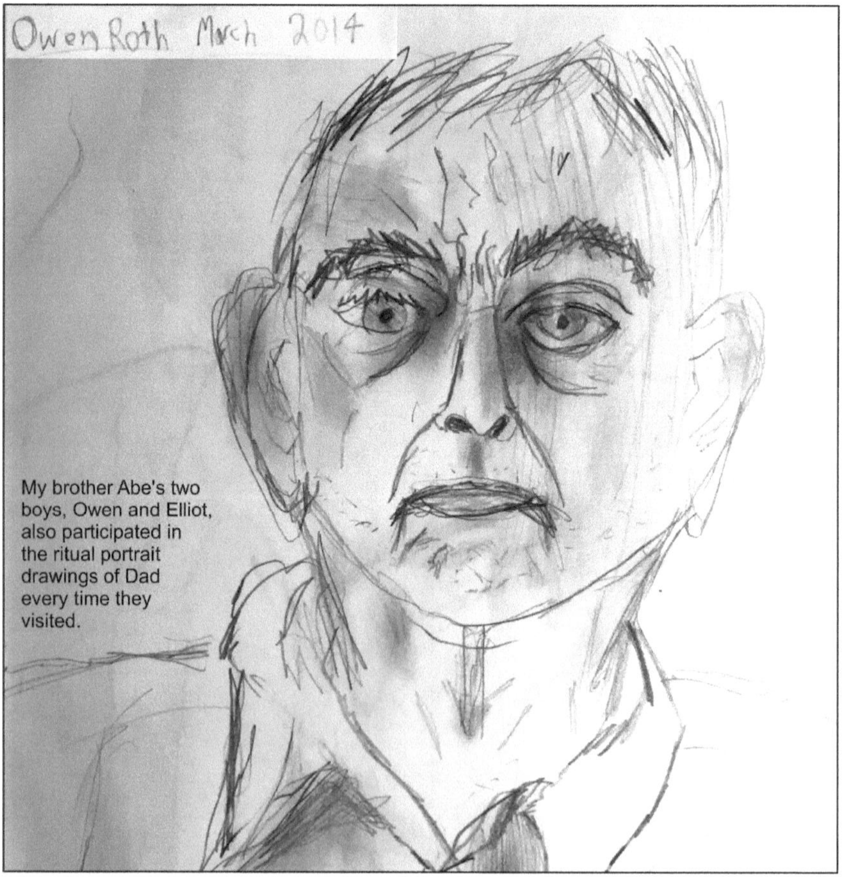

My brother Abe's two boys, Owen and Elliot, also participated in the ritual portrait drawings of Dad every time they visited.

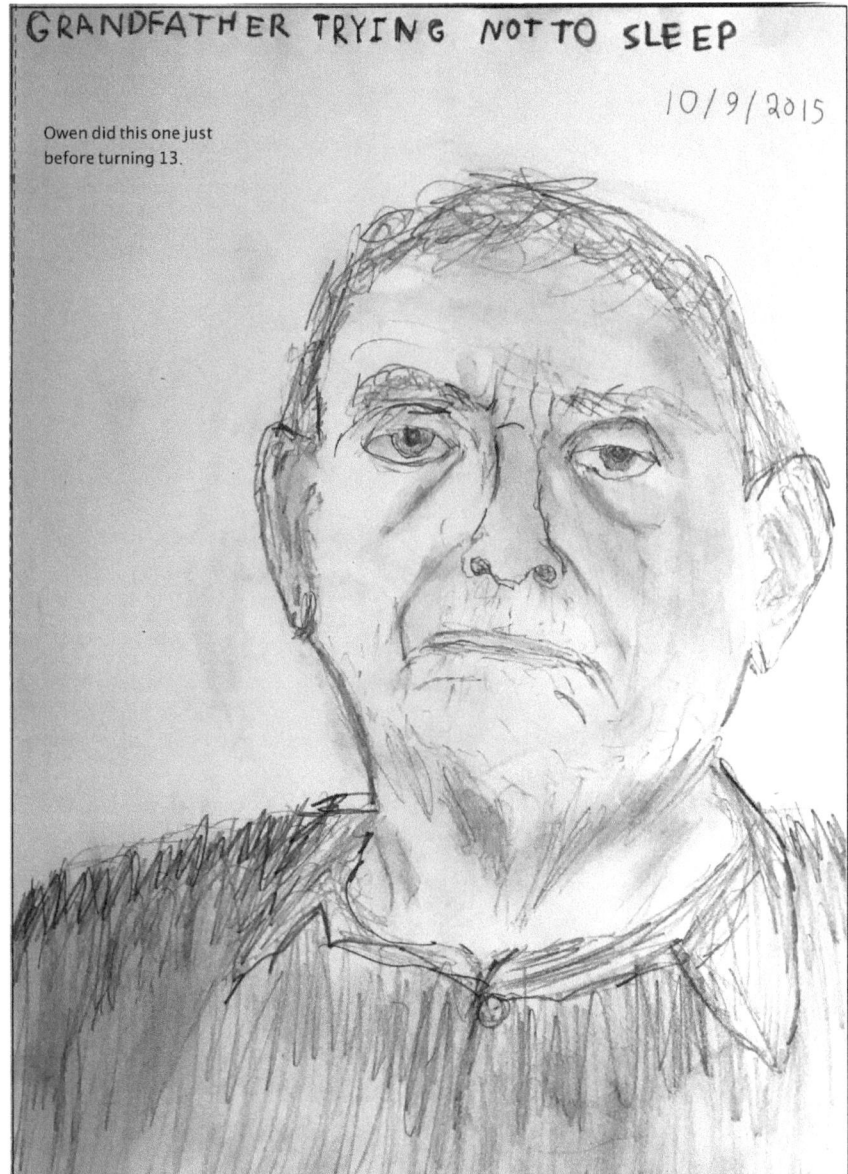

Owen did this one just before turning 13.

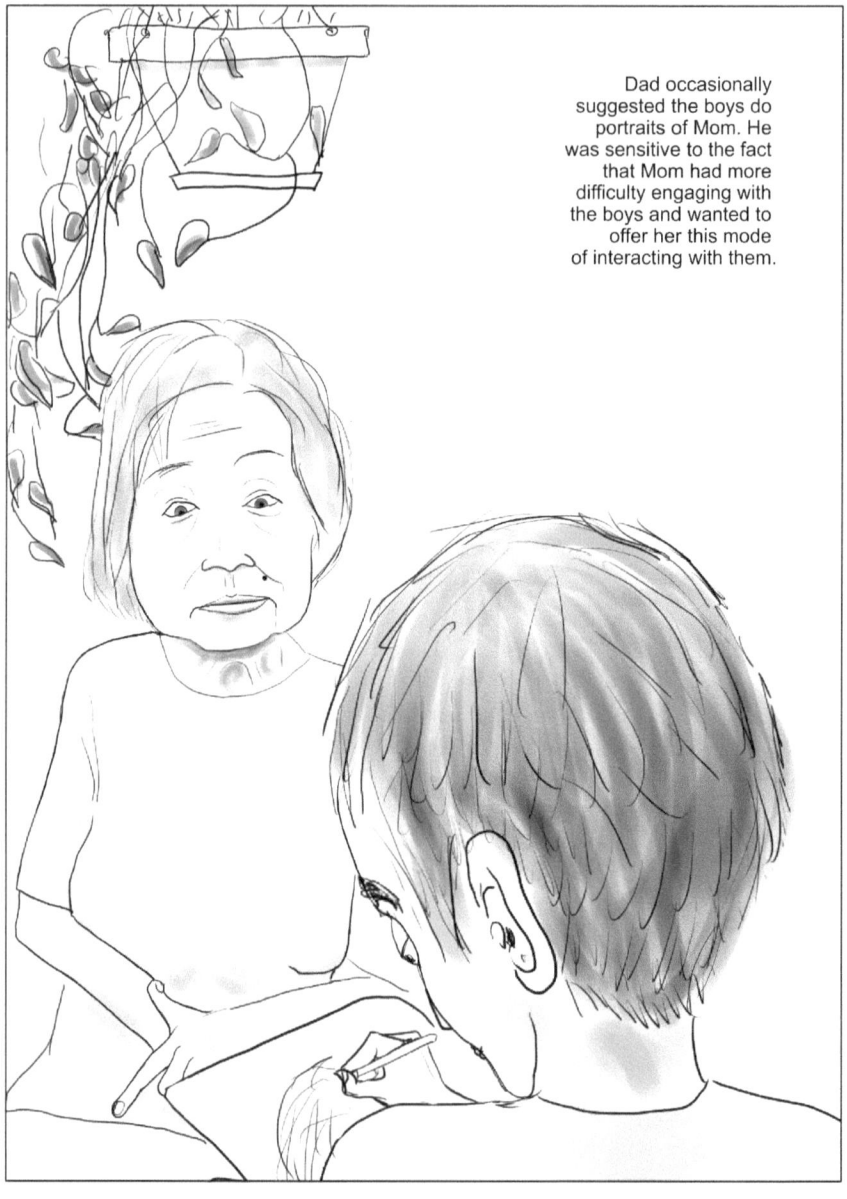

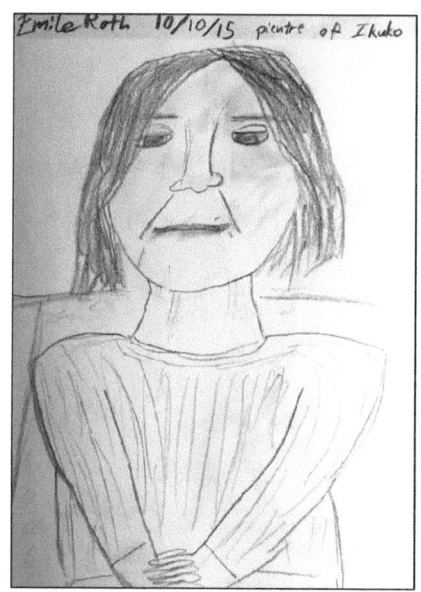
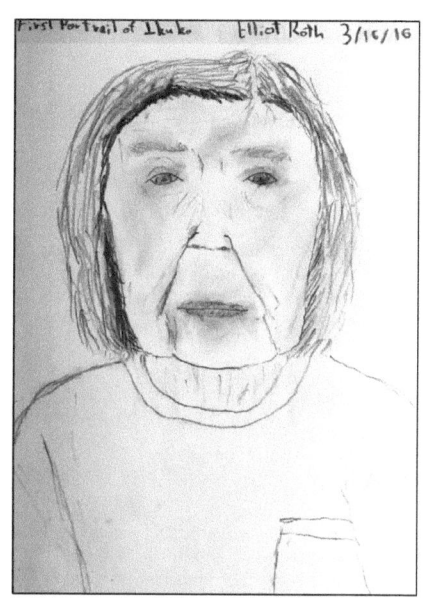
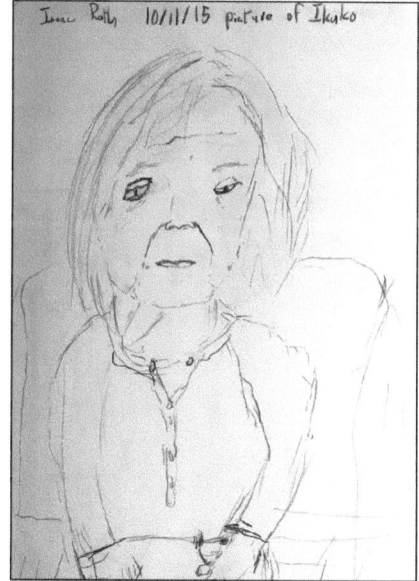
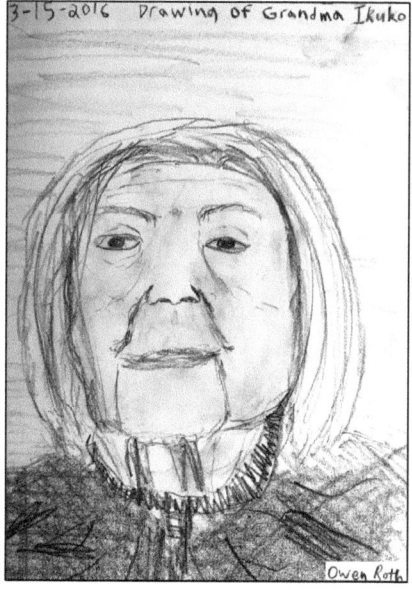

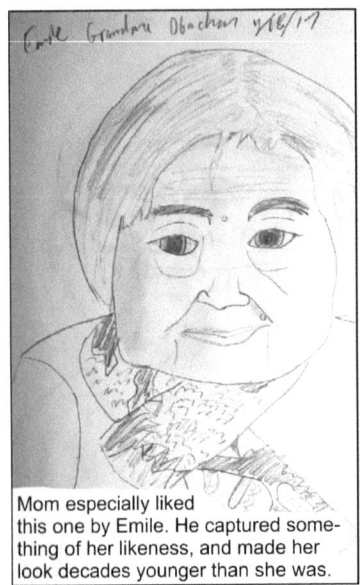

Mom especially liked this one by Emile. He captured something of her likeness, and made her look decades younger than she was.

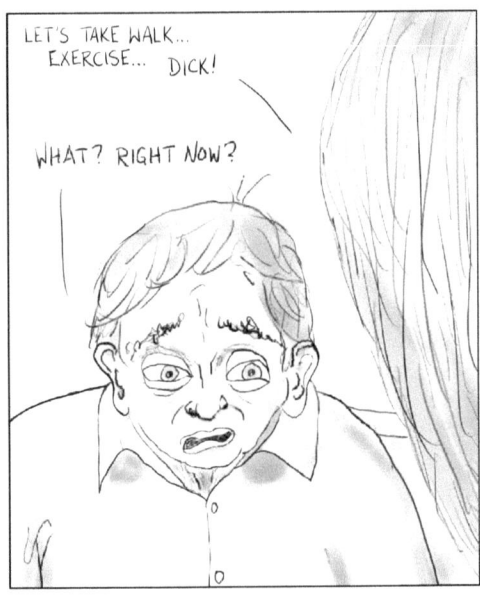

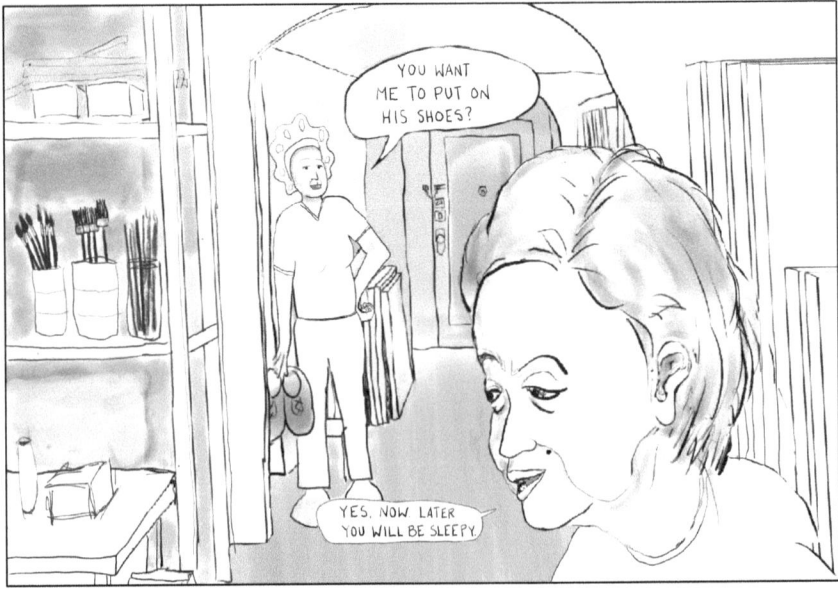

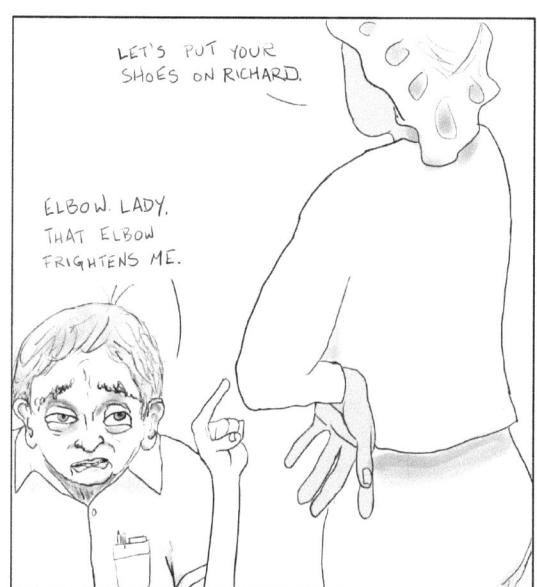
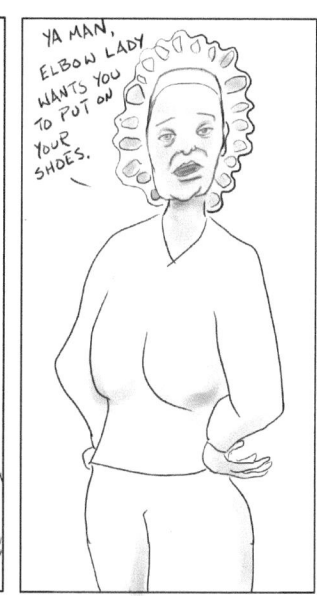
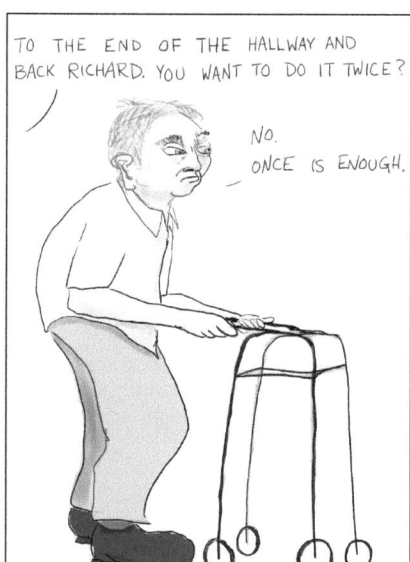
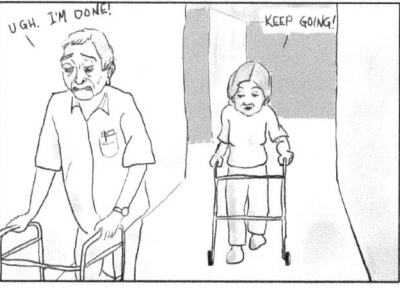
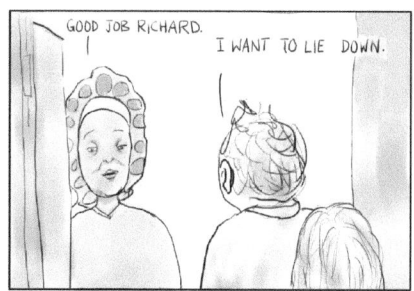

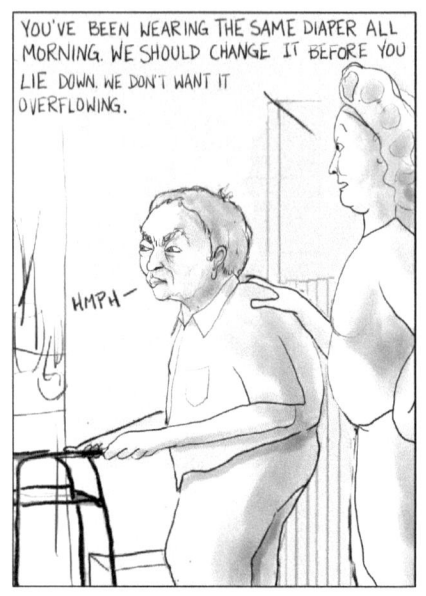
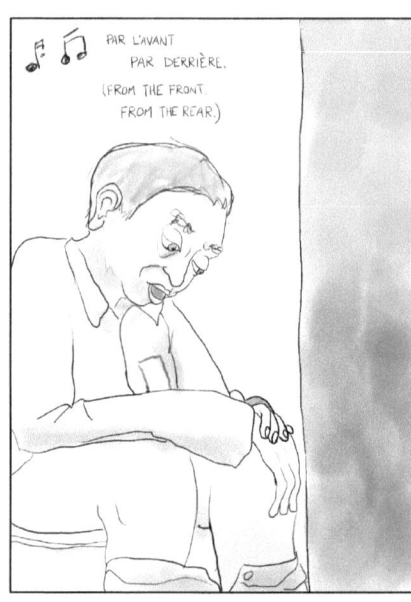
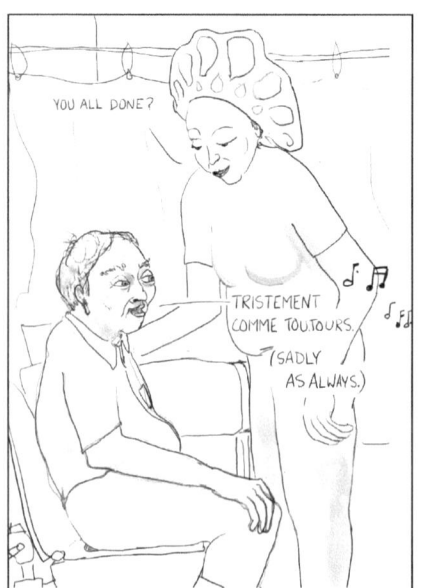
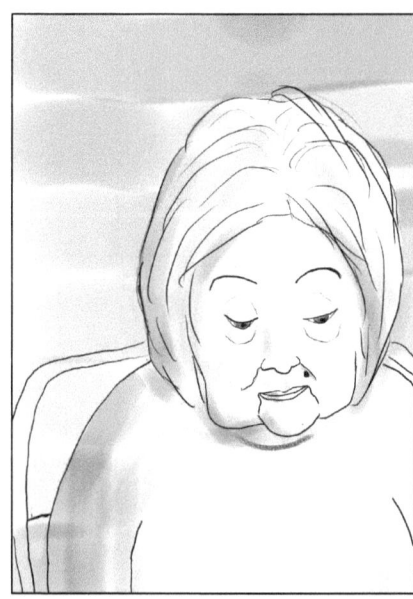

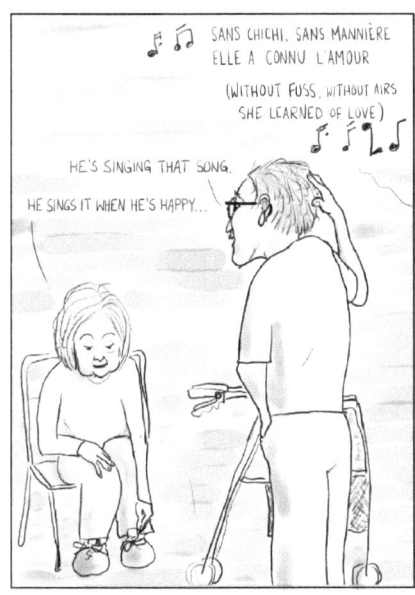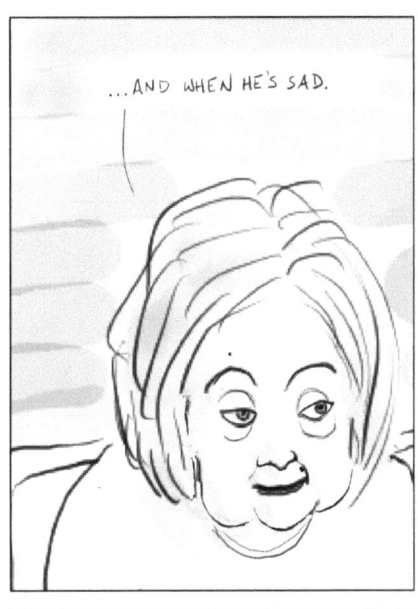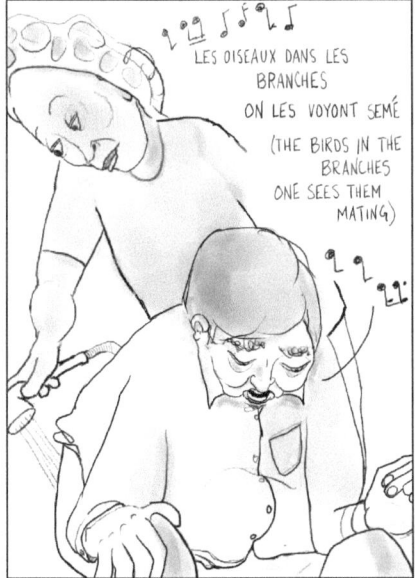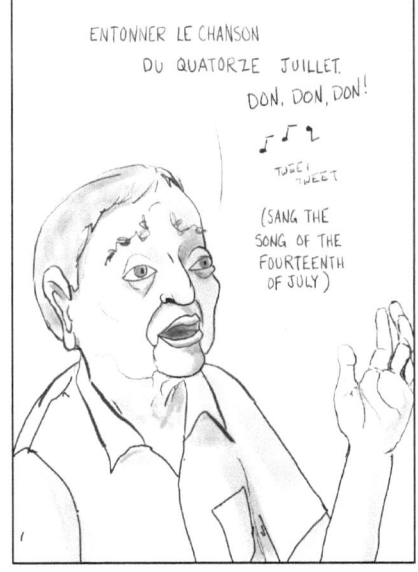

Dad has been able to maintain a positive attitude confronted with the daily assaults on his dignity by his own progressing decrepitude, a decrepitude that he himself has documented in his self-portraits, and that he has had his grandchildren document in their portraits of him over time.

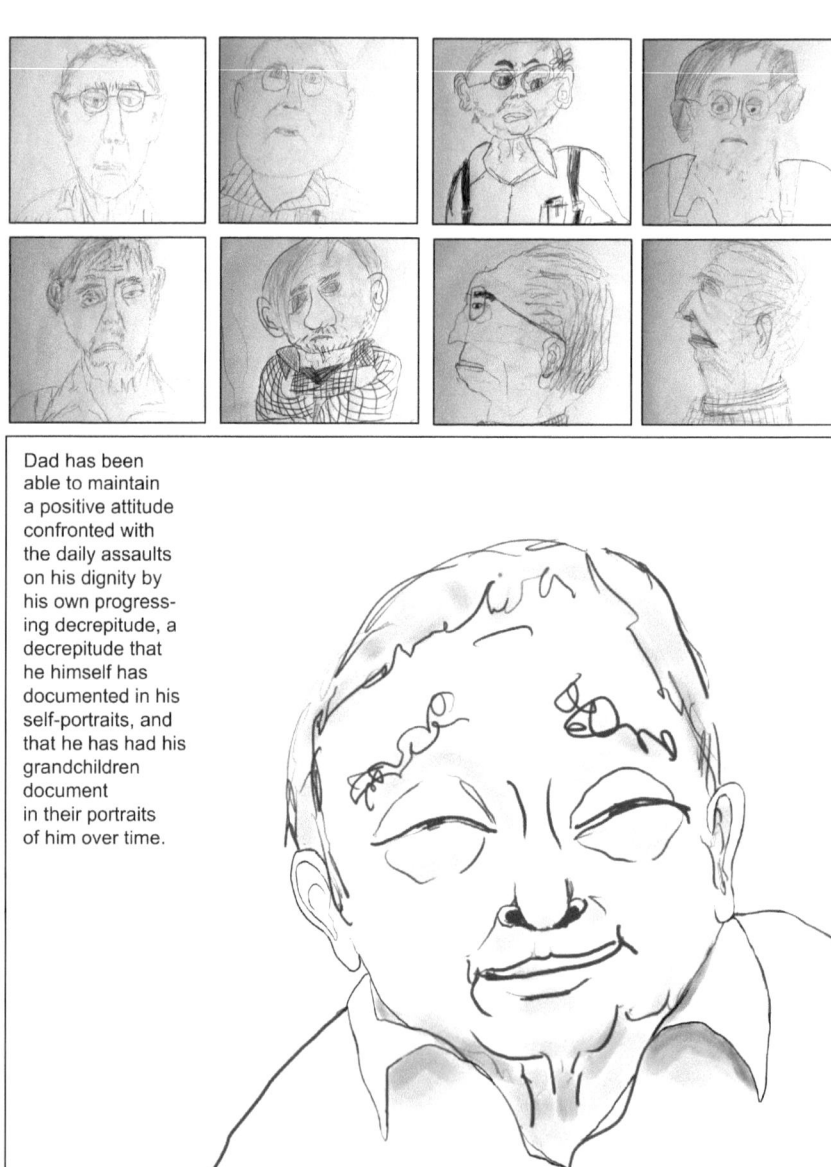

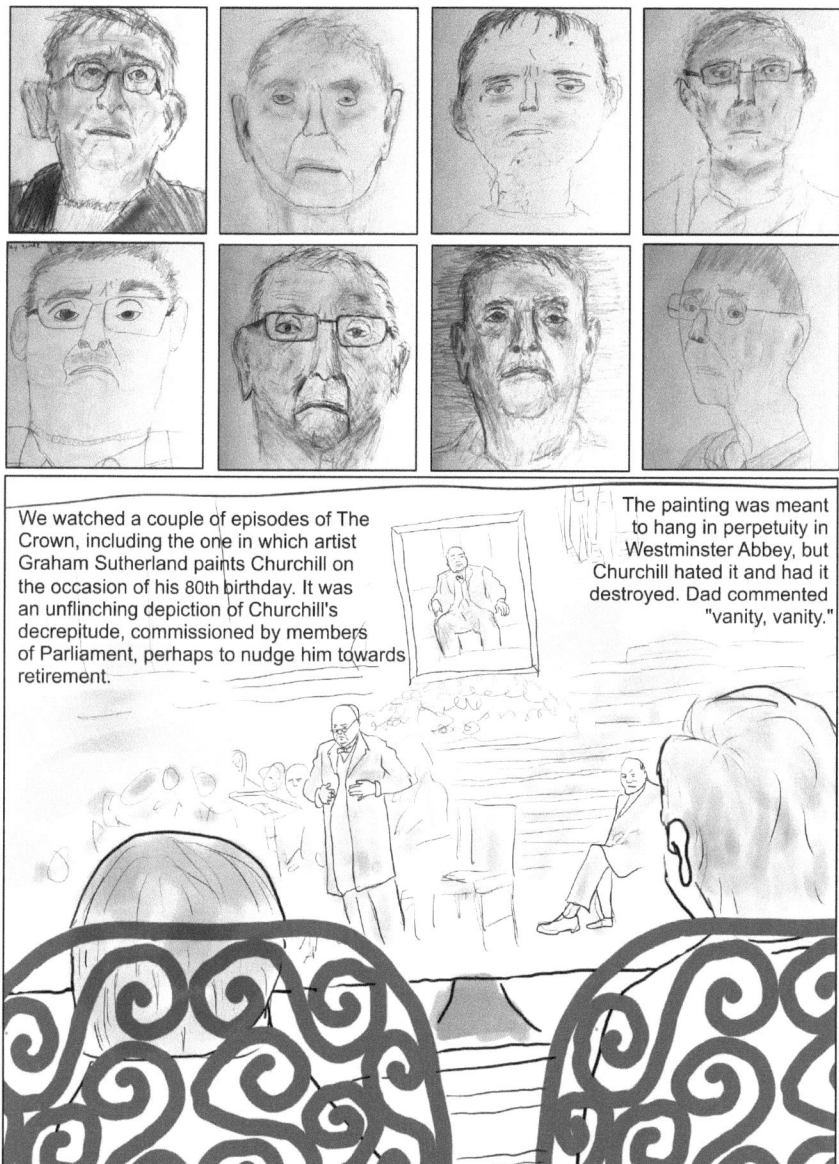

We watched a couple of episodes of The Crown, including the one in which artist Graham Sutherland paints Churchill on the occasion of his 80th birthday. It was an unflinching depiction of Churchill's decrepitude, commissioned by members of Parliament, perhaps to nudge him towards retirement.

The painting was meant to hang in perpetuity in Westminster Abbey, but Churchill hated it and had it destroyed. Dad commented "vanity, vanity."

What Am I Doing Here?

Chapter 9

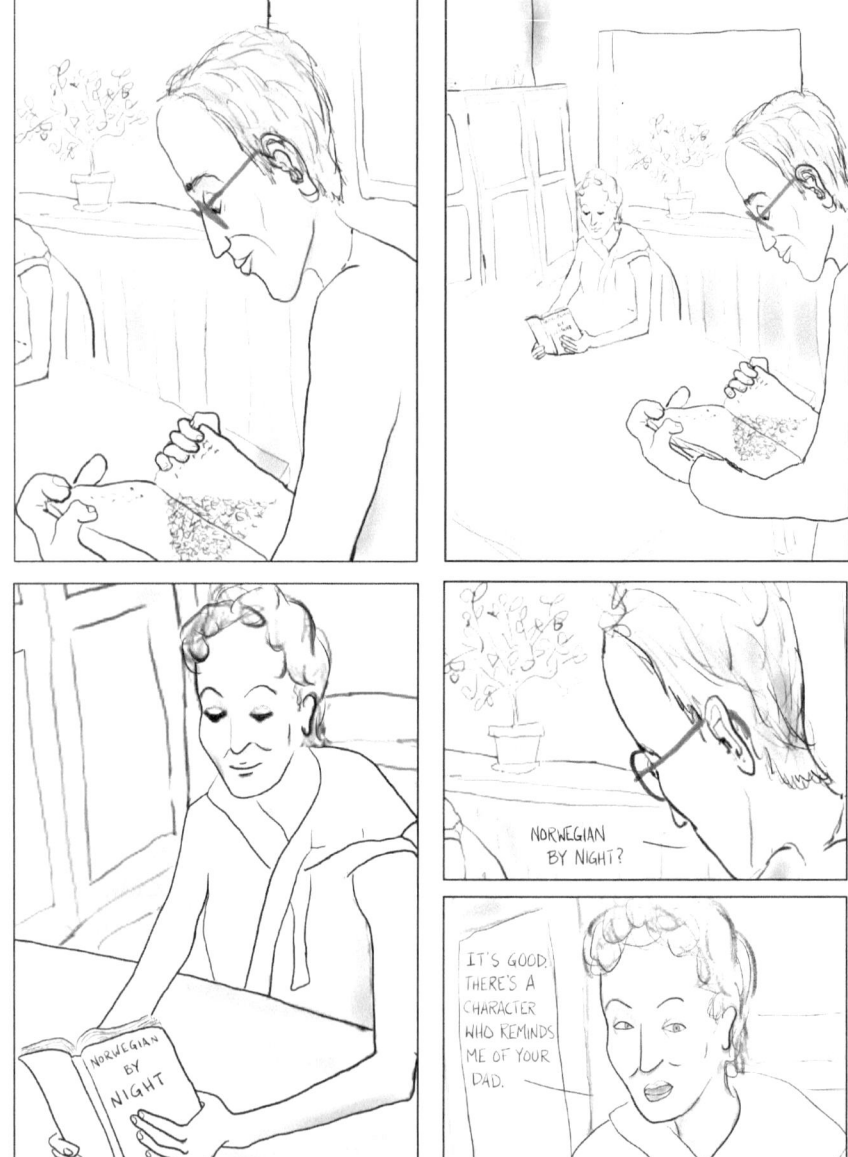

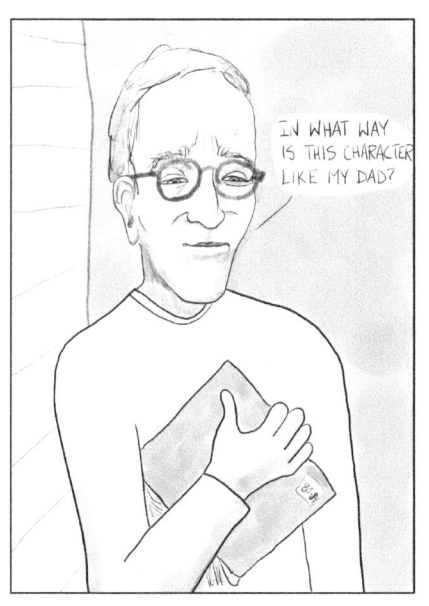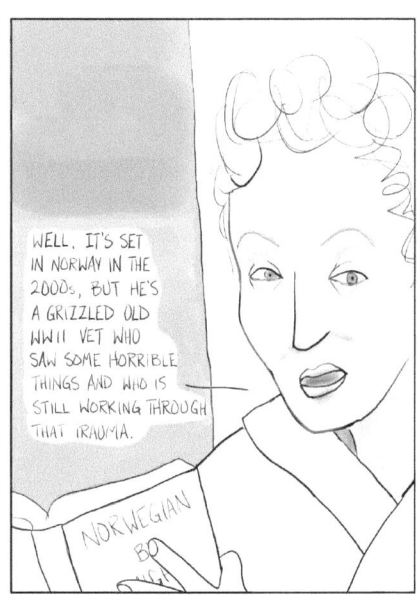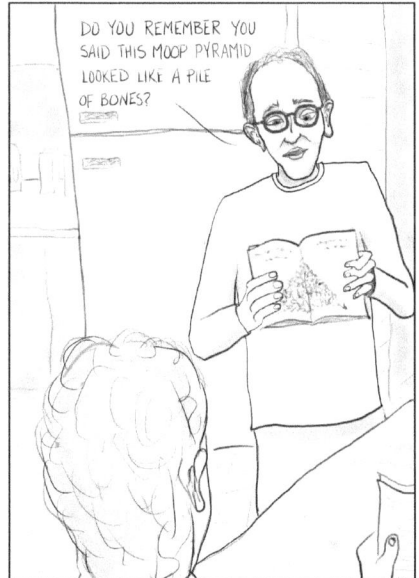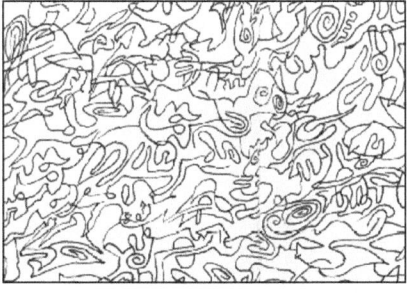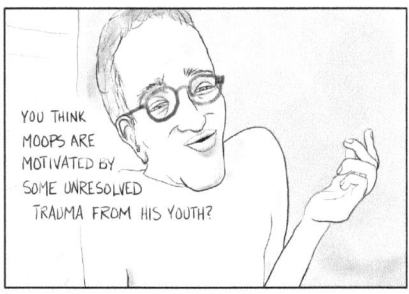

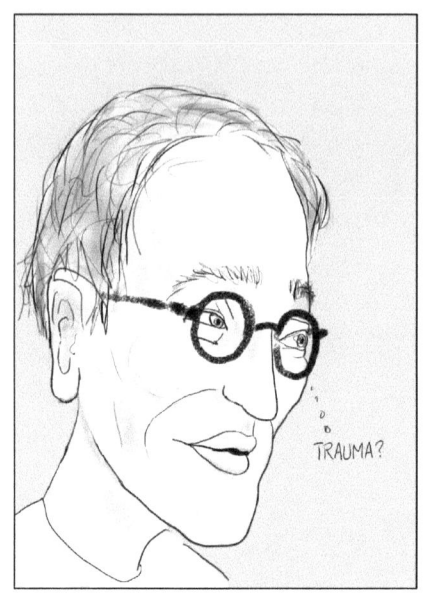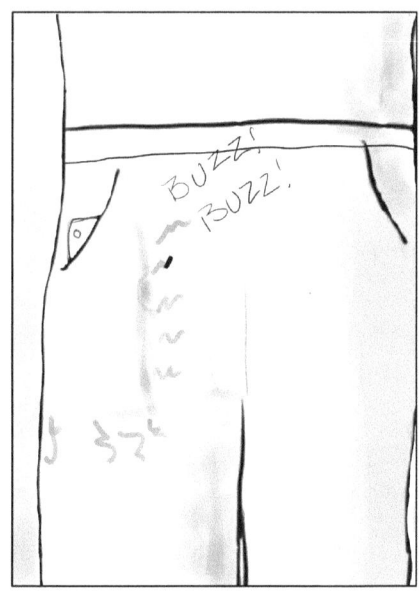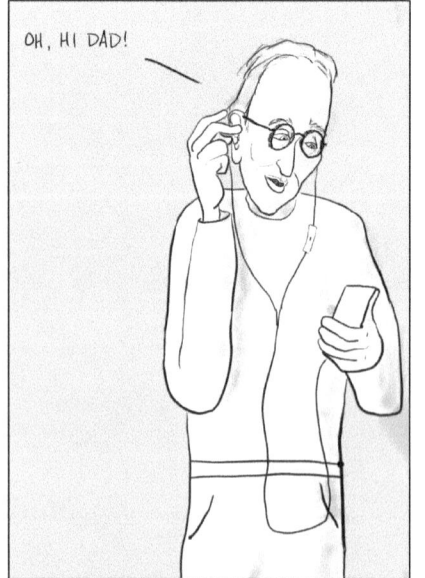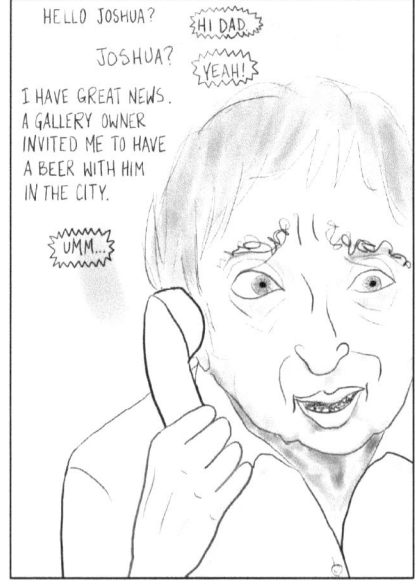

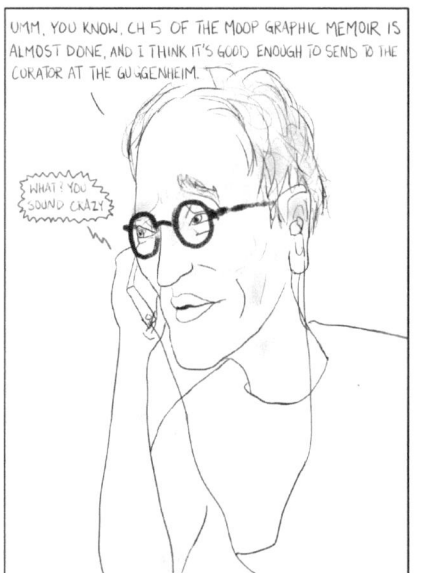
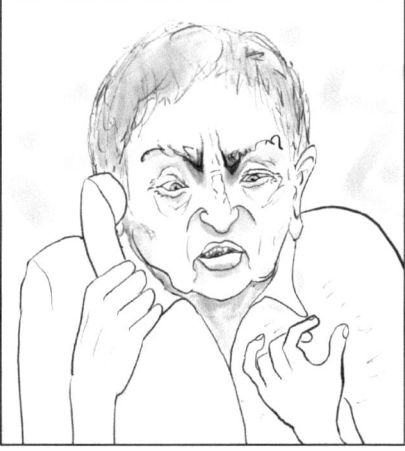
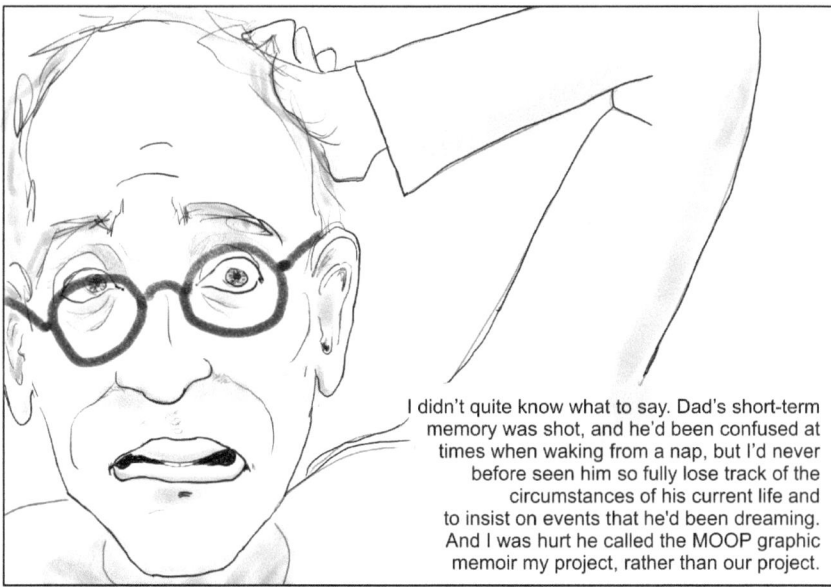

I didn't quite know what to say. Dad's short-term memory was shot, and he'd been confused at times when waking from a nap, but I'd never before seen him so fully lose track of the circumstances of his current life and to insist on events that he'd been dreaming. And I was hurt he called the MOOP graphic memoir my project, rather than our project.

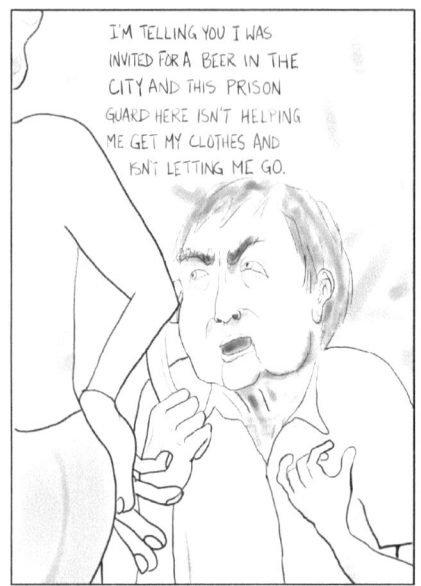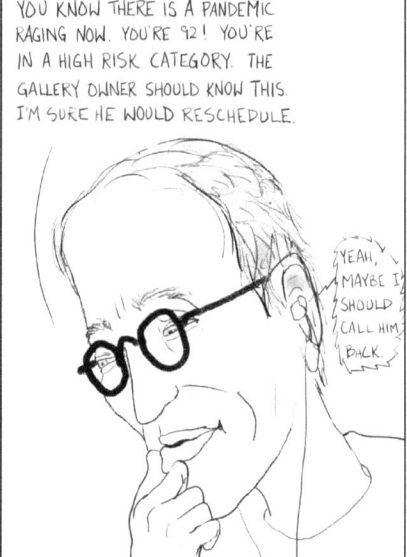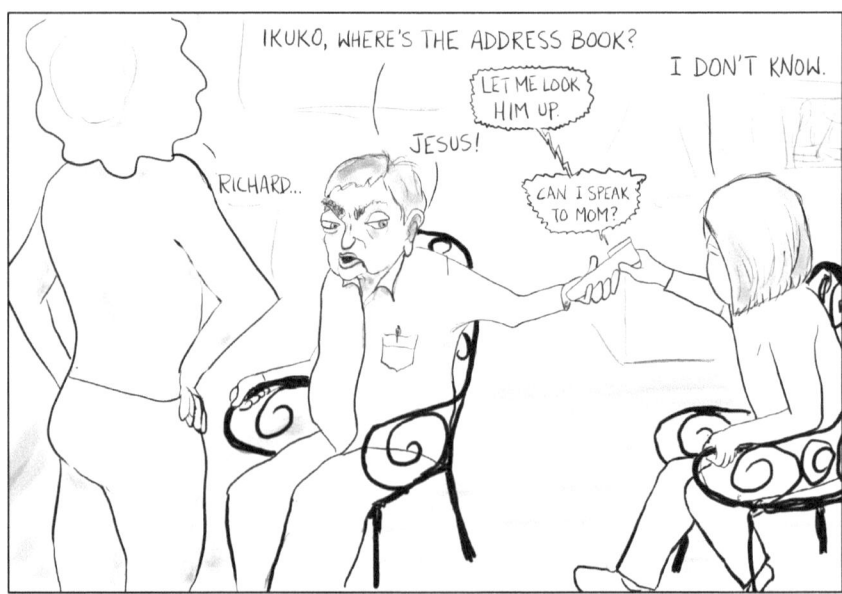

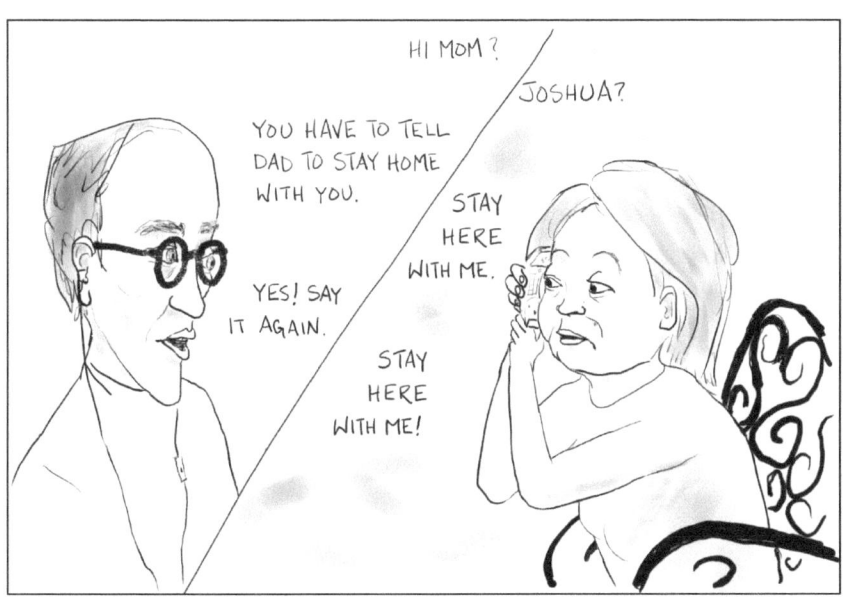
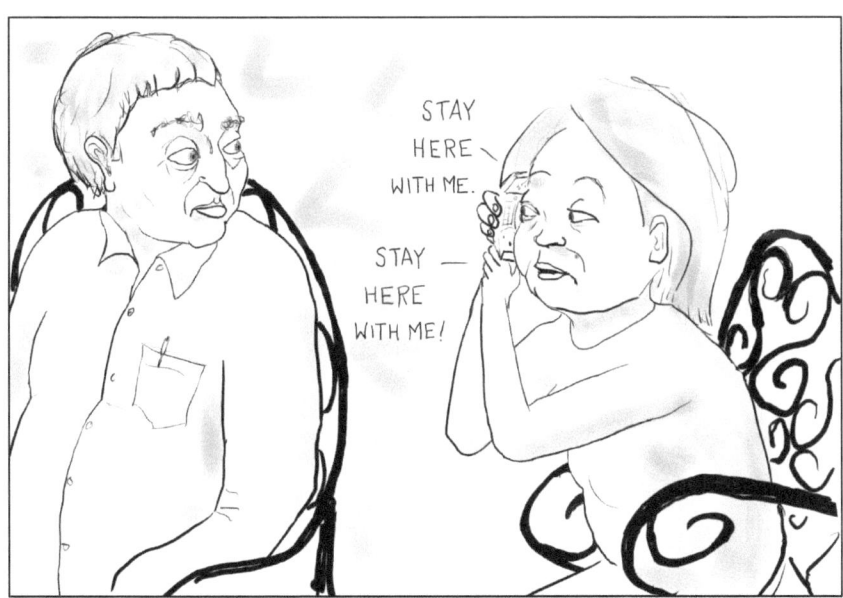

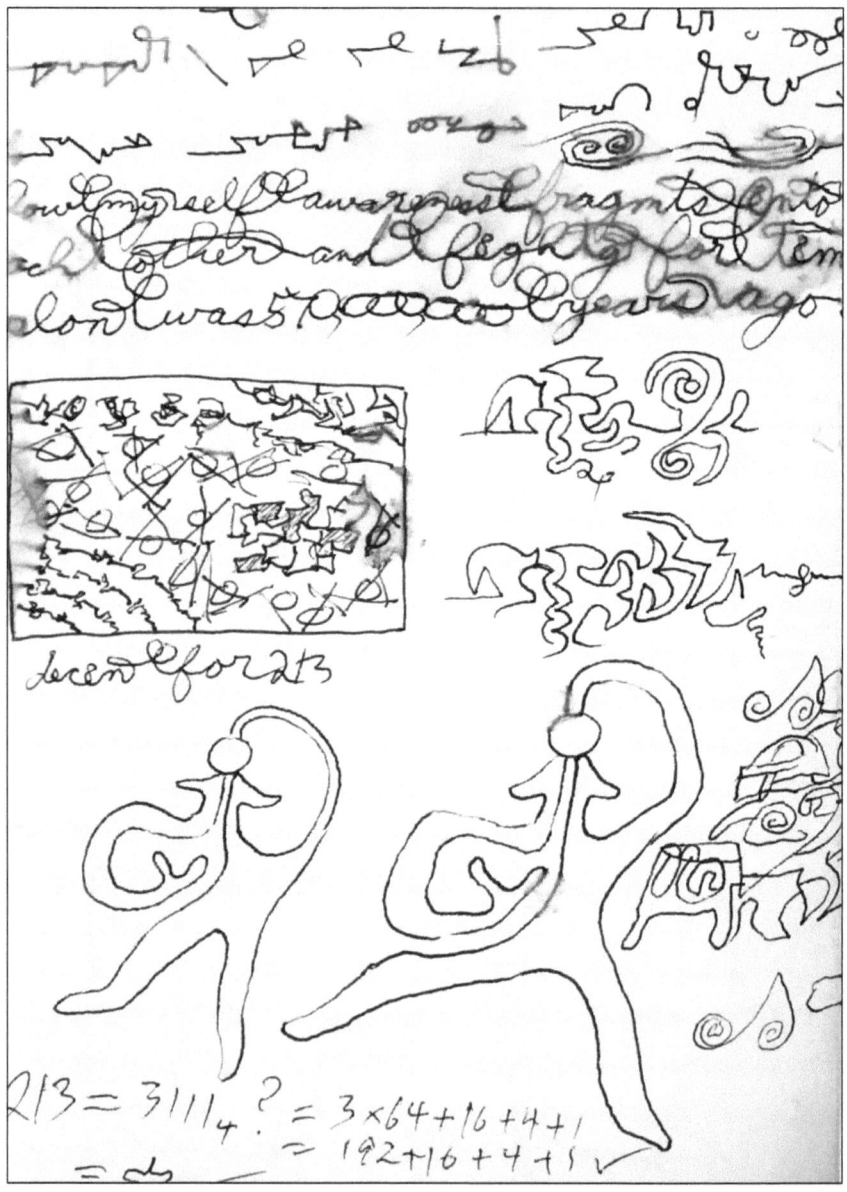

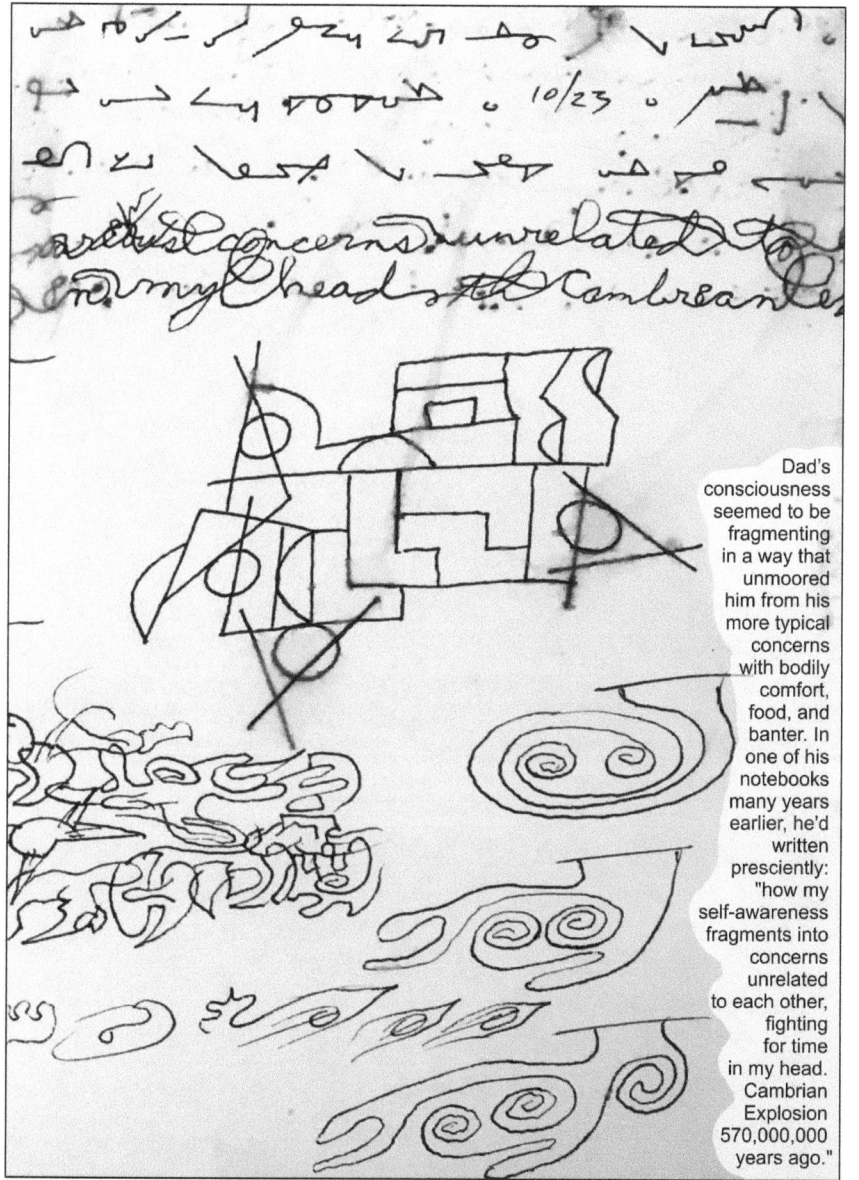

Dad's consciousness seemed to be fragmenting in a way that unmoored him from his more typical concerns with bodily comfort, food, and banter. In one of his notebooks many years earlier, he'd written presciently: "how my self-awareness fragments into concerns unrelated to each other, fighting for time in my head. Cambrian Explosion 570,000,000 years ago."

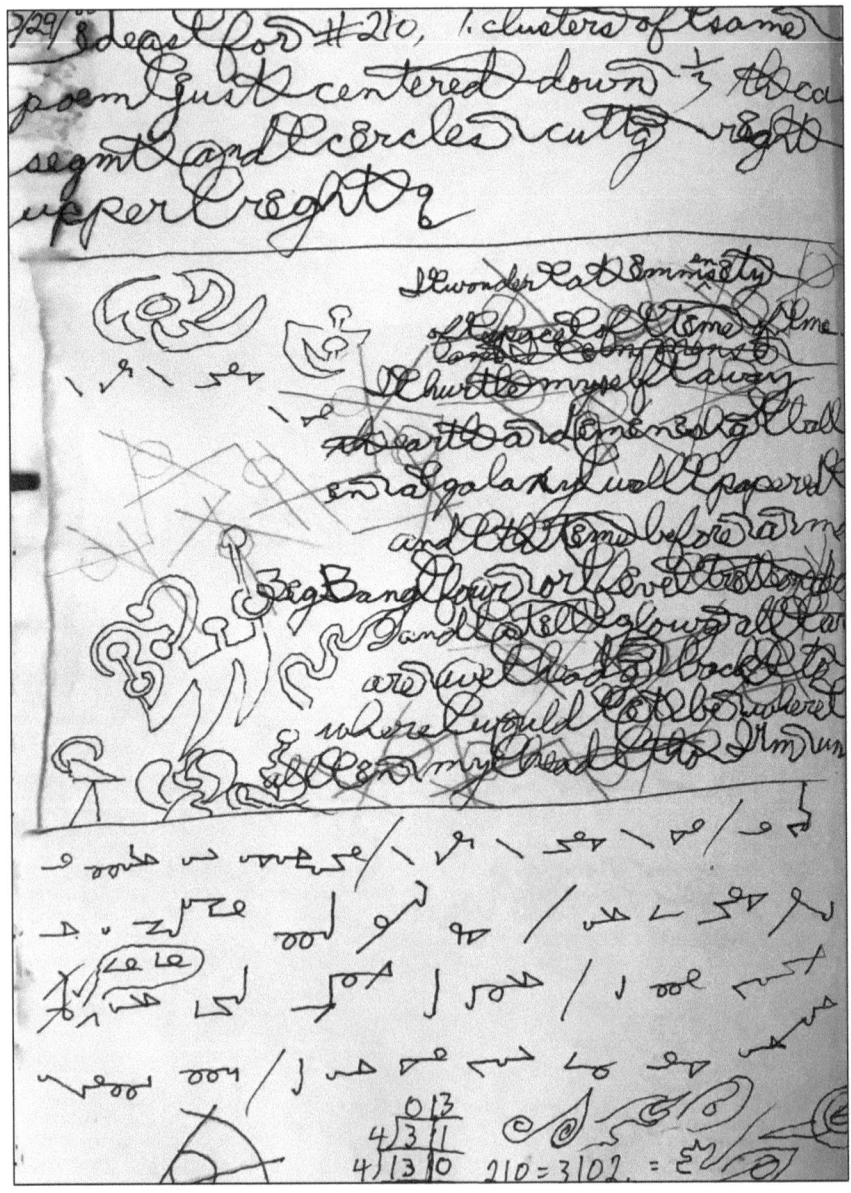

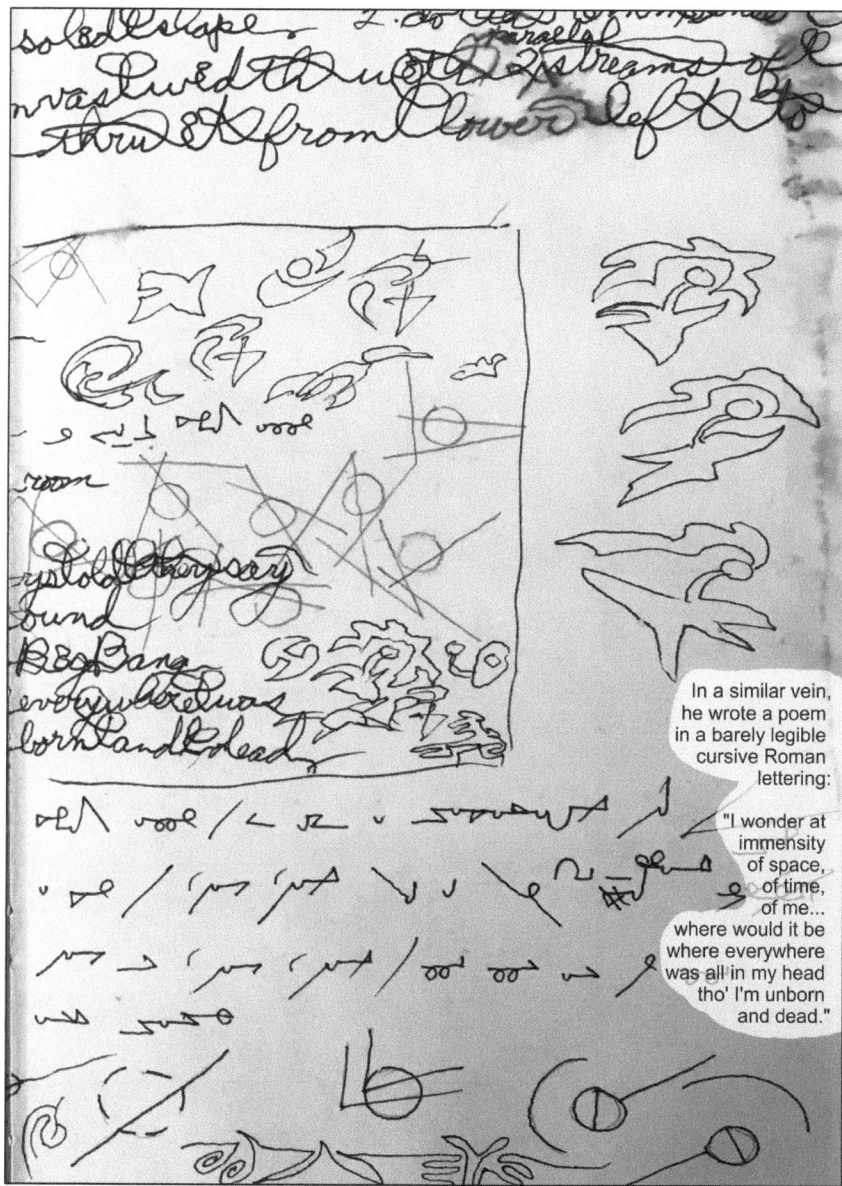

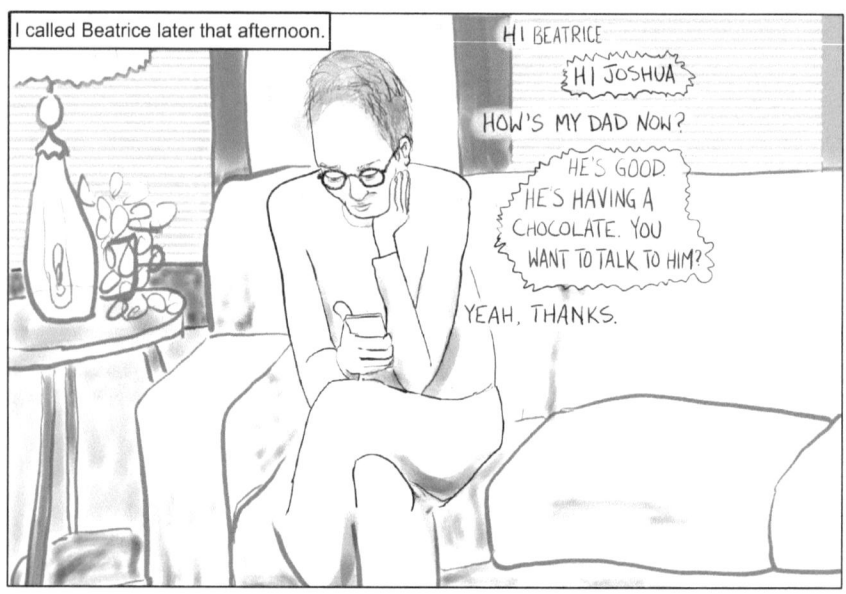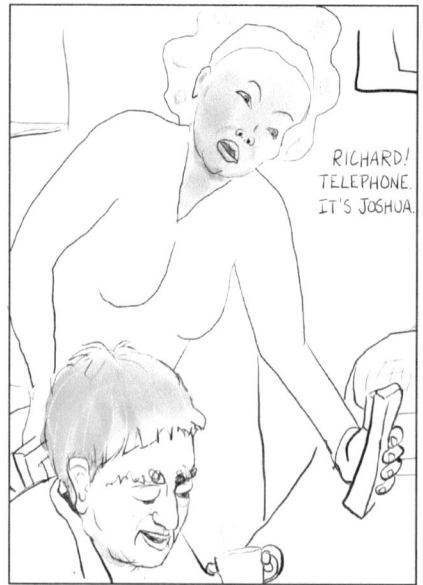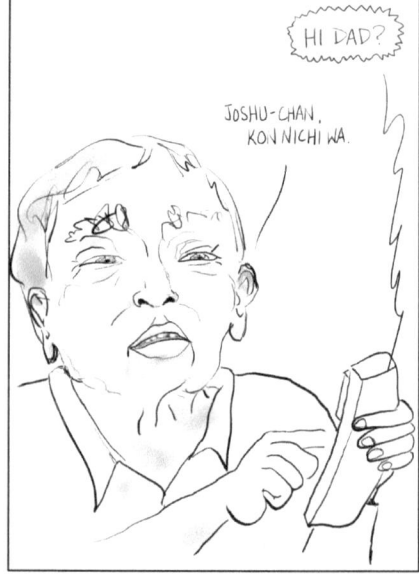

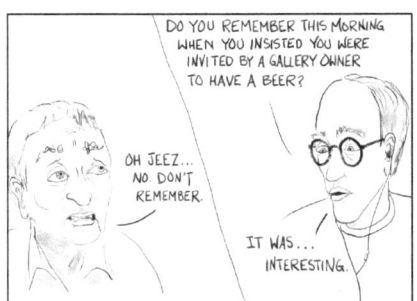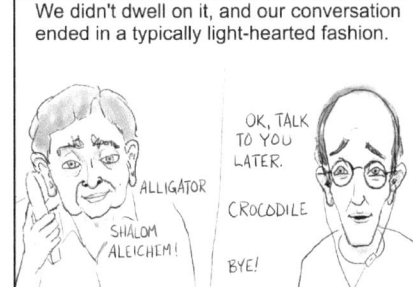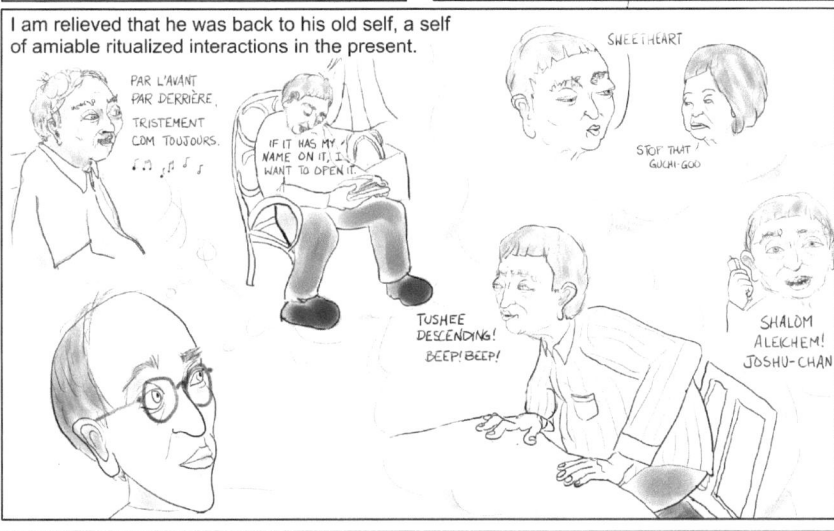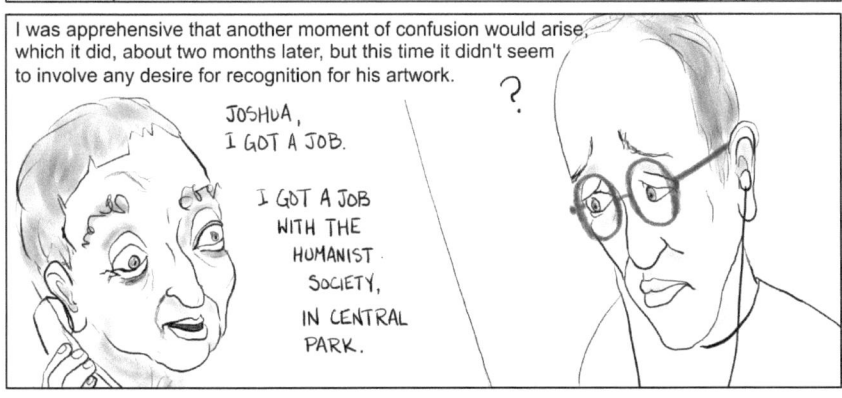

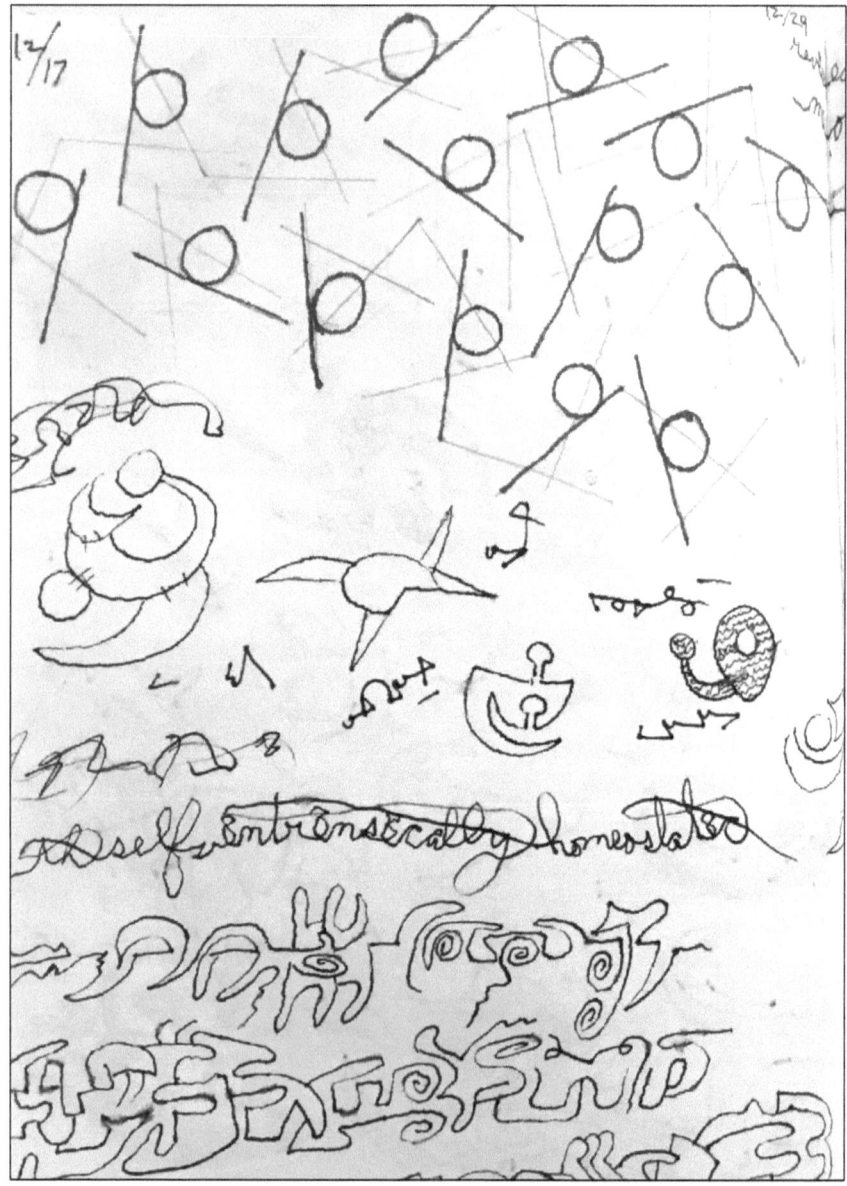

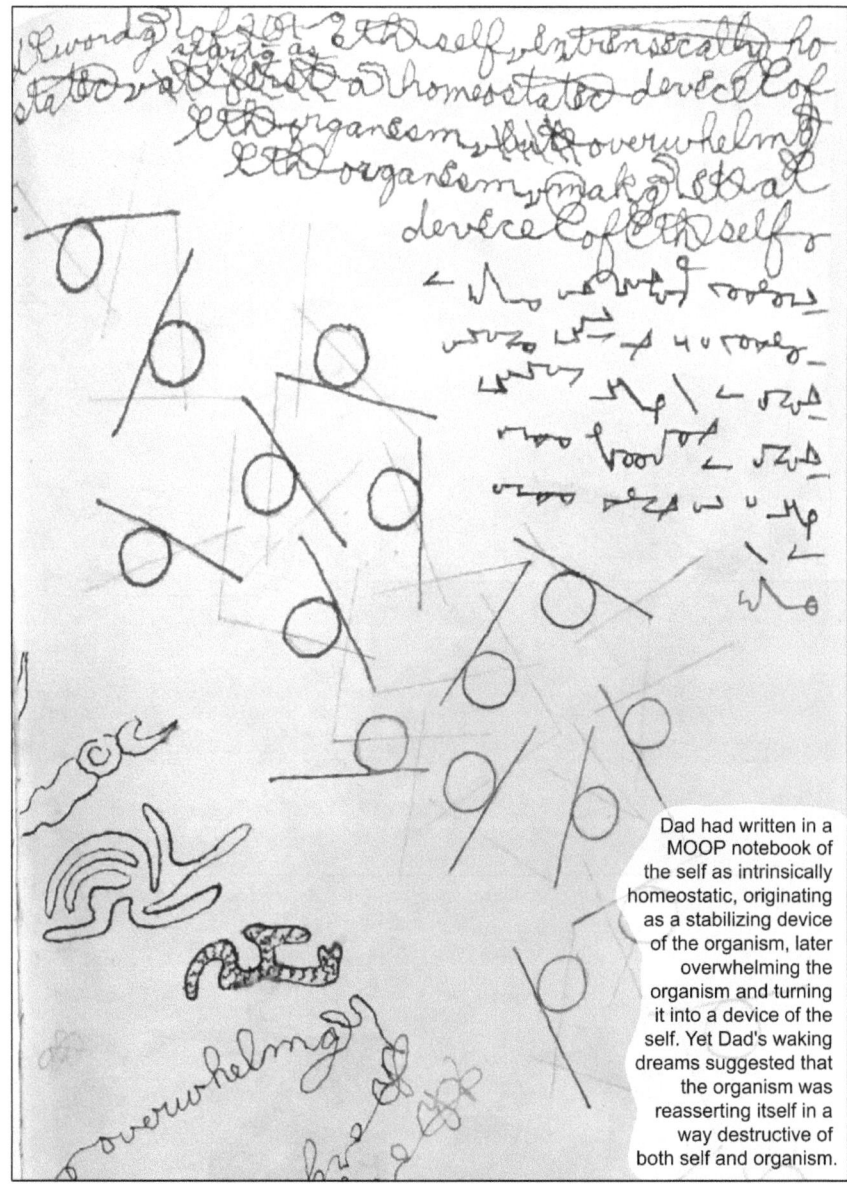

Dad had written in a MOOP notebook of the self as intrinsically homeostatic, originating as a stabilizing device of the organism, later overwhelming the organism and turning it into a device of the self. Yet Dad's waking dreams suggested that the organism was reasserting itself in a way destructive of both self and organism.

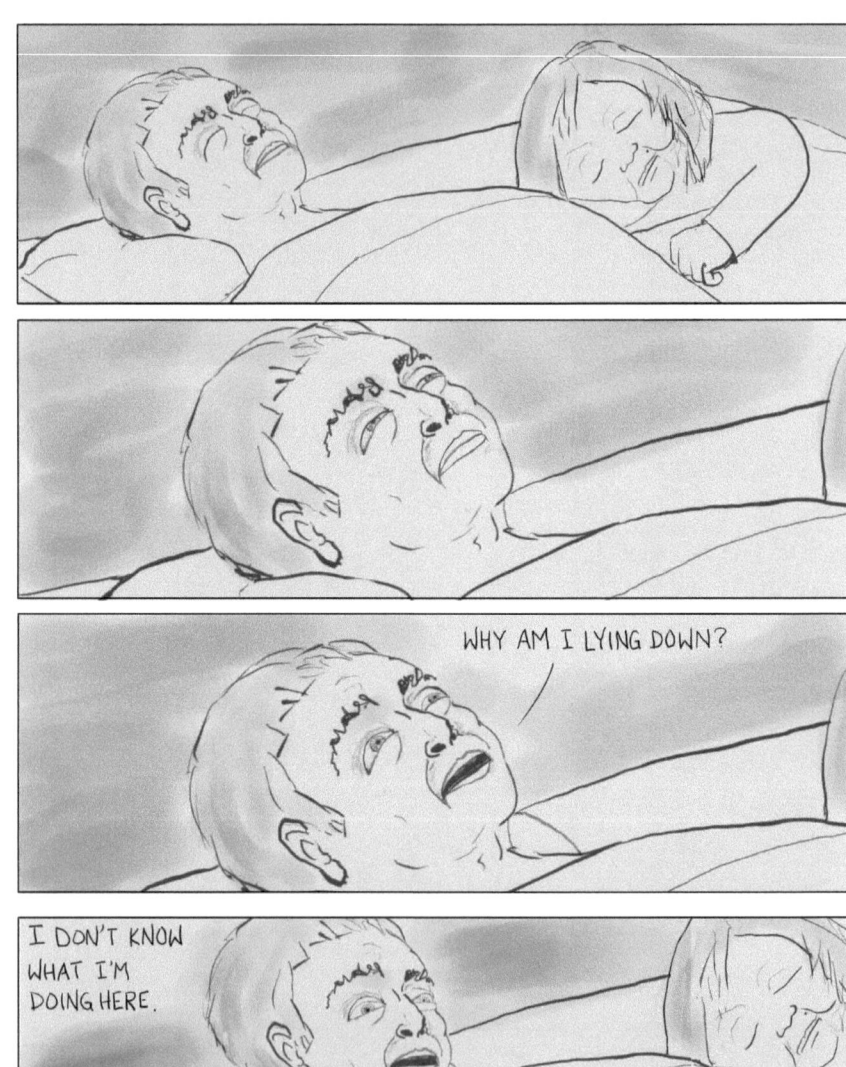

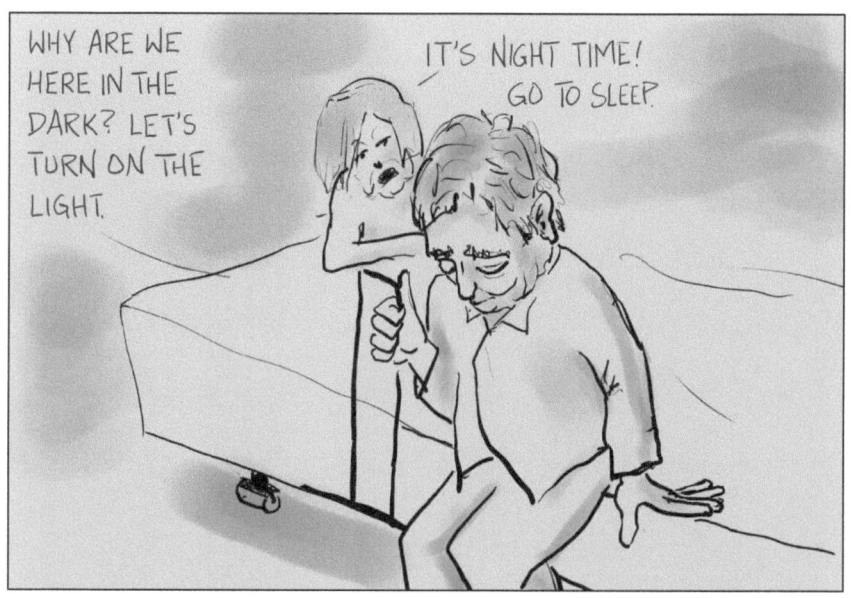
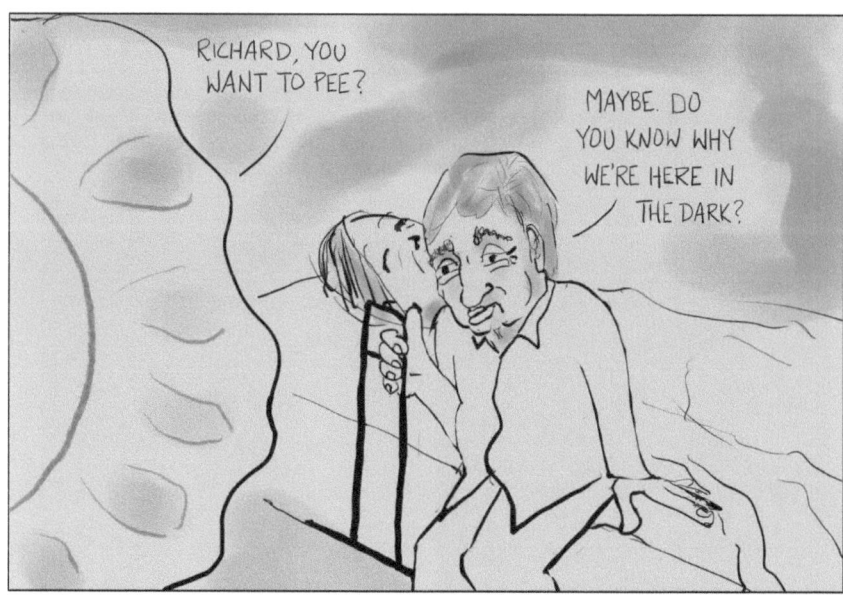

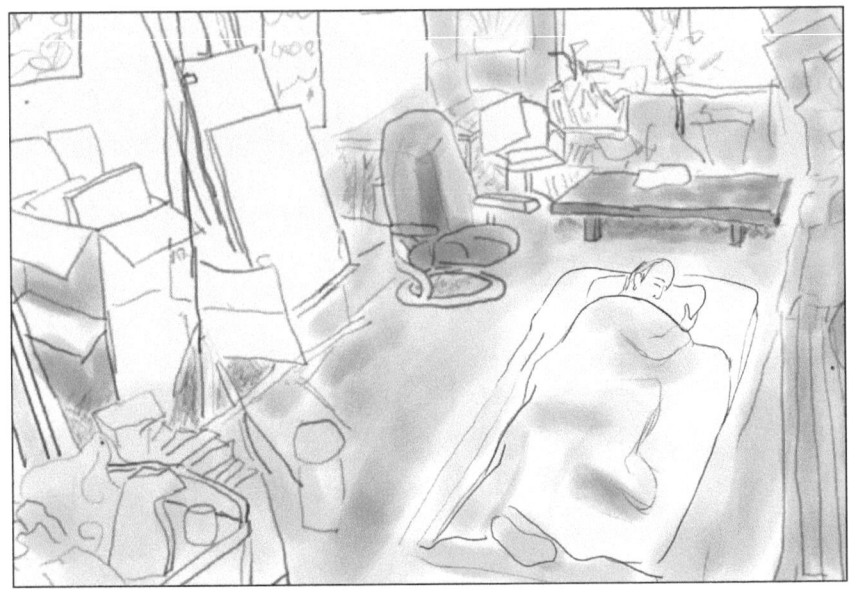

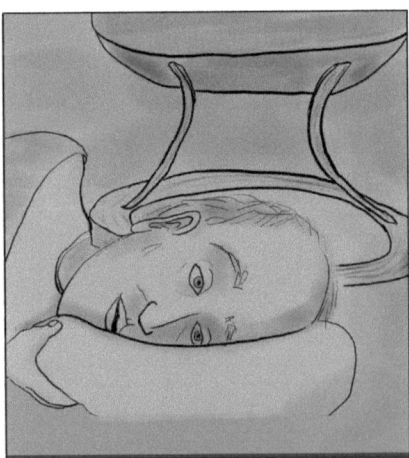

I rarely slept well at my parents'. Dad would often wake up at odd hours and start talking to Mom, or call the care worker to help him go pee. At other times, he would just yell out something I couldn't make out.

Our other care worker, Viola, works from Friday morning to Monday morning. She slept lightly, seldom more than three or four hours at a stretch before she heard something and checked in on Dad and Mom.

RICHARD, HE HAS SOME DREAMS. SOMETIMES HE SHOUTING SO IT WAKES ME UP. ONE TIME HE FIGHTING PIGS, LIKE IT WAS WAR, WAR WITH THE PIGS.

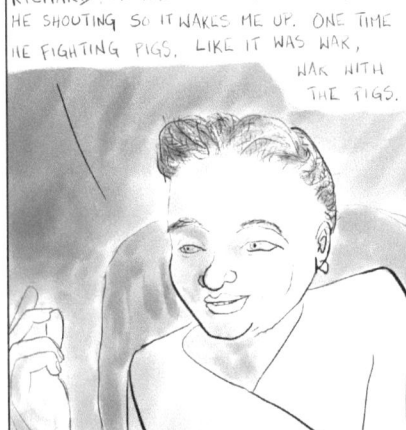

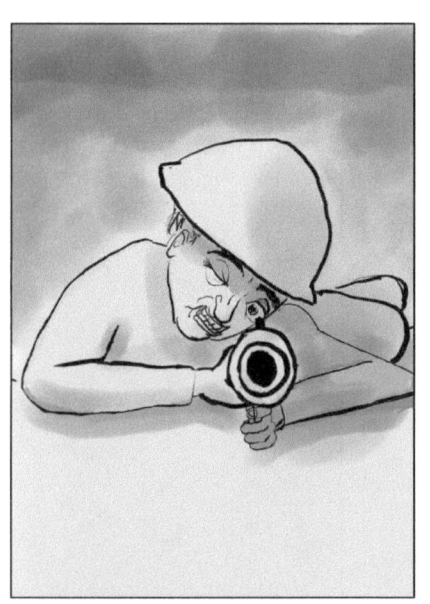
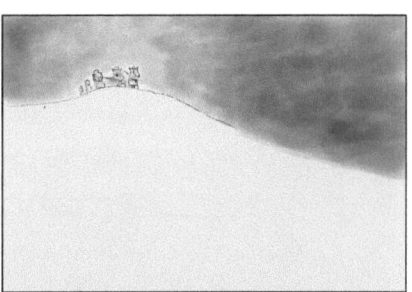
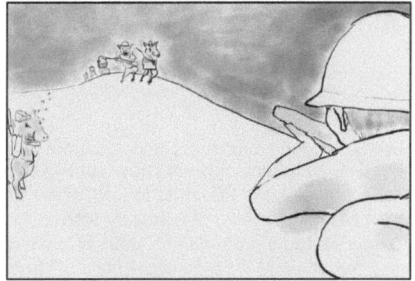
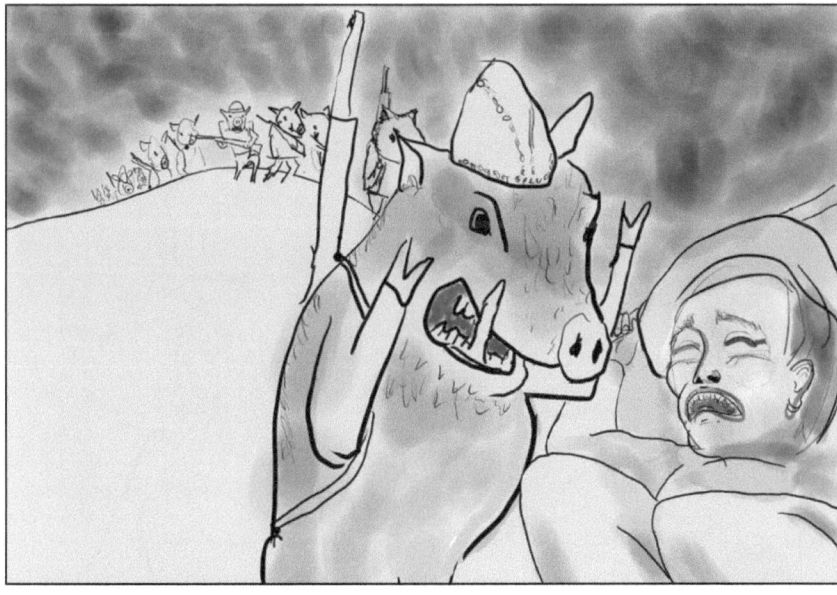

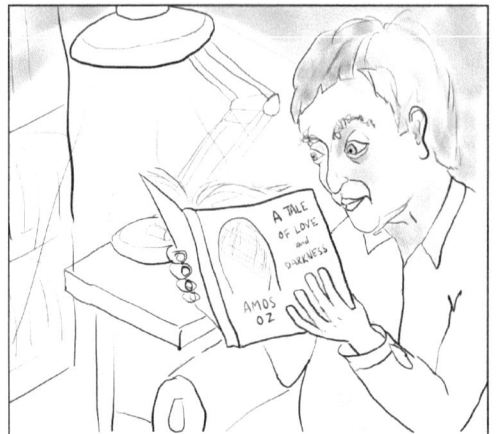
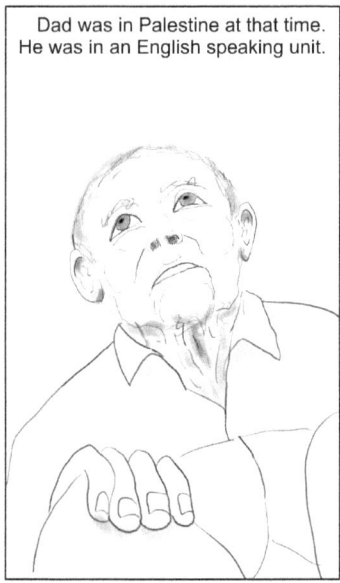

Dad was in Palestine at that time. He was in an English speaking unit.

I don't know the source of Dad's recurring nightmares. But it reminded me of when I gave Amos Oz's memoir *A Tale of Love and Darkness* to Dad for his birthday. It's a brooding coming of age story set in a Zionist community during the waning years of British mandate for Palestine and the birth of the state of Israel in 1948.

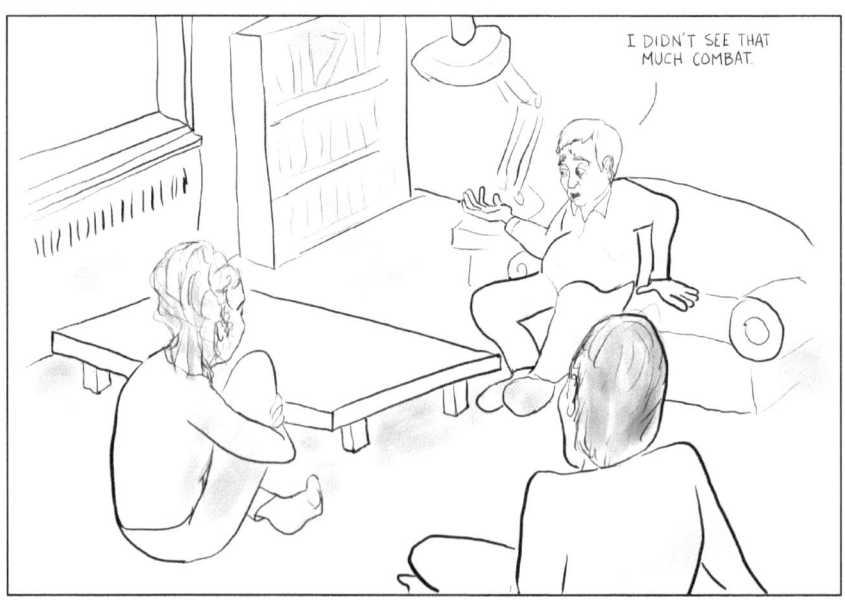

I DIDN'T SEE THAT MUCH COMBAT.

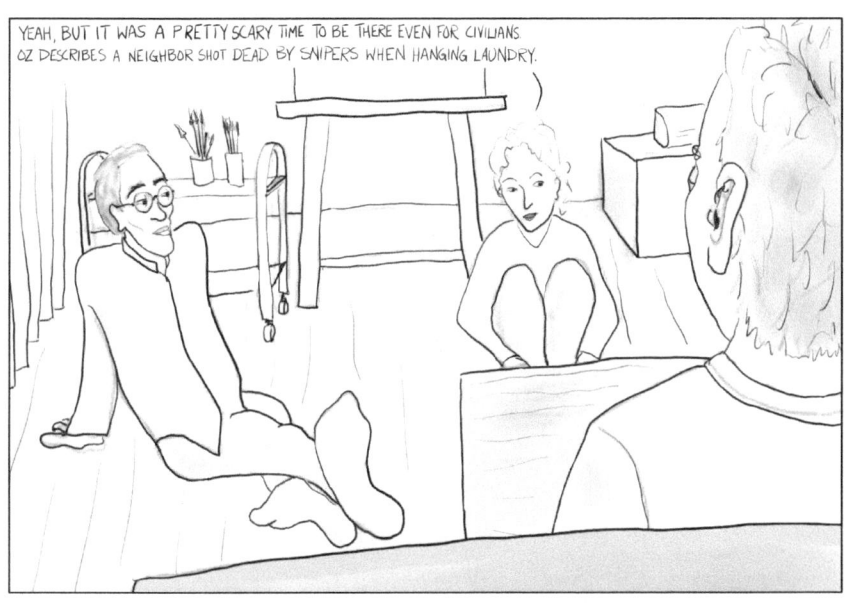

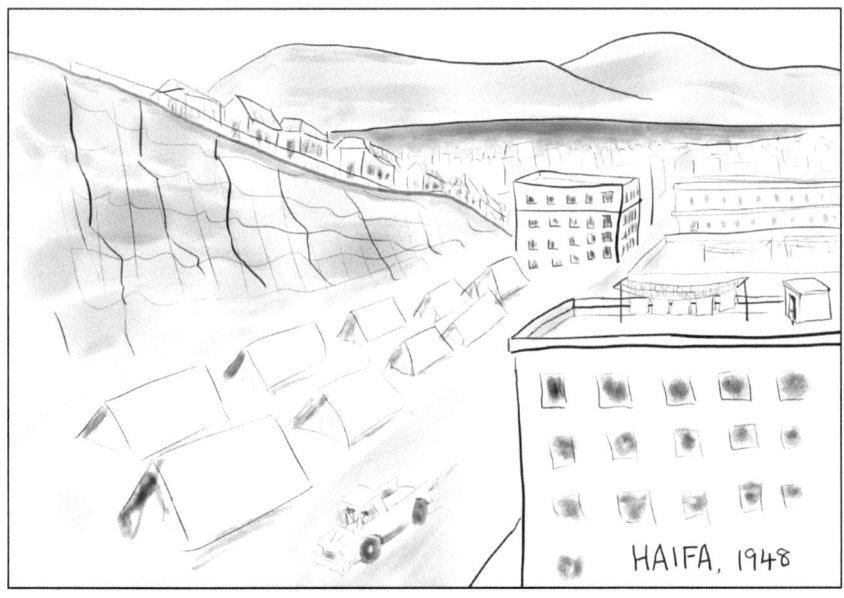

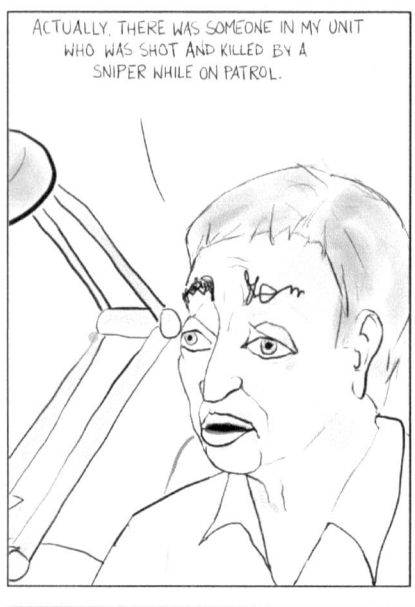

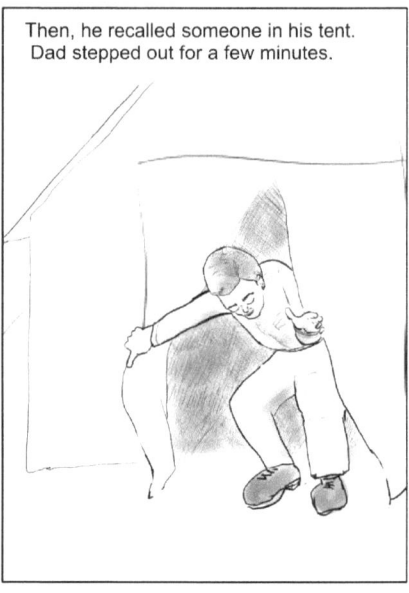

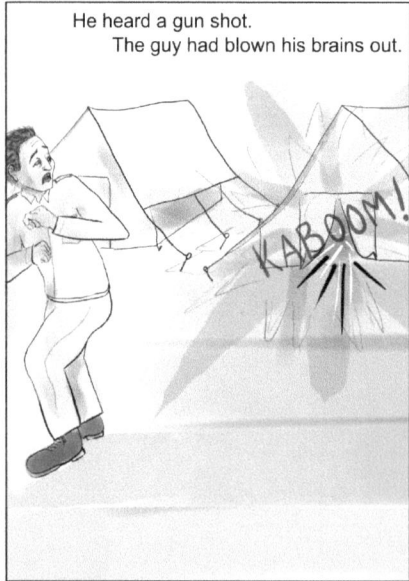

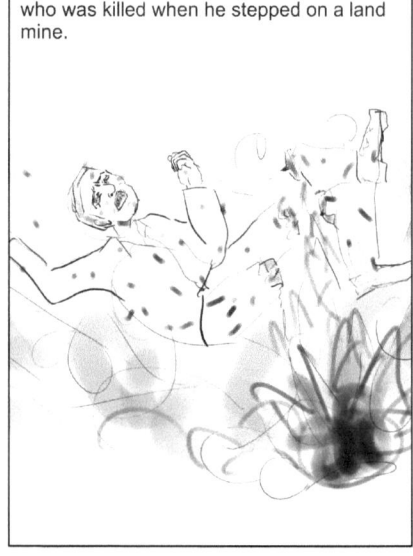

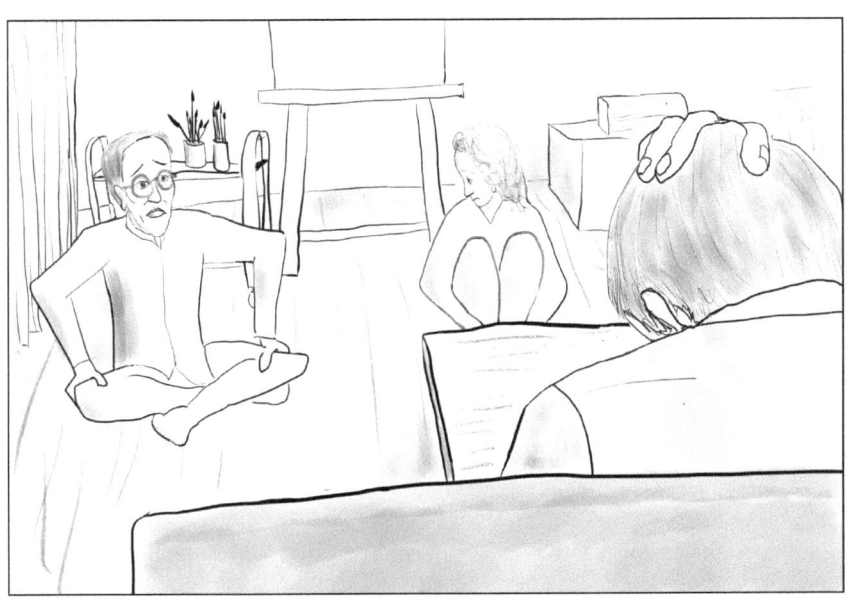

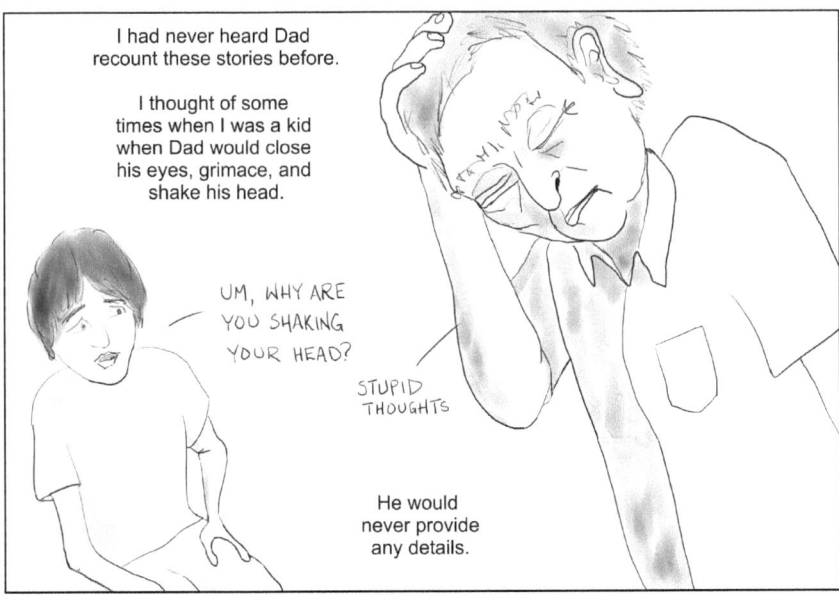

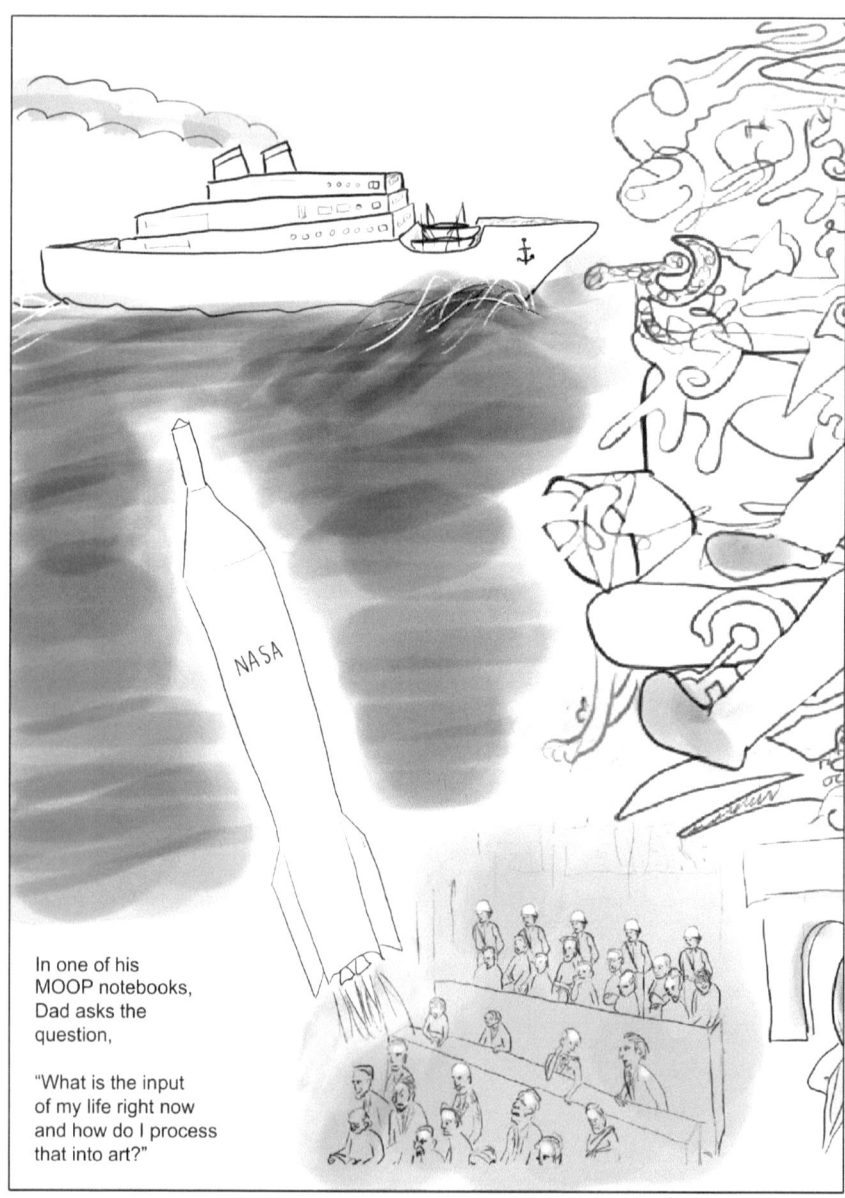

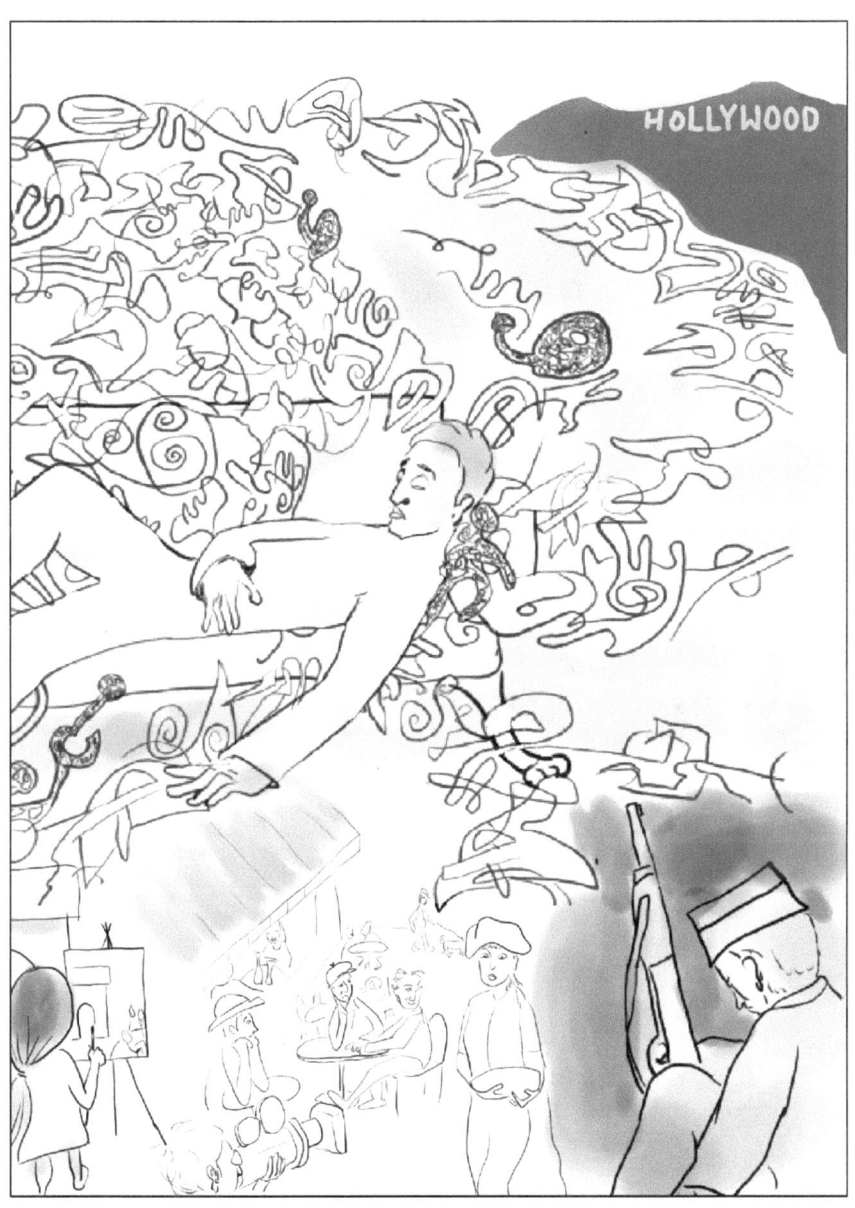

Does some of Dad's trauma manifest in his artwork?

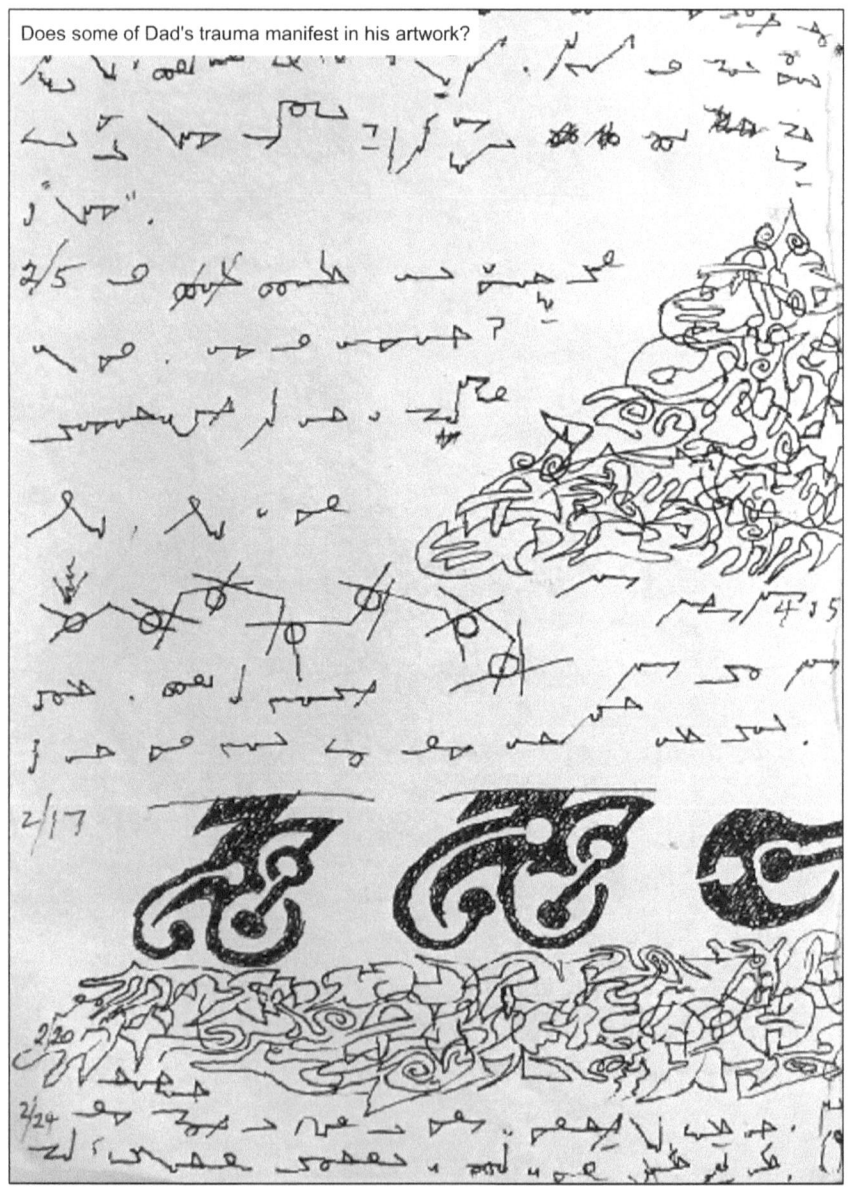

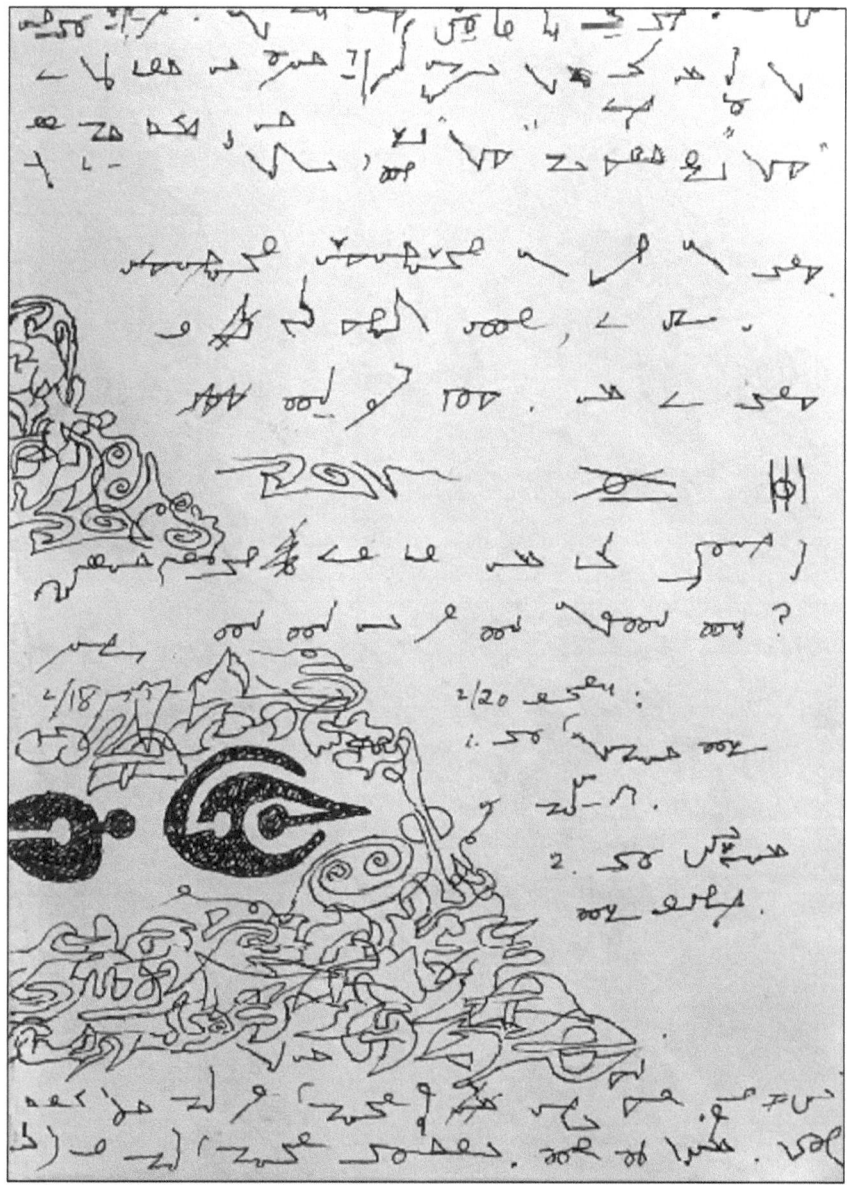

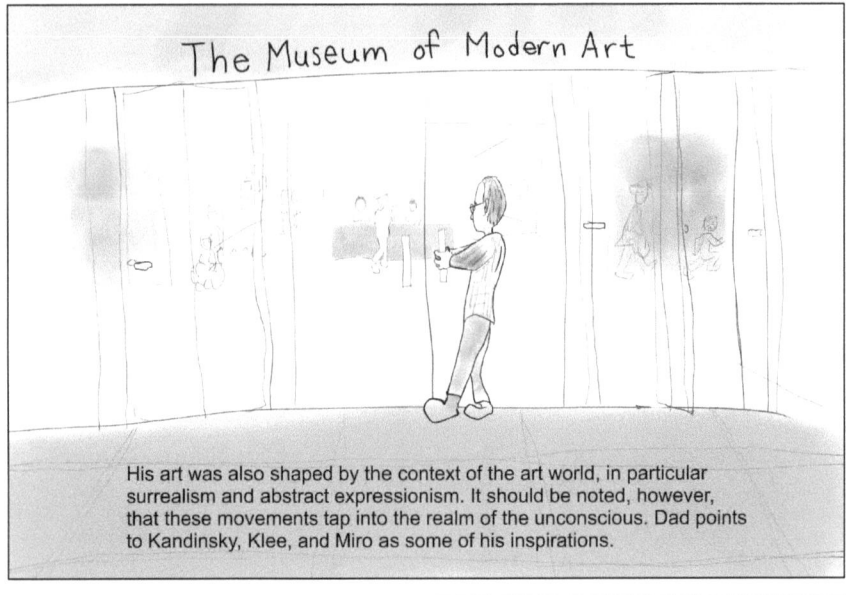

His art was also shaped by the context of the art world, in particular surrealism and abstract expressionism. It should be noted, however, that these movements tap into the realm of the unconscious. Dad points to Kandinsky, Klee, and Miro as some of his inspirations.

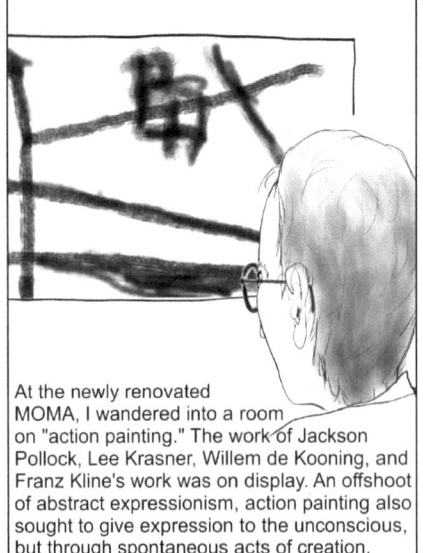

At the newly renovated MOMA, I wandered into a room on "action painting." The work of Jackson Pollock, Lee Krasner, Willem de Kooning, and Franz Kline's work was on display. An offshoot of abstract expressionism, action painting also sought to give expression to the unconscious, but through spontaneous acts of creation.

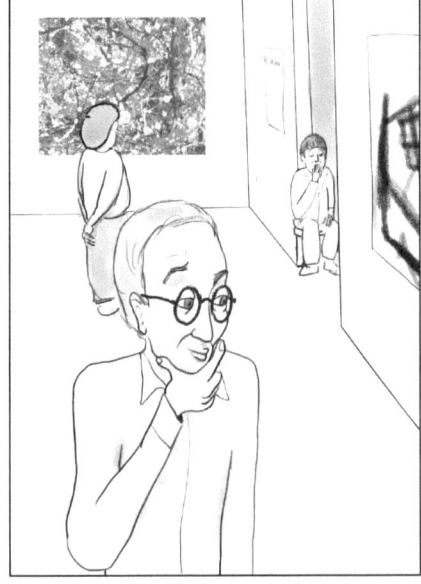

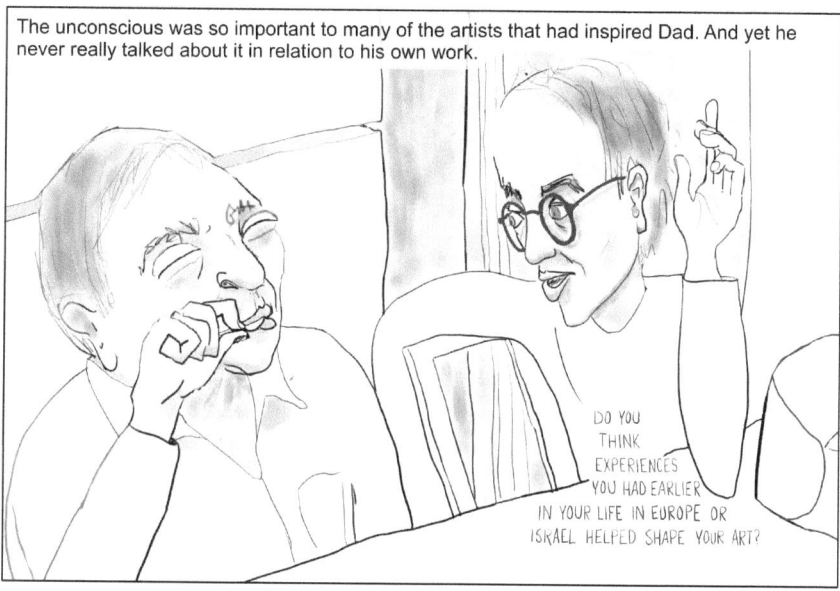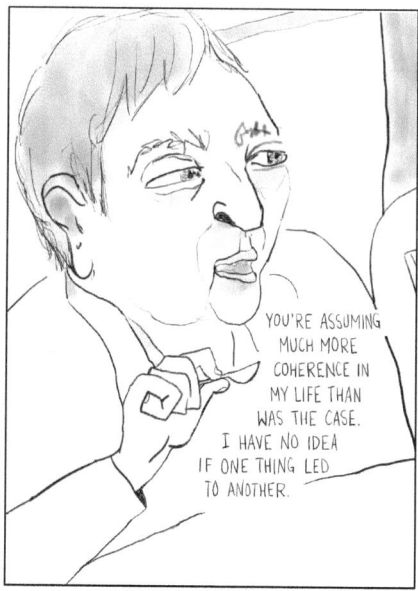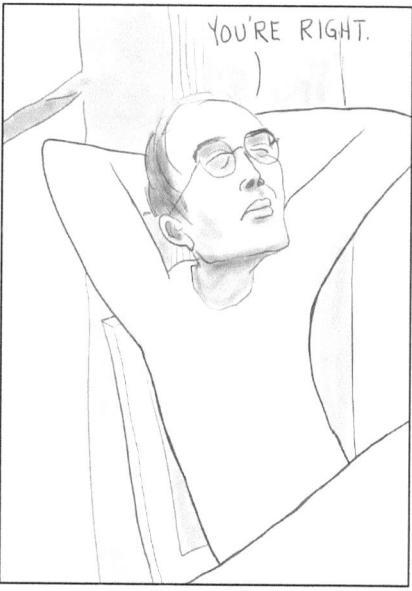

Sometime later I found an old spiral bound notebook at the bottom of Dad's dresser drawer, its pages yellow with age, its cover torn and frayed and mended with tape.

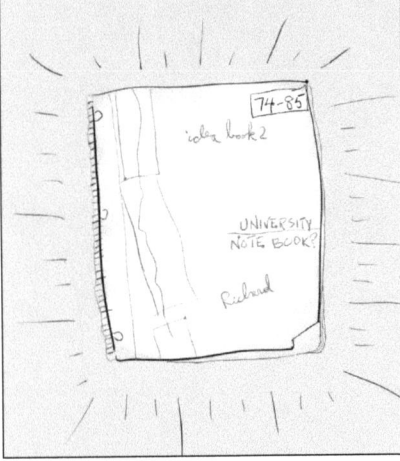

This one consisted mostly of writing—ideas for new projects, reflections, statements for possible use in upcoming paintings.

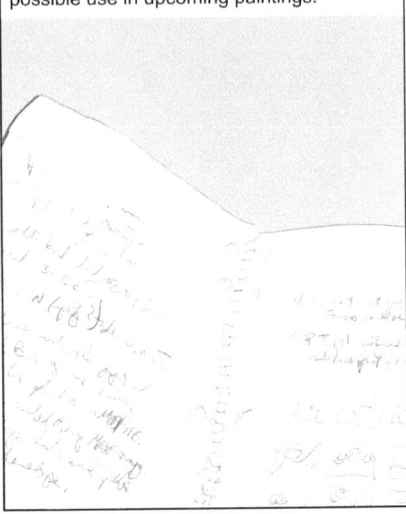

There were also some quick sketches testing compositional ideas for various paintings.

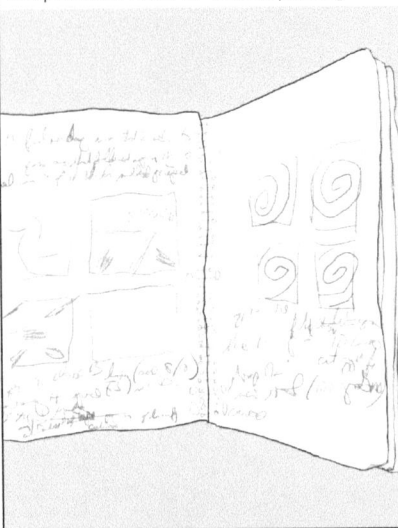

Towards the end of it, I noticed several little pyramid drawings. One of them was filled with tiny text in English cursive script. A note indicated that this was the "wording for MOOP #203." This entry was dated 9/27/86.

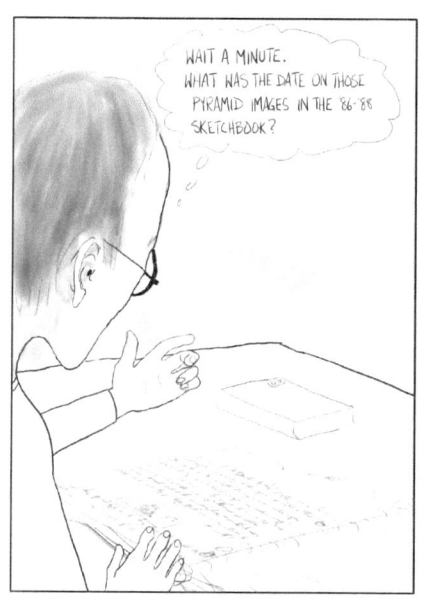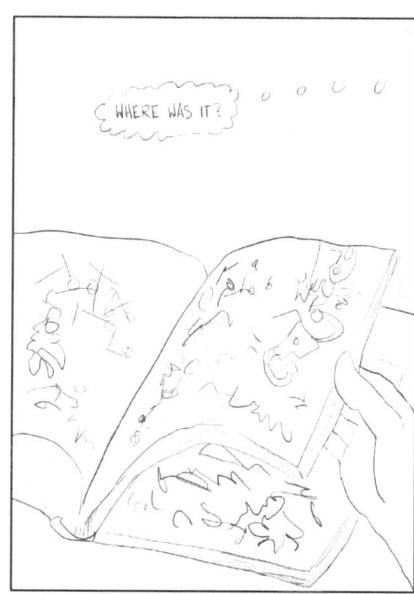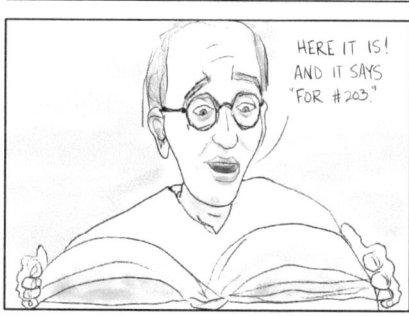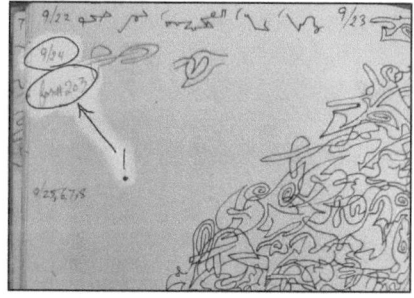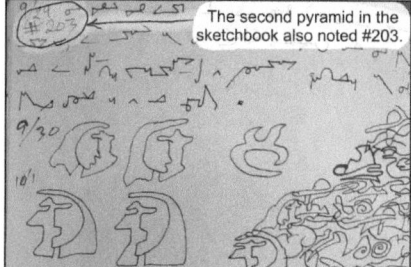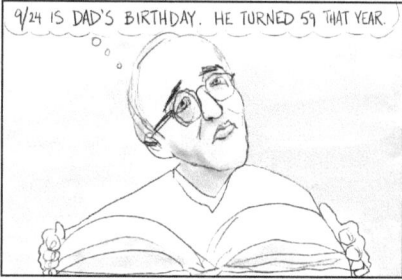

Picasso - "Charnel House" mostly simple bll [?]
dk grey lines drawn on a greyish wht BG
some grey + blk areas painted in, numerous erased
but still visible lines — should I use a stubby
brush + try: 400P ptg on [struck] canvas attached
to 1 wall?

9/27 words for #203

[boxed draft:]
what turned my thoughts this way?
1 trashpile   how   on 1 shoulders
of history   1 dead live
            w us - 1   of giants
            recently dead their tragedy
            in 1 dead of our
            time enmeshed in our living memor-
            ies + feelings + 1 further, past dead
            depends on 1 religious historical + poetic
            riches of our minds + 1 dead who live
            watg in we living, + our own death ling w us

Another possibility w 1 big triangle would be to have 1
regions filled in a horizontal stripes
1 squeezed acrylic color

[enlarged version of boxed draft:]
what turned my thoughts this way?
1 trashpile   how   on 1 shoulders
of history   1 dead live
            w us - 1   of giants
            recently dead their tragedy
            in 1 dead of our
            time enmeshed in our living memor-
            ies + feelings + 1 further, past dead
            depends on 1 religious historical + poetic
            riches of our minds + 1 dead who live
            watg in we living, + our own death ling w us

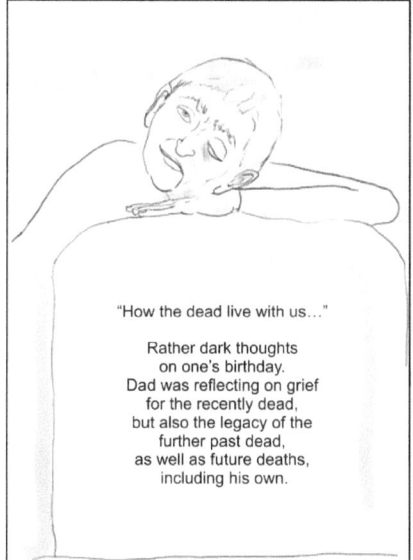

"How the dead live with us…"

Rather dark thoughts on one's birthday. Dad was reflecting on grief for the recently dead, but also the legacy of the further past dead, as well as future deaths, including his own.

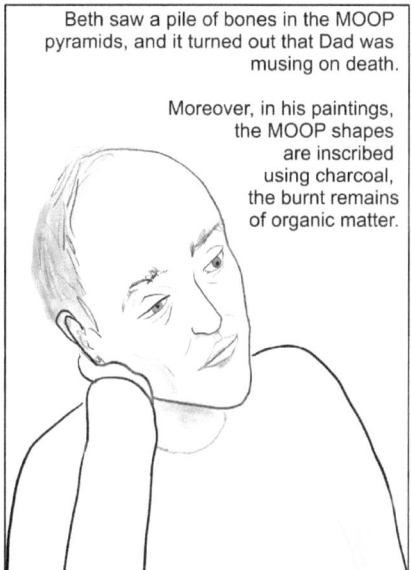

Beth saw a pile of bones in the MOOP pyramids, and it turned out that Dad was musing on death.

Moreover, in his paintings, the MOOP shapes are inscribed using charcoal, the burnt remains of organic matter.

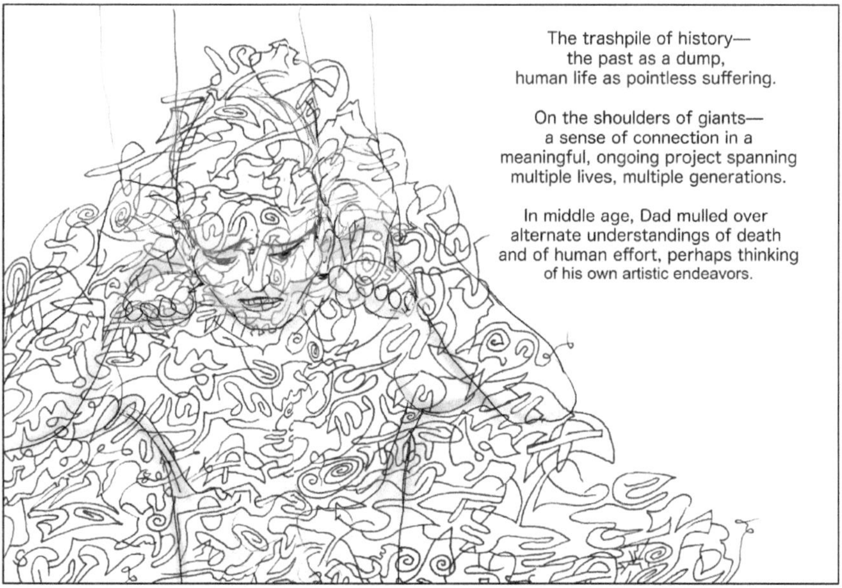

The trashpile of history— the past as a dump, human life as pointless suffering.

On the shoulders of giants— a sense of connection in a meaningful, ongoing project spanning multiple lives, multiple generations.

In middle age, Dad mulled over alternate understandings of death and of human effort, perhaps thinking of his own artistic endeavors.

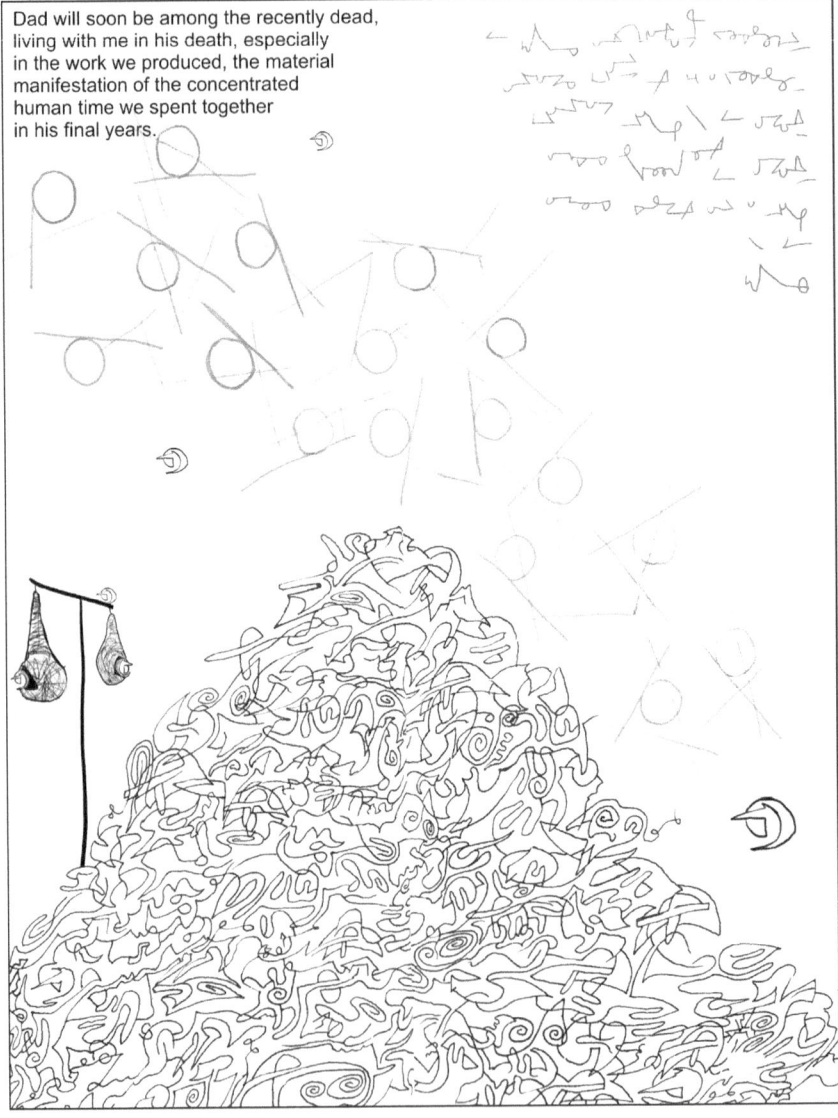

Dad will soon be among the recently dead, living with me in his death, especially in the work we produced, the material manifestation of the concentrated human time we spent together in his final years.

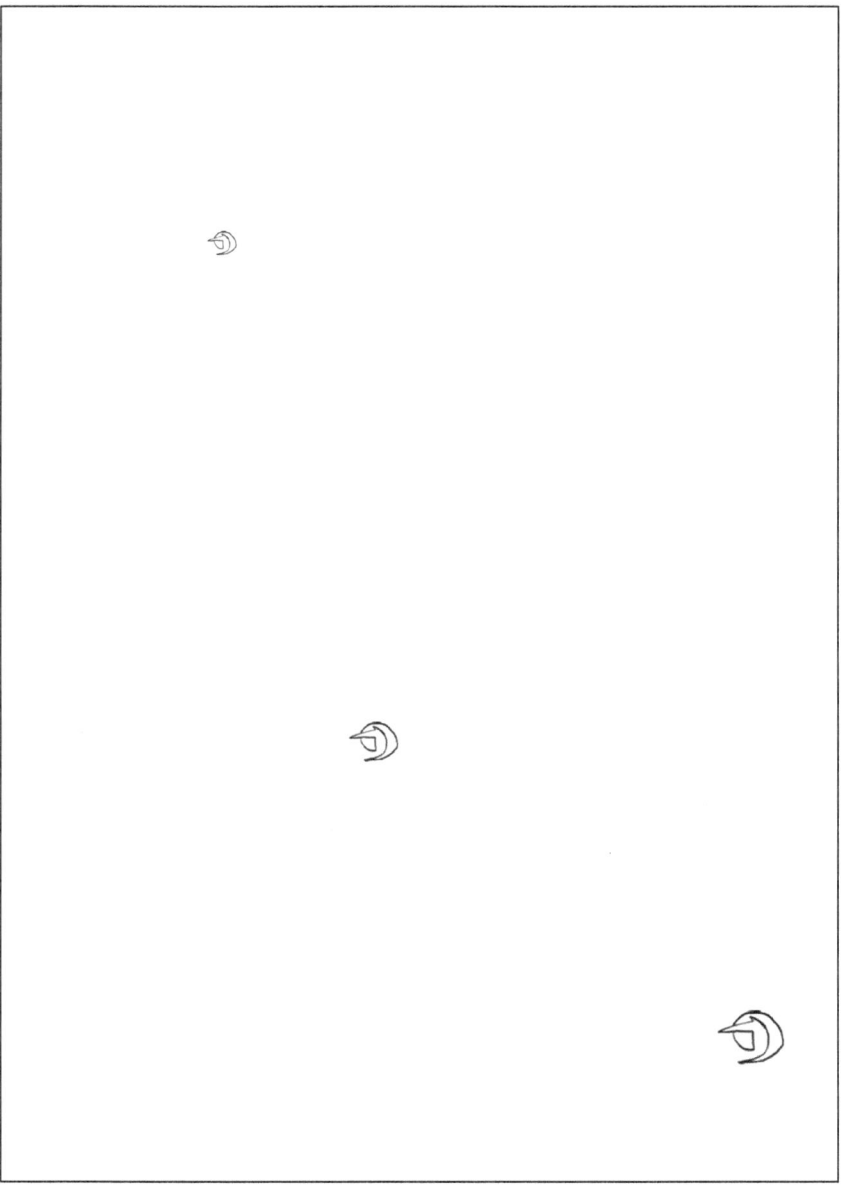

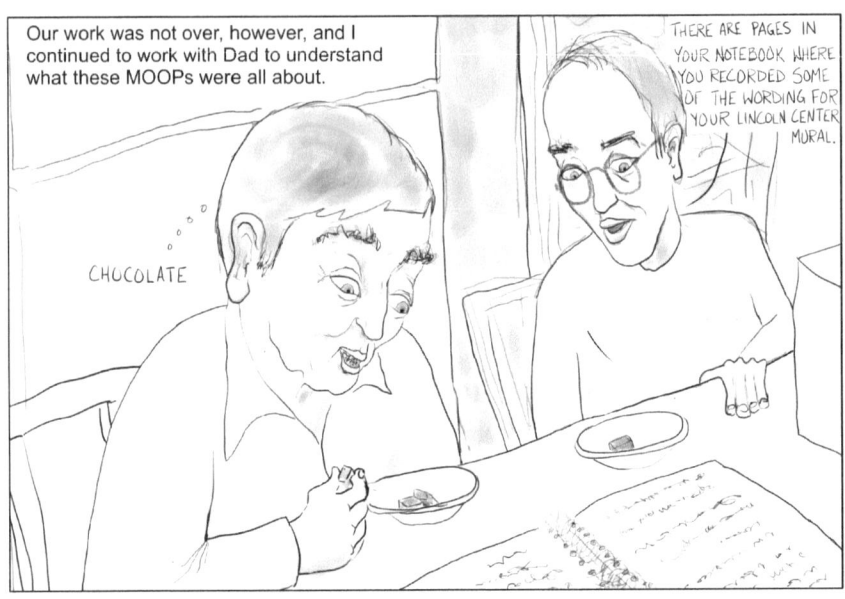
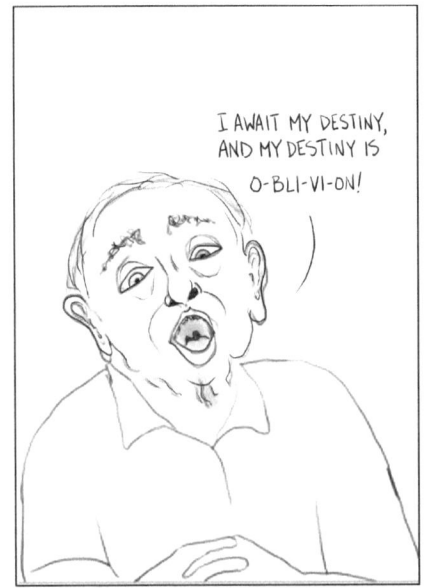
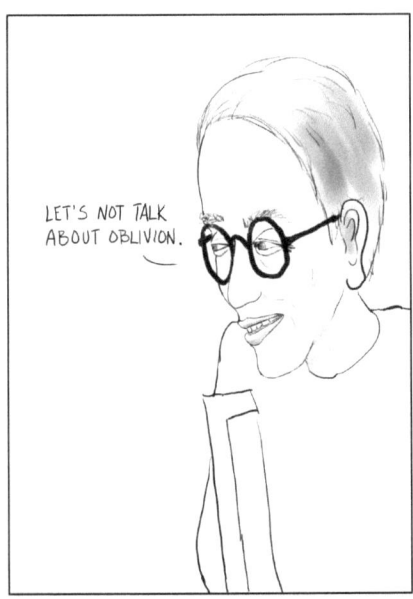

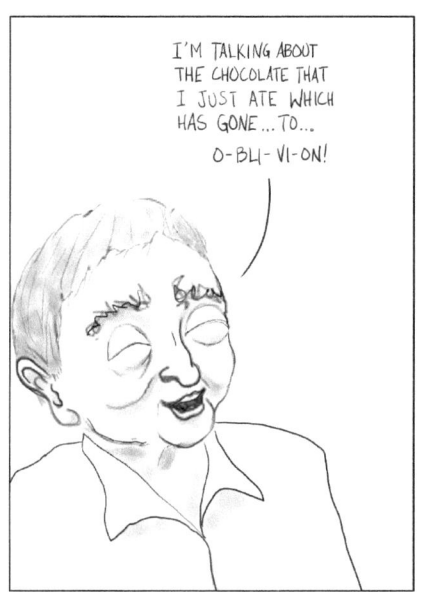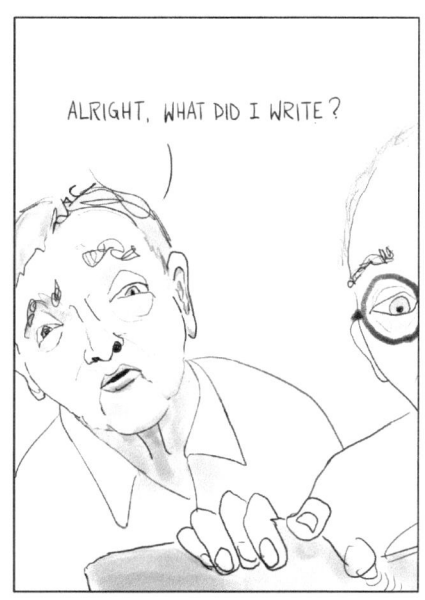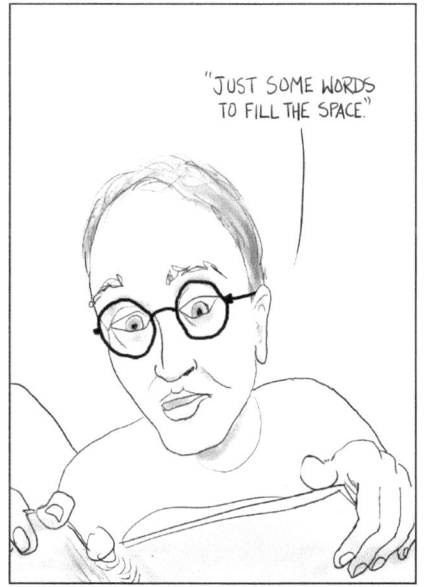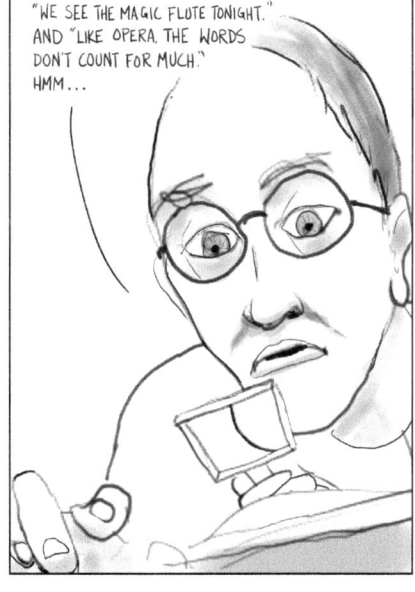

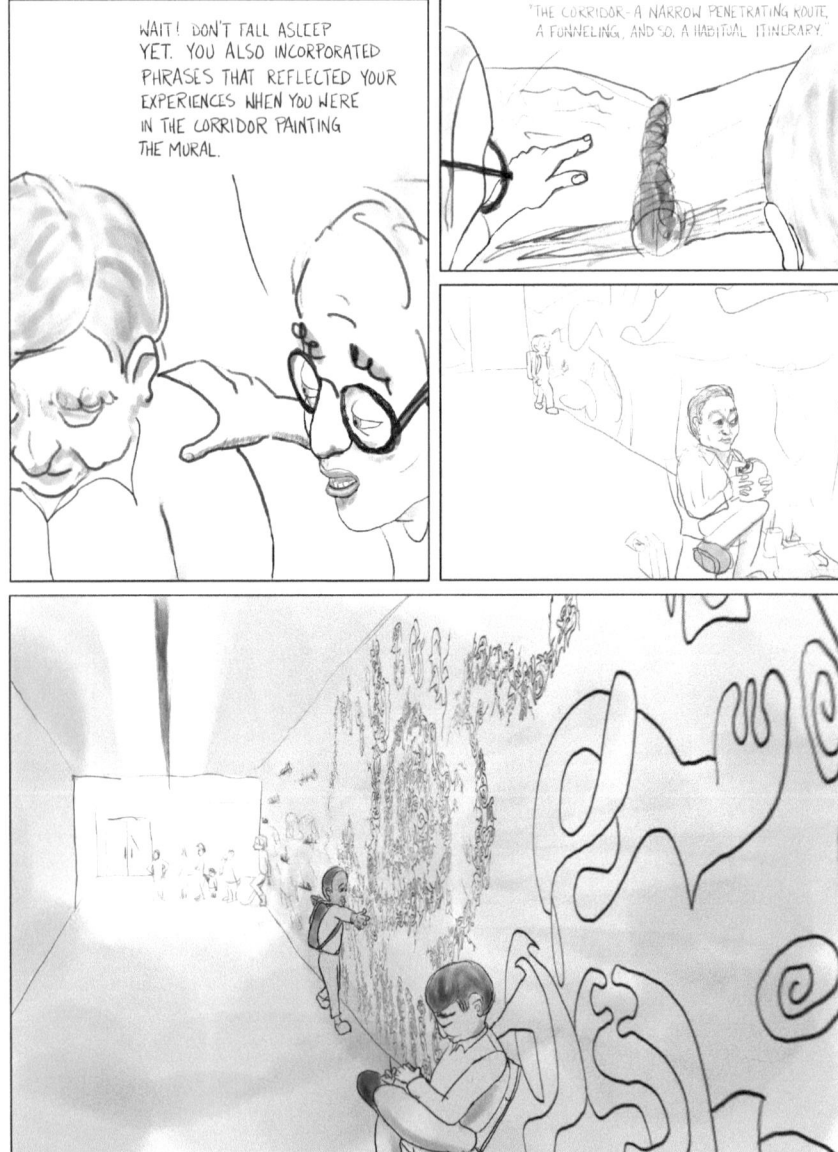

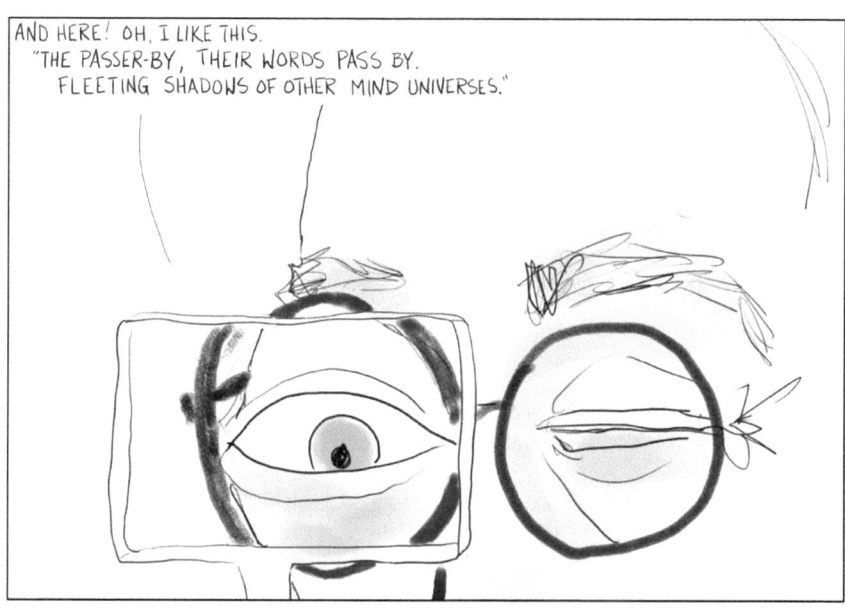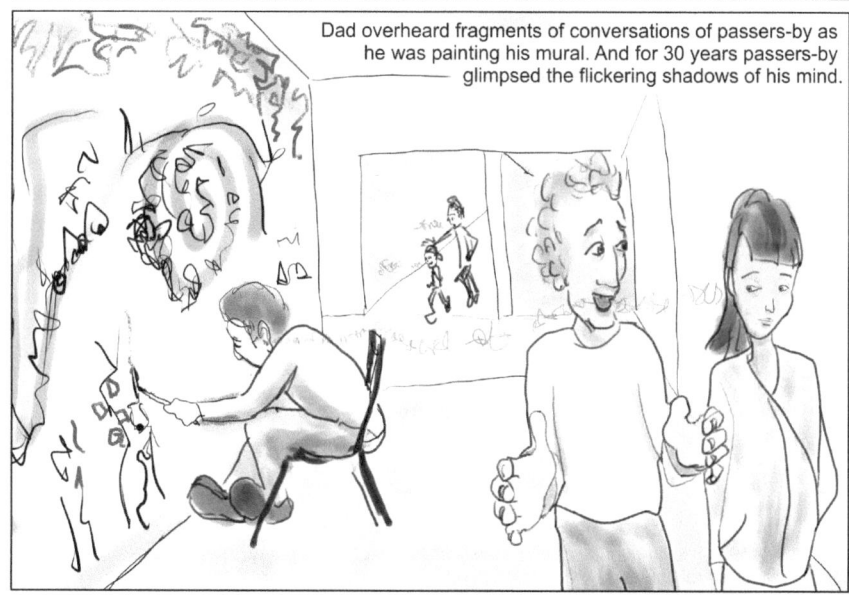

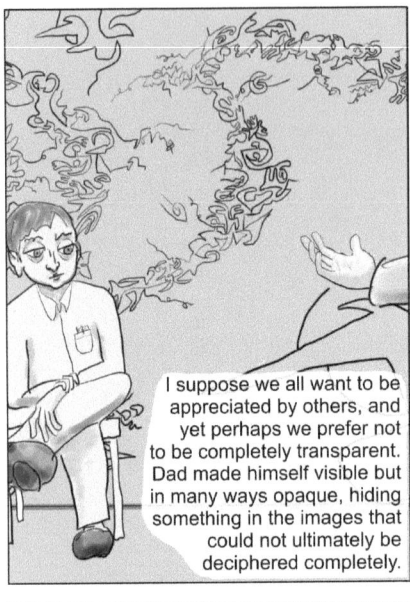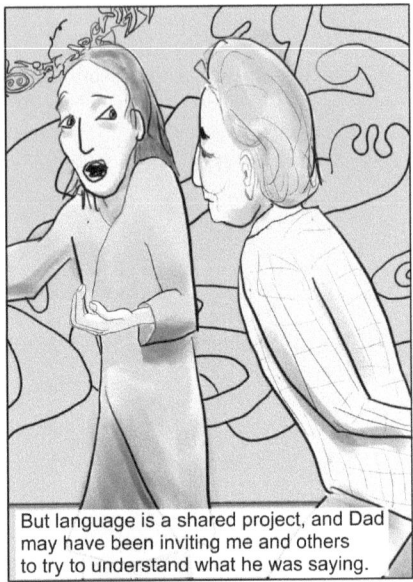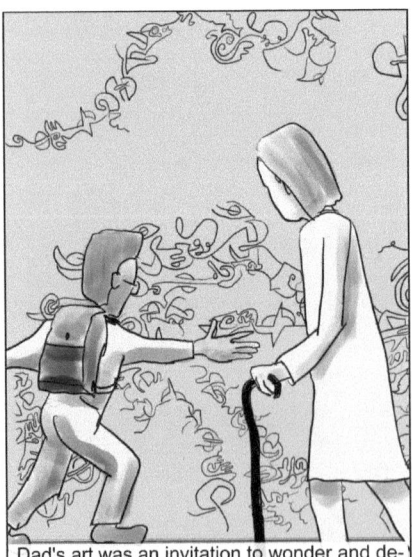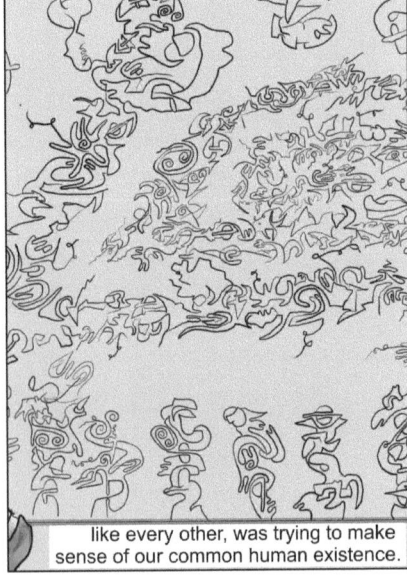

Epilogue

Chapter 10

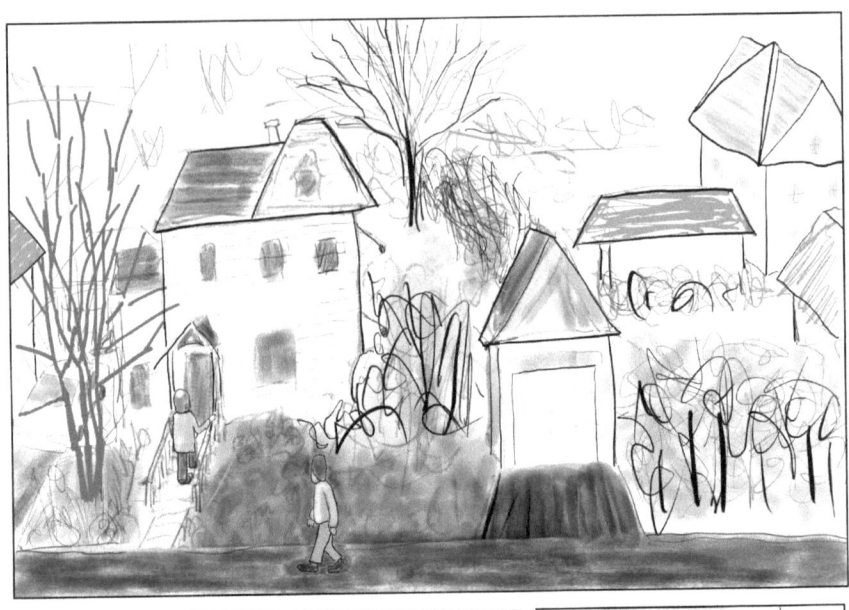
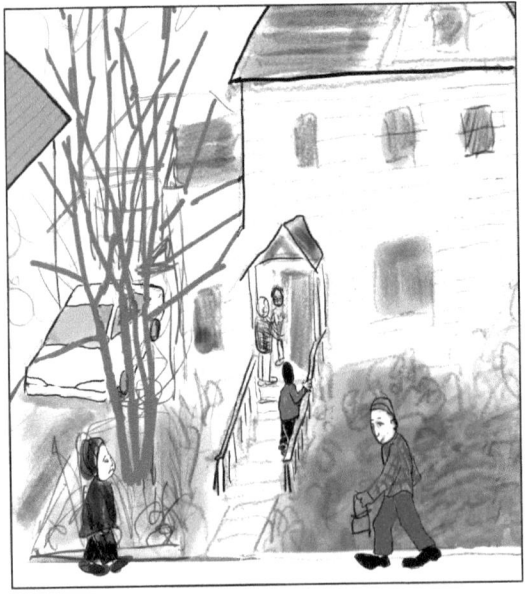
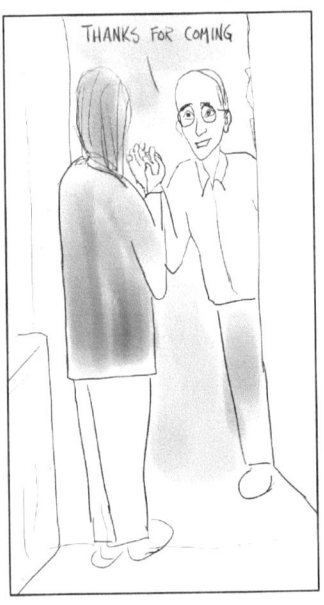

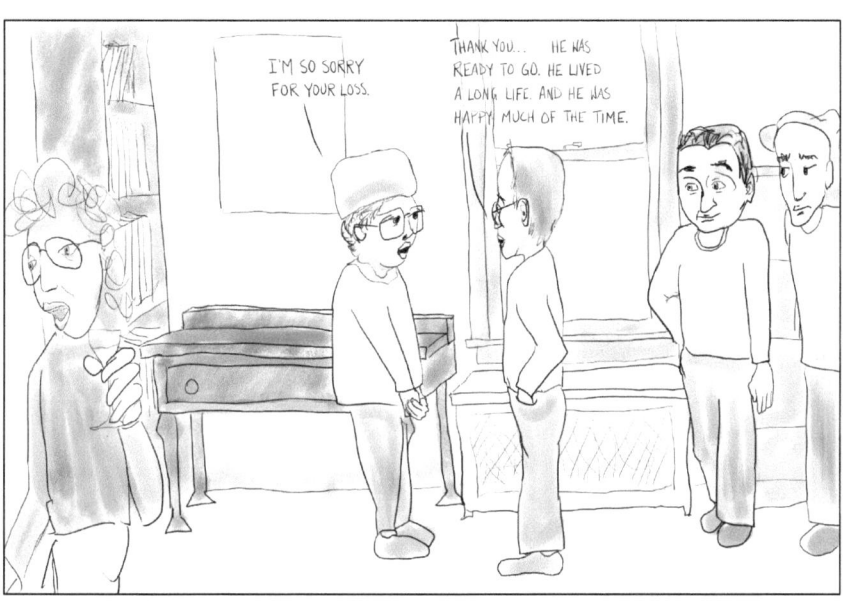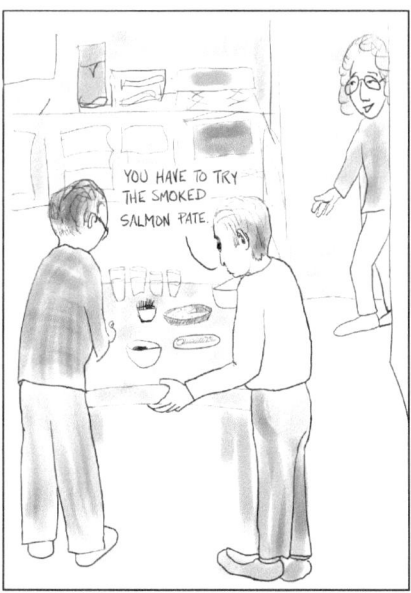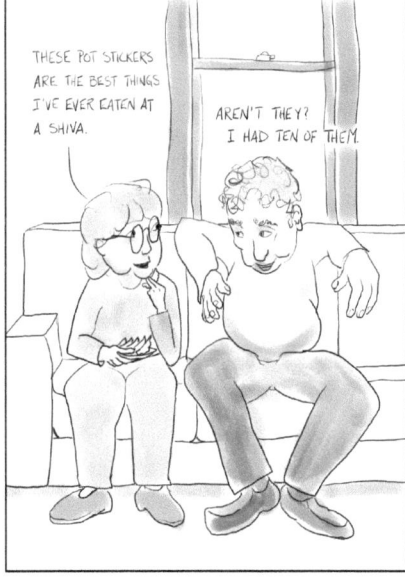

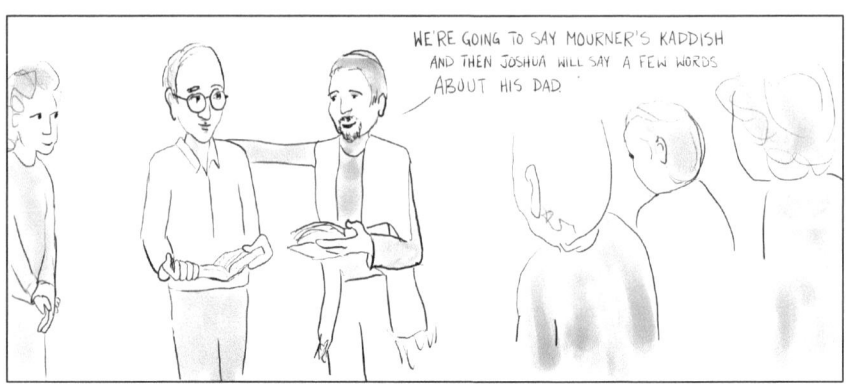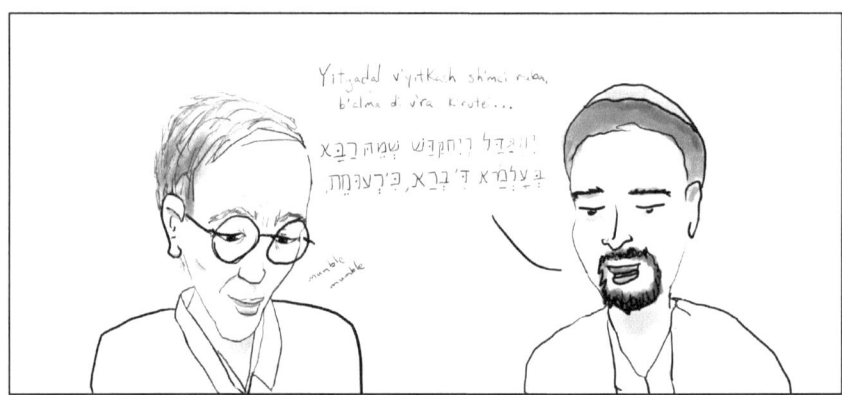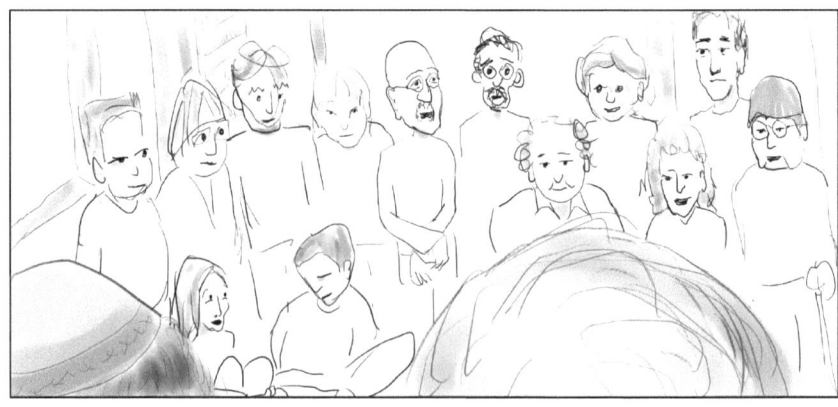

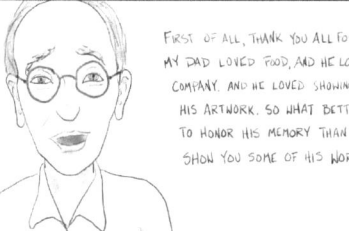

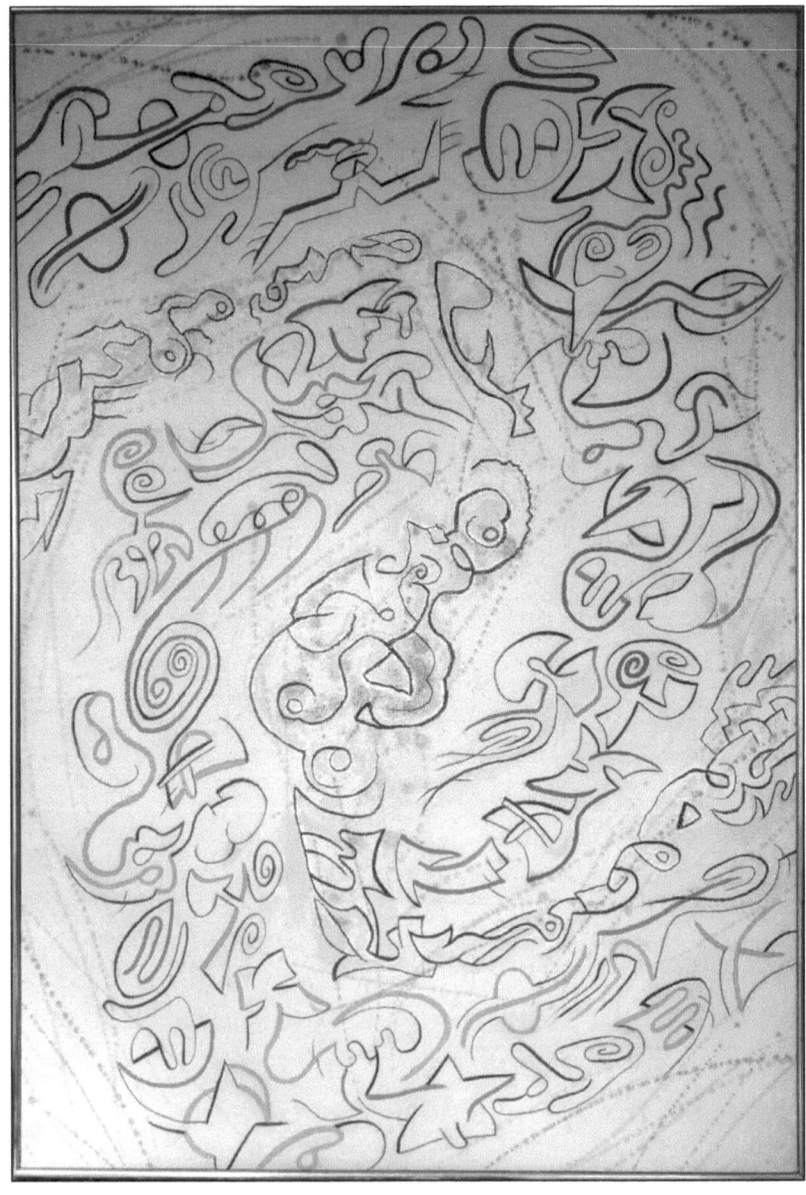

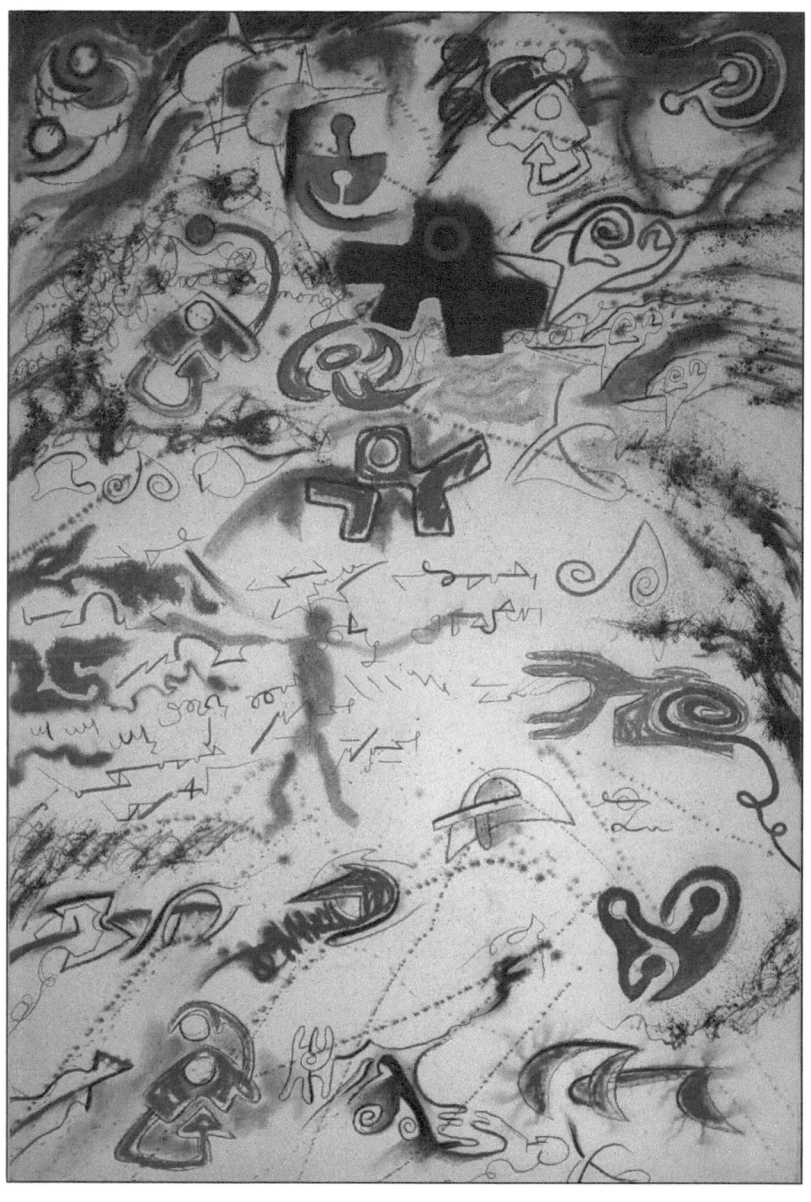

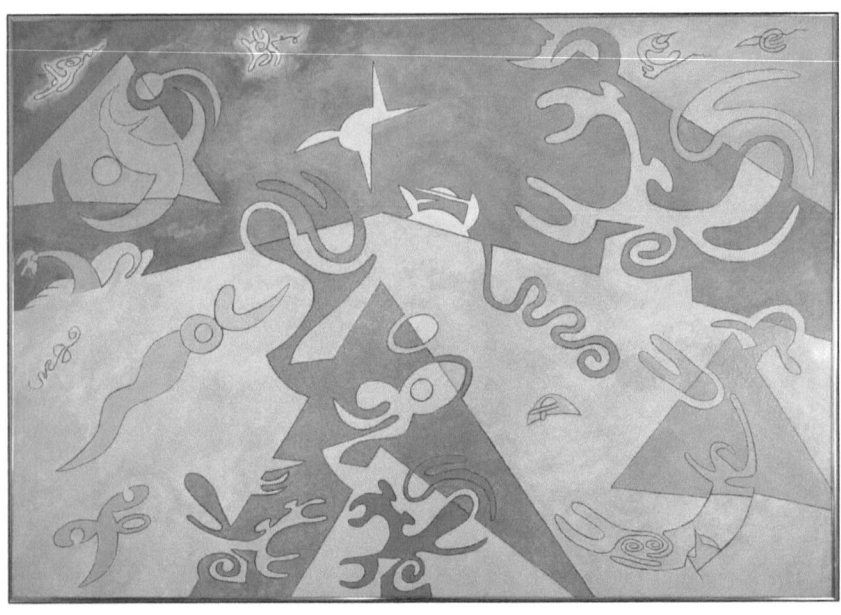
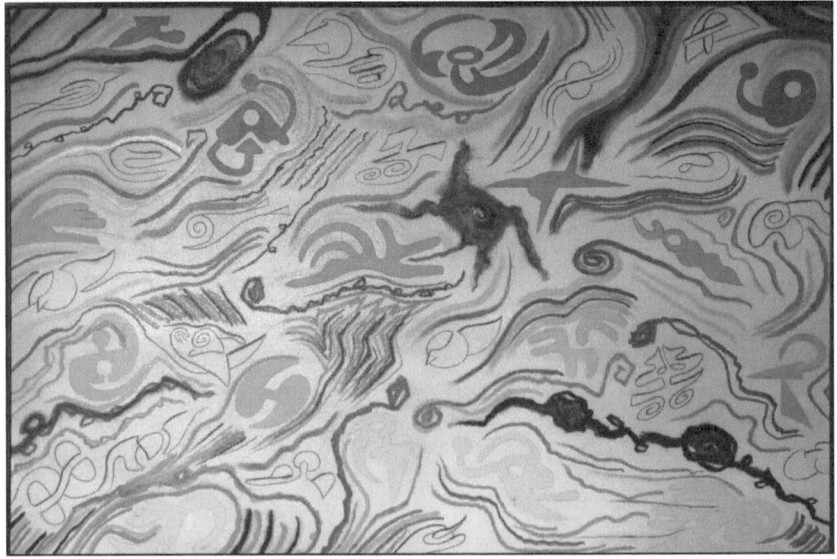

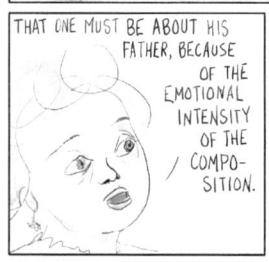

Afterword

Not everyone got it right, but a good number felt the force of the emotion behind the images, and the game kept people focused on the paintings with a sense of wonder that Dad would have appreciated. Likewise, the game of figuring out the connections between Dad's life and his art kept me occupied and engaged with Dad for years, and became a form of care in itself — a "reciprocal distributed interactional achievement" where I benefitted as much as Dad, where we both acted as givers and recipients of care. Of course, Mom was an enormous comfort to Dad, even when she was no longer able to really look after him, up until her death from cancer, a year before Dad.

And the kind of care I provided was not sufficient in itself to sustain Dad in his final years. That depended heavily on the three care workers that attended to the needs of daily living — bathing, dressing, feeding, and toileting, but they did so much more too. They engaged with him, conversing and joking while attending to those needs of daily living. They became essential members of his community of care, one that was infused with love.

But I recognize that there are limits to what we can expect in care giving relationships. After Dad died, Viola told me that Dad would be her last long-term patient. The emotional burden of love was too great. She wanted a more professional relationship, one that allowed her to do her job without creating the bonds of affection that make the inevitable loss that much harder to bear. If anything, Beatrice took the loss hardest of all. She was visibly shaken when Dad died, sobbing in the apartment when the coroner and police came to ascertain the cause of death.

According to Viola, Dad was ready to die a week before he did, but he waited for my brother Abe and I to be with him. He could no longer see or speak, but he felt our presence, his ears pricking up when I sang him his favorite song. Once he died, we called 911, and were visited by a parade of police, detectives, the fire department, medical examiner, and finally the funeral home. After Dad's body was taken away, the police sealed the apartment, a process meant to prevent individual members of the family from taking things at will. But the immediate effect was to leave Abe and me, just orphaned, homeless, or without our home base in New York City, the apartment that we had grown up in.

Viola invited us to stay the night in her apartment, which was very generous, but we decided to rent a room. I visited Viola at her apartment a couple of weeks later, after I filed the necessary paperwork at housing court to have the apartment unsealed. Two of Mom's paintings hung on the wall in Viola's living room.

Viola mentioned that Beatrice was returning that day from a trip back to Jamaica. Her housing situation was uncertain, and we discussed the possibility of her staying in my parents' apartment while she figured out a more permanent arrangement.

We may be writing another chapter about the community of care that had formed around my parents.

Acknowledgments

Even before I realized that I could draw well enough to carry out this project, Paul Lopes and Michelle Bigenho told me that I could. Debbora Battaglia, Joe and Jessica Bacal, and Bill Girard provided valuable feedback at the early stages. Thanks go to Felicity Aulino, a colleague at Mount Holyoke College and the University of Massachusetts, who co-organized a panel with me on care at the American Anthropological Association meeting in 2019 when I was first starting on this project, and who, along with graduate student Adrian Godboldt, invited me to present at the anthropology colloquium at UMass in 2025 when the manuscript was almost complete. Thanks to my students Lilly Ann Brown, Hitomi Nakamura, Emma Schein, Yian Wang, and Grace Wan who showed up for that talk!

Anne Brackenbury provided essential orientation on overall structure, suggestions about pacing and the relationship of text and image, as well as valuable detailed comments on each chapter. Mitra Emad, David Syring, Jerome Crowder, and other organizers and participants of the Visual Research Conference in 2022 provided a stimulating venue to workshop my project. At later stages I received insightful perspectives from Andy Lass, Mark Auslander, Barbara Yngvesson, Michelle Bigenho, Julie Hemment, Beth Notar, Lynn Morgan, Kathleen Zane, and Calvin Collins, and so many of my colleagues in Anthropology, Sociology, Art Studio, and Asian Studies at Mount Holyoke College, including Elif Babul, Patricia Banks, Jinhwa Chang, Benjamin Gebre-Medhin, Lisa Iglesias, Amanda Maciuba, Naoko Nemoto, Megan Saltzman, Sabra Thorner, Eleanor Townsley, Kenneth Tucker, Matthew Watson, and Ayca Zayim.

I'm very grateful to Lohit Jagwani, my acquisitions editor and advocate at the University of Toronto Press, for believing in my project and shepherding it through the publication process, and to Leah Connor, Aditi Parikh, and the entire team at UTP. Thanks also to Mount Holyoke College for a grant for the purchase of a digital drawing pad, and a subvention towards the costs of publication.

Naomi Tannen, organizer of a care givers' group, along with members Ron Ackerman, Susan Adelson, Deborah Epstein, Judy Katz, Deb Novitch, Laura Pravitz, Eric Roth, Eileen Rutman, Corrie Trattner, Elise Young were willing to listen to my trials and tribulations on a monthly basis even as they were going through their own. They demonstrated how valuable communities of support can be for those who spend so much time and energy giving to others.

Thanks go to my kids Isaac and Emile, and nephews Owen and Elliot, for allowing me to use the wonderful portraits they made of Dad and Mom, and to my brother Abe for the use of his quick sketch of himself he left with Dad nagging him to exercise.

Thanks go to my mom for her loving support as well as her vocal admonitions throughout my life. And of course, thanks go to the care workers who gave so much to dad and mom, and to me, over a period of five years. Thanks also to Beth Notar for her insights and encouragement throughout the entire process, as well as to Russ and Ellen Notar. And thanks to Parbatie Gulcharran, Ophelia Jerrett-Little, and Diane Ramsay for everything!

Thanks go to my dad most of all, for being willing to share images from his unpublished sketchbooks, and for being a playful collaborator in this project. I hope I did him and his work justice.

References

Allison, Anne. 2023. *Being Dead Otherwise*. Durham: Duke University Press.
Auslander, Mark. 2011. *The Accidental Slaveowner: Revisiting a Myth of Race and Finding an American Family*. Athens: The University of Georgia Press.
Chatzidakis, Andreas, Jamie Hakim, Jo Littler, Catherine Rottenberg, and Lynne Segal. 2020. "Caring Kinships." In *The Care Manifesto: The Politics of Interdependence*. London: Verso.
Danely, Jason. 2014. *Aging and Loss: Mourning and Maturity in Modern Japan*. New Brunswick, NJ: Rutgers University Press.
Fisher, Berenice, and Joan Tronto. 1990. "Toward a Feminist Theory of Caring." In *Circles of Care: Work and Identity in Women's Lives*, edited by Emily K. Abel and Margaret K. Nelson, 35–62. New York: State University of New York Press.
Garcia-Sanchez, Inmaculada. 2018. "Children as Interactional Brokers of Care." *Annual Review of Anthropology* 47: 167–84. https://doi.org/10.1146/annurev-anthro-102317-050050.
Gawande, Atul. 2014. *Being Mortal: Medicine and What Matters in the End*. New York: Metropolitan Books.
Kawano, Satsuki. 2005. *Nature's Embrace: Japanese Aging Urbanites and New Death Rites*. Honolulu: University of Hawai'i Press.

Kleinman, Arthur. 2009. "Caregiving: The Odyssey of Being More Human." *The Lancet* 373. https://doi.org/10.1016/s0140-6736(09)60087-8.

Lamb, Sarah. 2014. "Permanent Personhood or Meaningful Decline: Toward a Critical Anthropology of Successful Aging." *Journal of Aging Studies* 29: 41–52. https://doi.org/10.1016/j.jaging.2013.12.006.

Lamb, Sarah, ed. 2017. *Successful Aging as a Contemporary Obsession: Global Perspectives*. New Brunswick, NJ: Rutgers University Press.

Long, Susan Orpett. 2005. *Final Days: Japanese Culture and Choice at the End of Life*. Honolulu: University of Hawai'i Press.

Mol, Annemarie, Ingunn Moser, and Jeannette Pols. 2010. "Care: Putting Practice into Theory." In *Care in Practice: On Tinkering in Clinics, Homes and Farms*, edited by Annemarie Mol, Ingunn Moser, and Jeannette Pols, 7–26. Bielefeld, Germany: Transcript Verlag.

Radtke, Kristen. 2021. *Seek You: A Journey Through American Loneliness*. New York: Pantheon Books.

Shohet, Merav. 2013. "Everyday Sacrifice and Language Socialization in Vietnam: The Power of a Respect Particle." *American Anthropoligist* 115: 203–17. https://doi.org/10.1111/aman.12004.

Stevenson, Lisa. 2014. *Life Beside Itself: Imagining Care in the Canadian Arctic*. Berkeley, CA: University of California Press.

Taylor, Janelle S. 2010. "On Recognition, Caring, and Dementia." In *Care in Practice: On Tinkering in Clinics, Homes and Farms*, edited by Annamarie Mol, Ingunn Moser, and Jeannette Pols, 27–56. Bielefeld, Germany: Transcript Verlag.

Traphagan, John W. 2000. *Taming Oblivion: Aging Bodies and the Fear of Senility in Japan*. New York: State University of New York Press.

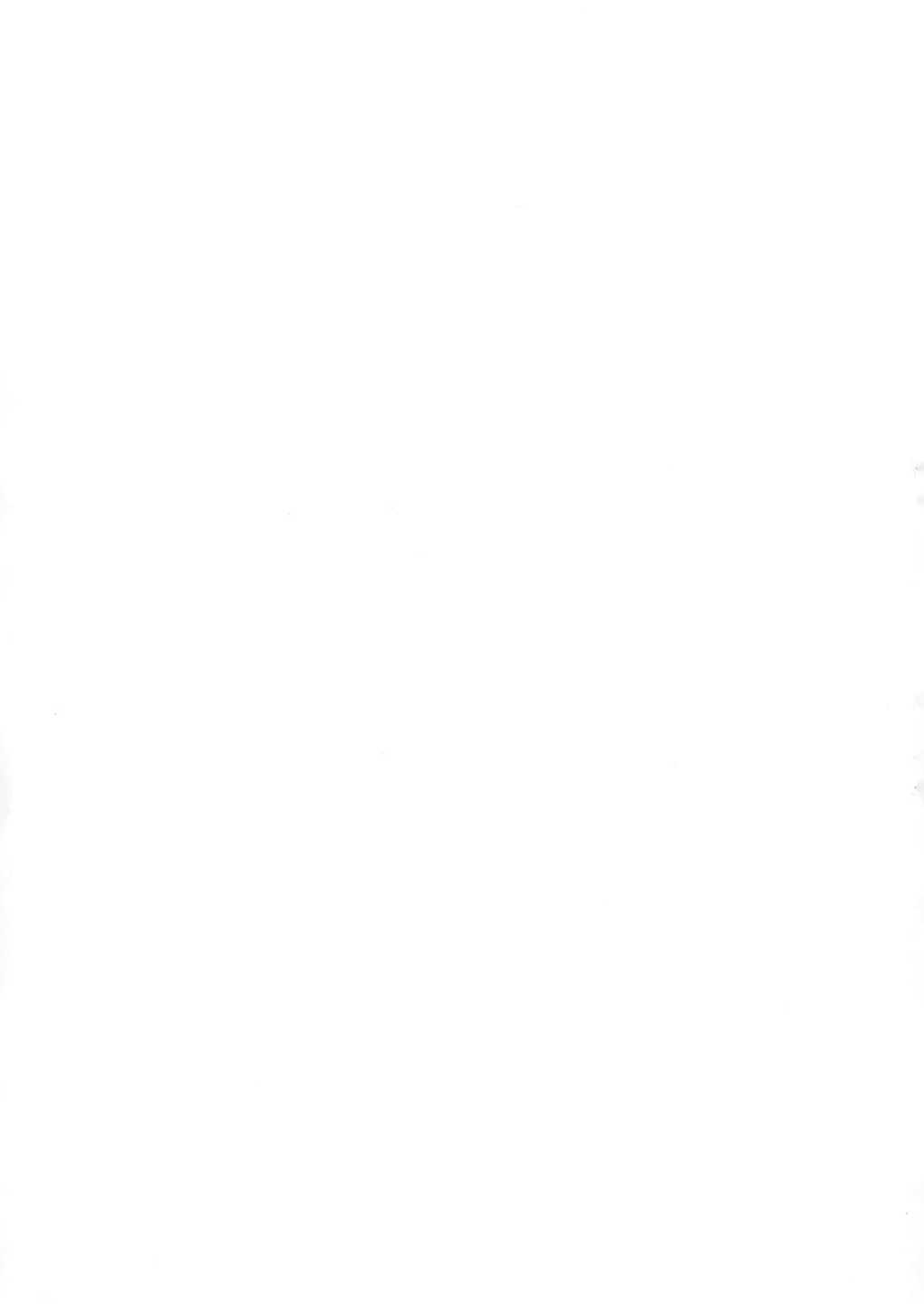